T0200210

THE WASHINGTON MANUAL® OF ECHOCARDIOGRAPHY

Second Edition

Editor

Nishath Quader, MD, FACC, FASE
Assistant Professor of Medicine
Cardiovascular Division
Washington University School of Medicine
St. Louis, Missouri

Associate Editors

Majesh Makan, MD, FACC, FASE
Associate Professor of Medicine
Associate Director of Echocardiography
Division of Cardiology
Washington University School of Medicine
St. Louis, Missouri

Julio E. Pérez, MD, FACC, FASE, FACP, FAHA
Professor of Medicine
Director of Echocardiography
Cardiovascular Division
Barnes-Jewish Hospital
Washington University School of Medicine
St. Louis, Missouri

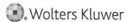. Wolters Kluwer

Philadelphia • Baltimore • New York • London
Buenos Aires • Hong Kong • Sydney • Tokyo

Executive Editor: Julie Goolsby
Senior Product Development Editor: Andrea Vosburgh
Production Project Manager: Bridgett Dougherty
Marketing Manager: Rachel Mante Leung
Design Coordinator: Elaine Kasmer
Senior Manufacturing Coordinator: Beth Welsh
Prepress Vendor: Aptara, Inc.

9 8 7

Printed in the U.S.A.

978-1-49632-128-2
Library of Congress Cataloging-in-Publication Data
availabel upon request

LWW.com

Dedication

To the Washington University Cardiology Fellowship Program and Barnes Jewish Hospital Cardiac Diagnostic Laboratory.

Contributors

Suzanne V. Arnold, MD, MHA
Assistant Professor
Department of Internal Medicine
Saint Luke's Mid America Heart Institute
University of Missouri—Kansas City
Kansas City, Missouri

Mirnela Byku, MD, PhD
Fellow, Cardiovascular Disease
Washington University School of Medicine
St. Louis, Missouri

Pedro M. Calderón-Artero, MD, MS
Cardiology Fellow
Barnes-Jewish Hospital
Washington University School of Medicine
St. Louis, Missouri

Daniel H. Cooper, MD
Assistant Professor of Medicine
Associate Program Director for
* Electrophysiology*
Cardiovascular Division, Department of
* Medicine*
Clinical Cardiac Electrophysiologist
Barnes-Jewish Hospital
Washington University School of Medicine
St. Louis, Missouri

Sharon Cresci, MD
Assistant Professor
Departments of Medicine and Genetics
Washington University School of Medicine
St. Louis, Missouri

Rafael S. Garcia-Cortes, MD
Cardiology Fellow
Barnes-Jewish Hospital
Washington University School of Medicine
St. Louis, Missouri

Jacob S. Goldstein, MD
Cardiology Fellow
Barnes-Jewish Hospital
Washington University School of Medicine
St. Louis, Missouri

Justin Hartupee, MD, PhD
Cardiology Fellow
Department of Medicine
Washington University School of Medicine
St. Louis, Missouri

Christopher L. Holley, MD, PhD
Instructor of Medicine
Cardiovascular Division
Department of Internal Medicine
Washington University School of Medicine
St. Louis, Missouri

Kathryn J. Lindley, MD
Assistant Professor of Medicine
Cardiovascular Division
Washington University School of Medicine
St. Louis, Missouri

Brian R. Lindman, MD, MSCI
Assistant Professor of Medicine
Cardiovascular Division
Washington University School of Medicine
St. Louis, Missouri

Jose A. Madrazo, MD, FASE
Assistant Professor of Medicine
Johns Hopkins School of Medicine
Baltimore, Maryland

Majesh Makan, MD, FACC, FASE
Associate Professor of Medicine
Associate Director of Echocardiography
Division of Cardiology
Washington University School of Medicine
St. Louis, Missouri

Deana Mikhalkova, MD
Fellow
Department of Cardiology
Barnes-Jewish Hospital
Washington University School of Medicine
St. Louis, Missouri

Michael E. Nassif, MD
Fellow
Division of Cardiology
Washington University School of Medicine
St. Louis, Missouri

Olusegun Olusesi, MD
Cardiac Electrophysiology Fellow
Division of Cardiology
Washington University School of Medicine
St. Louis, Missouri

**Julio E. Pérez, MD, FACC, FASE,
FACP, FAHA**
Professor of Medicine
Director of Echocardiography
Cardiovascular Division
Barnes-Jewish Hospital
Washington University School of Medicine
St. Louis, Missouri

Nishath Quader, MD, FACC, FASE
Assistant Professor of Medicine
Cardiovascular Division
Washington University School of Medicine
St. Louis, Missouri

Praveen K. Rao, MD
Cardiology Fellow
Barnes-Jewish Hospital
Washington University School of Medicine
St. Louis, Missouri

David S. Raymer, MD
Cardiology Fellow
Barnes-Jewish Hospital
Washington University School of Medicine
St. Louis, Missouri

Justin S. Sadhu, MD, MPHS, FACC
Instructor of Medicine
Cardiovascular Division
Department of Internal Medicine
Washington University School of Medicine
St. Louis, Missouri

Marc Sintek, MD
Interventional Fellow
Cardiovascular Division
Washington University School of Medicine
St. Louis, Missouri

Nishtha Sodhi, MD
Interventional Fellow
Cardiovascular Division
Washington University School of Medicine
St. Louis, Missouri

Tyson E. Turner, MD, MPH
Fellow
Cardiovascular Division
Washington University School of Medicine
St. Louis, Missouri

Justin M. Vader, MD
Assistant Professor of Medicine
Cardiovascular Division
Washington University School of Medicine
St. Louis, Missouri

Michael Yeung, MD
Assistant Professor
Department of Cardiology
University of North Carolina
Chapel Hill, North Carolina

Foreword

It is a pleasure to be able to write the forward for the second edition of the Washington Manual of Echocardiography. The second edition hues closely to the same guiding principles that formed the basis for the first edition: namely, to provide a handheld, easy-to-use manual that serves as a quick reference for physicians on call, in the emergency room, on the wards, or in the intensive care unit. Certainly there are a number of excellent, comprehensive textbooks on echocardiography that are available; however, these books are too big to fit into your pocket and take with you, and hence are less useful in the middle of the night when one is faced with diagnosing a critically ill patient rapidly. Increasingly cardiology fellows, intensive care physicians, and emergency room physicians are being placed in the situation of having to perform and interpret echocardiograms, and to utilize this diagnostic information in real time, in order to make split-second management decisions that have life or death consequences. This book was written for you!

Dr. Nishath Quader, who is the new lead editor for the book, and Drs. Makan and Perez have done a masterful job in updating the second edition of the Washington Manual of Echocardiography. The second edition is more than an update, it is re-envisioning of the excellent first edition. For example, the second edition has been completely reformatted in an "easy-to-read" layout with many new and updated figures. The second edition has also been modernized and includes a new chapter on imaging cardiac circulatory assist devices, which is playing an increasingly important role in managing critically ill patients. The second edition also features extensive updates in the section on transesophageal echocardiography, including new information on three-dimensional imaging of mitral and aortic valves. Finally, the second edition is written to reflect the latest American College of Cardiology/American Heart Association (ACC/AHA) and American Society of Echocardiography (ASE) guidelines, so that it serves as a useful resource for trainees who are interested in board certification.

I am quite certain that the second edition of the Washington Manual of Echocardiography will prove to be a useful and reliable source of information for physicians and sonographers who provide care for patients afflicted with cardiovascular disease. I am proud to endorse this book, which I believe will not only prove to be a worthy successor of the first edition, but will also be of great help to health care providers who are on the front lines of cardiovascular care.

Douglas L. Mann, MD

Preface

You are a first year cardiology fellow and the pager goes off; it's the ICU asking for a "stat" echo for assessment of a pericardial effusion and possible tamponade. You have only been a cardiology fellow for a short amount of time, so you want to quickly review the echo findings of tamponade before making your way up to the ICU with the echo machine. The only problem is, you didn't bring your 785-page echo textbook with you while you are on call!

The above scenario, in which cardiology fellows have to make complex decisions at night, which are based, at least in part, on echo images is becoming increasingly more common. Fellows are faced with the daunting task of not only performing a quality diagnostic echo but also interpreting it accurately. Even though there are several excellent, comprehensive textbooks on echocardiography available, our fellows have frequently commented that they need a "handheld," easy-to-carry book, that they can use as a quick reference when important questions came up while on call or on different cardiology rotations.

The goal of this book is to provide an introduction to echocardiography, as well as highlight some of the critical echocardiographic findings in the normal heart and in different disease states. Thus, not only will cardiology fellows find this book helpful, but so will anesthesia fellows and cardiac sonographers who utilize echocardiography on a daily basis. In addition, intensive care and emergency department physicians who also have been increasingly utilizing hand-held ultrasound will find that this book provides a succinct overview of disease states frequently encountered by them.

After the wonderful feedback that we received from the first edition of this book, it was clear that a second edition was needed in order to keep pace with the rapid changes in the field. In keeping with the purpose of the first edition (i.e., to provide a succinct overview of various topics in echocardiography), the second edition again focuses on critical aspects of interpreting echocardiograms in different disease states. Although some of the sections retain the same structure, each of the chapters has been revised extensively. Moreover, this second edition is completely re-formatted in an "easy-to-read" layout with multiple updated and additional figures. This edition also features brand new chapters on hypertrophic cardiomyopathy and cardiac devices (LVAD, IABP, Impella). These chapters are designed with the latest American College of Cardiology/American Heart Association (ACC/AHA) and American Society of Echocardiography (ASE) guidelines in mind. In addition, the chapter on LV systolic and diastolic function now has integrated the updated chamber quantification guidelines by the ASE. The chapters on valve assessment have incorporated the recent valvular heart disease guidelines published by the ACC/AHA. This edition also features several updates to the TEE section with a special focus on the mitral valve and three-dimensional echocardiography.

The editors of this book would like to thank all the authors who made the production of this book possible. We would also like to thank our cardiology fellows who conceived the original idea for this book. Without their relentless efforts to learn, provide great clinical care to patients with complex diseases, and to provide a unique perspective from a trainee's standpoint, this book would not have become a reality. Finally, we would like to thank our cardiac sonographers who constantly strive to learn and improve their echocardiographic skills and knowledge, and who provided the spectacular images used in this book.

Nishath Quader
Majesh Makan
Julio Pérez

Contents

1

Introduction to Echocardiographic Principles

Jose A. Madrazo and Suzanne V. Arnold

HIGH-YIELD CONCEPTS

- Pulsed-wave (PW) Doppler is **range** specific but is limited in the peak velocity it can measure.
- Continuous-wave (CW) Doppler is able to measure **high** velocities but cannot localize the origin along its beam.
- M-mode has high **temporal** resolution but is limited by oblique imaging of structures of interest.

KEY FORMULAS

- **Simplified Bernoulli equation: $\Delta P \text{(mm Hg)} = 4 \times V^2$ (V = m/sec)**
- LVOT area $= \pi \times \text{(LVOT diameter in cm/2)}^2$
- SV = (LVOT area) × (LVOT VTI)
- QP/QS = (RVOT area) × (RVOT VTI)/(LVOT area) × (LVOT VTI)
- **Continuity principle for aortic valve area = (LVOT area) × (LVOT VTI)/(AoV VTI)**
  Where AoV = aortic valve, LVOT = left ventricular outflow tract, QP/QS = pulmonary to systemic flow ratio, RVOT = right ventricular outflow tract, SV = stroke volume, and VTI = velocity time integral.

GENERAL PRINCIPLES

Echocardiography uses sound waves to create images of the heart and other structures.
- Sound waves are mechanical vibrations described in terms of frequency or Hertz (Hz) = the number of cycles per second.
- The frequency used by the ultrasound transducer affects image resolution and tissue penetration.
  - High frequency = high-resolution image, low tissue penetration
  - Low frequency = low-resolution image, high tissue penetration
- Ultrasound refers to sound waves with 20 kHz or higher.
  - Adult echocardiography typically uses frequencies of 2–7 MHz.
- Transthoracic echocardiography employs low-frequency transducers (2–4 MHz), which allows deeper penetration through the chest wall but at the expense of reduced resolution.

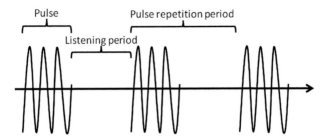

Figure 1-1. Description of ultrasound waves using standardized nomenclature.

- Transesophageal echocardiography does not require deep tissue penetration and can use higher frequency transducers (3.5–7 MHz) to produce higher resolution images.
- Piezoelectric elements are crystals that convert electrical energy into mechanical sound waves and vice versa. These crystals are in the transducer and their properties, number, and movement determine the characteristics of the images obtained.
- **Harmonic imaging:** Tissue and contrast bubbles not only reflect ultrasound at the transmitted frequency but also resonate at multiples of that frequency (harmonic frequencies). Harmonic imaging refers to setting the transducer to receive frequencies at multiples of the emitted frequency (e.g., transmit at 3 MHz and receive at 6 MHz, the second harmonic). Harmonic imaging improves signal-to-noise ratio and the delineation of the endocardial border.
- **Mechanical index (MI):** A measure of the mechanical pressure exerted on tissues by the ultrasound waves. It is important to **lower the MI during contrast echocardiography** so as not to burst the contrast bubbles quickly.
- **Frame rate:** The number of still images displayed sequentially per unit of time. Multiple still images displayed sequentially lead to the perception of motion; thus, higher frame rates lead to better temporal resolution but may sacrifice image quality and vice versa.
- **Pulse repetition period:** A pulse of ultrasound of a given frequency is sent by the transducer, followed by a prespecified "listening period" before the transducer senses waves of the same frequency and generates an image. The duration of the pulse, plus the time spent listening, is referred to as the pulse repetition period. The longer the duration of this period, the deeper the images obtained (Fig. 1-1).

- **Key Points:**
  1. *It is sometimes useful to decrease the transducer frequency in obese patients so as to improve image quality.*
  2. *Shallower imaging and narrower imaging sector can be easily adjusted to allow for higher frame rates and better temporal resolution.*

IMAGING MODALITIES

M-Mode Echocardiography

- M-mode echocardiography depicts the structures along the path of a single line of the ultrasound beam. The still image of these structures is continuously updated over time on the "x" axis. Thus, the structures along the line of the ultrasound beam are depicted as they change with time (Fig. 1-2).
- Because of its high sampling frequency (up to 1000 pulses per second), M-mode has excellent axial resolution and is useful in identifying the relative location of structures and measuring range of motion.

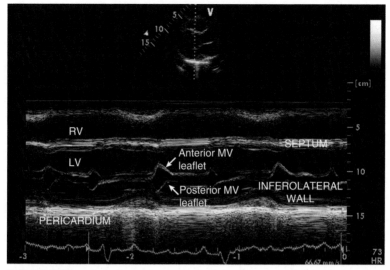

Figure 1-2. M-mode providing an "ice-pick" view of changes in cardiac structures seen in the parasternal long-axis view over time. LV, left ventricle; MV, mitral valve; RV, right ventricle.

- **M-mode also has better temporal resolution than two-dimensional (2D) imaging,** and thus subtle abnormalities in motion and timing may be better appreciated with M-mode. For example, systolic anterior motion of the mitral valve in hypertrophic cardiomyopathy (HCM) and right ventricular (RV) diastolic collapse in cardiac tamponade may be better appreciated by M-mode.

- Key Points:
  1. *It may be useful to visualize the M-mode transducer as a virtual ice-pick with the structures along its path depicted on the screen and updated horizontally over time.*
  2. *M-mode has higher temporal resolution than 2D echocardiography.*
  3. *M-mode is very useful in identifying mitral valve prolapse, systolic anterior motion of mitral leaflet, and RV diastolic collapse in tamponade.*

Two-dimensional Echocardiography

- The cardiac structures in the plane defined by the transducer position are depicted in two dimensions on the screen and the screen is updated continuously (see frame rate mentioned previously), thus producing a "movie."
- In adult echocardiography, structures closest to the transducer are displayed at the top of the screen, and the side of the ultrasound plane that corresponds to the **notch** on the transducer is on the **right** side of the screen.
- Imaging the heart in multiple 2D planes allows for the reconstruction and visualization of all the parts of a three-dimensional (3D) structure.

Three-dimensional Echocardiography

- Multiple 2D planes can be pieced together to recreate a 3D structure. Modern 3D echocardiography transducers accomplish this by imaging along a pyramidal ultrasound beam.

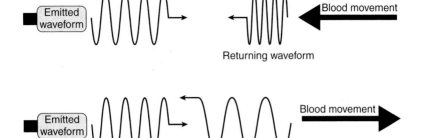

Figure 1-3. Diagram showing how the direction and speed of movement of an object change the frequency of the reflected ultrasound wave (Doppler shift).

DOPPLER PRINCIPLES AND APPLICATIONS

Doppler Effect

- Proposed in 1842 by Austrian physicist Christian Doppler, the Doppler effect is the change in frequency of a wave received by an observer (the reflected frequency) relative to the source of the wave (originating frequency).
- When sound is emitted from a source at a given frequency and is reflected from a static source, the waves return at the same frequency emitted.
- However, when sound is reflected from a moving source, the received frequency is shifted proportionally to the source's velocity.
  - If the object is moving toward the transducer, the resulting frequency is higher than the originating frequency and there is a "positive Doppler shift."
  - If the object is moving away from the transducer, the resulting frequency is lower than the originating frequency and there is a "negative Doppler shift" (Fig. 1-3).
- The angle at which the object is moving relative to the observer influences the magnitude of the Doppler shift—that is, the measured velocity of the blood is related to both the true velocity of the blood and the angle at which it is measured.
  - From a mathematical perspective, the Doppler shift is proportional to the cosine of the angle between the sound emitter and the moving object: $\text{velocity}_{measured} = \text{cosine of angle} (\Theta) \times \text{velocity}_{true}$ (Fig. 1-4).

> - **Key Point:** *So as to not underestimate the velocity of a jet, it is important that the ultrasound beam is as parallel as possible to the direction of blood flow (i.e., cosine of zero degrees equals one, meaning measured velocity is equal to true velocity). This is accomplished by using multiple views, nonimaging transducers, and guidance by color Doppler.*

Pulsed-wave Doppler

- In PW Doppler, the transducer sends pulses of ultrasound at a given frequency and interrogates for Doppler shift at a specific site defined in a 2D image (**sample volume**).
- **Pulse repetition frequency (PRF)** refers to the number of pulses in one second, and is therefore inversely proportional to pulse repetition period. A **low PRF is used to image deeper structures**.

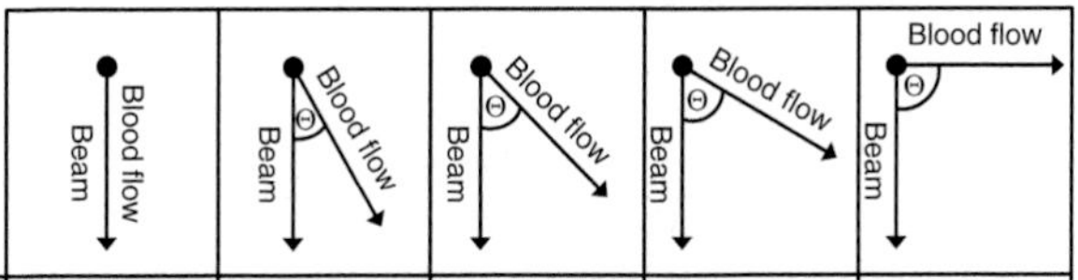

Angle (Θ)	0	30	45	60	90
Cosine of Θ	1	0.87	0.7	0.5	0
Measured velocity	5 m/s	4.35 m/s	3.5 m/s	2.5 m/s	0 m/s

Figure 1-4. The effect of angle of insonation in measuring a jet with a true velocity of 5 m/sec by Doppler echocardiography.

- The PRF determines the depth at which the Doppler shift is evaluated.
  - Lower PRF allows for longer "listening time" between the pulses and therefore interrogates at a deeper level and vice versa.
- **Nyquist limit:** Named after Swedish-American engineer Harry Nyquist, who discovered that the number of pulses per unit time is limited to twice the bandwidth of the channel, the Nyquist limit, in practical terms, is equivalent to one-half PRF.
  - If the velocity of blood flow exceeds the Nyquist limit, the direction and velocity are inaccurately displayed and appear to change direction, a phenomenon termed **aliasing**.
- PW is limited by the maximum velocity that can be measured, as the next pulse cannot be sent out before the signal is returned. The highest velocity that can be accurately measured is the Nyquist limit. Velocities greater than the Nyquist limit appear on the opposite side of the scale, aliasing (Fig. 1-5).

- **Key Points:**
  1. *PW allows for the determination of flow velocity at a specific point (sample volume) but is limited to measuring only lower velocities because of aliasing.*
  2. *Imaging shallower structures allows for the use of a higher PRF and therefore higher Nyquist limit. Use views that minimize the distance to the jet of interest if aliasing is a problem.*

Continuous-wave Doppler
- In CW Doppler, the transducer has some crystals dedicated to constantly emitting ultrasound, while other crystals continuously "listen" for a shift in frequency.
- Because the ultrasound beam is continuous, CW is not limited by PRF in the velocities it detects (i.e., there is no aliasing). Hence, **CW can interrogate high-velocity flows**.
- Since the shift occurs anywhere along the path of the beam, **CW cannot localize the position along that beam where the highest velocity occurs** (Table 1-1).
- A *Pedoff* probe is a specialized nonimaging CW transducer that contains two elements—one element is always transmitting while the other is always receiving. It provides very accurate CW Doppler data and, as a result of its very small size, is useful for assessing peak velocities from high parasternal and suprasternal views and in patients with a challenging body habitus.

- **Key Point:** *CW allows for the determination of the highest flow velocity anywhere along the ultrasound beam but cannot localize the point of maximal velocity. It is not range specific.*

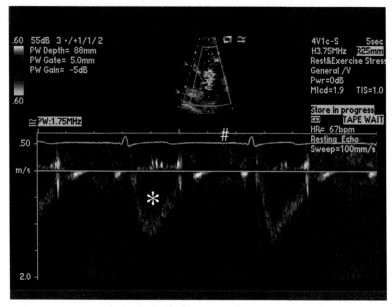

Figure 1-5. A spectral display from pulsed-wave (PW) Doppler in the left ventricular outflow tract shows aliasing of the high velocity aortic regurgitant jet (#). Lower-velocity flow in systole does not alias (*).

High-pulse Repetition Frequency (HPRF) Pulsed Doppler

- HPRF attempts to overcome the limitations of CW in depth ambiguity and PW in aliasing.
- HPRF is a variant of PW, where one or more new pulses are sent out before the echo from the first is received. This shortens the PRF and thereby increases the Nyquist limit and results in multiple sample volumes.

TABLE 1-1	Characteristics of the Different Doppler Modes		
	Advantages	**Disadvantages**	**Common uses**
CW	Measures high velocity flows	Cannot determine site of high velocity	Peak and mean aortic and mitral stenosis gradients, regurgitation jets
PW	Measures velocity at a specific location	Cannot assess high velocities	Ventricular outflow tract, mitral valve inflow, pulmonary veins
HPRF	Increased Nyquist limit	Cannot tell which sampling volume contains the high velocity	Left ventricular outflow obstruction

CW, continuous wave; HPRF, high-pulse repetition frequency; PW, pulsed wave.

- HPRF increases the accuracy of high velocity measurements at the cost of depth ambiguity, as it is unknown which sampling volume is the site of the highest velocity. Thus, it results in "partial depth ambiguity."

- **Key Point:** *HPRF is ideal for trying to determine where along a beam the high velocity occurs and is most often used in the setting of a dynamic LVOT obstruction (i.e., hypertrophic cardiomyopathy).*

Color Doppler

- Color Doppler is a variation in PW in which multiple sample volumes in a 2D plane are interrogated simultaneously. Each sample's velocity is assigned a color according to a prespecified scheme and superimposed on the underlying 2D image (Fig. 1-6).
- By convention, most echocardiography labs display flow going away from the transducer as blue and flow toward the transducer as red **(Blue-Away, Red-Toward)**.
- Higher-velocity flow shows progressively lighter shades of the same color until the Nyquist limit is reached, at which point aliasing occurs and the color changes to the opposite one (i.e., blue to red or red to blue).
- To highlight turbulence, many machines add a third color (such as green or yellow) to areas with a wide variability of flow velocities and directions. This feature (also called variance) can be turned off if needed to make the direction of blood flow more explicit.
- Color Doppler allows for a quick visual assessment of location, velocity, and turbulence of blood flow in a given region.

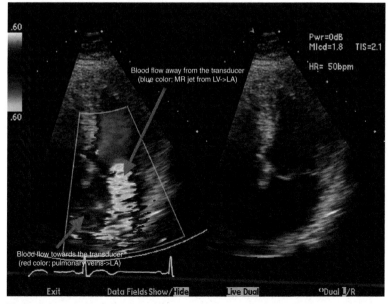

Figure 1-6. Color Doppler of blood flow in the left atrium (LA) and left ventricle (LV) during systole showing how the direction and velocity of flow are represented. MR, mitral regurgitation.

Tissue Doppler Imaging (TDI)

- TDI is a variation in PW Doppler that uses the principles of Doppler imaging to assess myocardial tissue velocity (typically <20 cm/sec), which is much lower than blood flow velocity (measured in m/sec).
- In conventional PW, the lower velocities generated by cardiac tissue are filtered out to focus on the higher velocities from moving blood cells. This filter is inactivated during TDI, allowing measurement of the higher-amplitude, lower-velocity signals of tissue motion.

- **Key Point:** *TDI is typically used in the assessment of diastolic function, RV function, and myocardial strain.*

USEFUL HEMODYNAMIC PRINCIPLES AND APPLICATIONS

Stroke Volume (SV) and Other Flow Volumes

- The volume of blood traveling through an orifice can be estimated by multiplying the area through which the blood travels by the velocity of blood flow through that orifice for the duration of the time period of assessment (Fig. 1-7).
- SV is defined as the volume of blood ejected from the LV per beat. A simple determination of SV can be made by measuring forward flow velocity in the LVOT and calculating the area of the LVOT.
- First, the LVOT cross-sectional area is determined by direct measurement of the LVOT diameter. Assuming the LVOT is circular, the area is calculated by the following formula:

$$\text{LVOT area in cm}^2 = \pi \times (\text{LVOT diameter in cm/2})^2$$

- *LVOT diameter is usually best measured in the parasternal long-axis (PLAX) view in early to mid systole using a magnified view.*
- If flow across an orifice is constant (like in a garden hose), then multiplying the velocity of the flow (cm/sec) by the orifice area (cm^2) calculates the flow rate (cm^3/sec). The flow rate multiplied by the ejection time equals the volume of flow. However, blood pumped by the heart is not only pulsatile, but the velocity of flow also varies throughout the systolic ejection period. To accurately determine the volume of blood pumped per beat, a sum of the velocities over the systolic ejection period must be calculated to create an average.

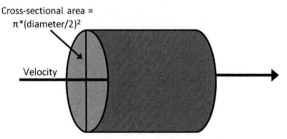

Figure 1-7. Diagram illustrating the assumption that blood flow through a cylinder approximates flow through a cardiac orifice.

- By integrating the flow velocity over time, the VTI, a measure of distance (cm), also termed stroke distance, is obtained.
  - From a conceptual point of view, the systolic LVOT VTI represents the distance a single blood cell would travel during one beat in a cylinder with a cross-sectional area equal to the LVOT.
  - The VTI is measured by obtaining a PW measurement at the LVOT and then tracing it on the screen. The computer calculates the area under the curve and reads out the VTI.
  - *LVOT VTI is best obtained from the apical five-chamber or apical long-axis view.*
- LVOT area (cm^2) multiplied by stroke distance (cm/beat) yields SV (cm^3/beat or mL/beat):

$$SV = (LVOT\ VTI) \times (LVOT\ area)$$

- Taking this concept further, SV can then be multiplied by heart rate to calculate cardiac output (CO):

$$CO\ (L/min) = SV\ (mL/beat)/1000 \times heart\ rate\ (beats/min)$$

- CO can then be divided by body surface area (BSA) to find the cardiac index (CI; divide by 1000 to convert from mL to L):

$$CI\ (L/min/m^2) = CO\ (L/min)/BSA\ (m^2)$$

- **This concept may be applied to any orifice to measure blood flow.**
- For example, this principle can be used to determine mitral regurgitation severity by a "volumetric method." Calculate how much blood flows into the LV using (mitral valve [MV] annulus area × diastolic VTI at that level) and comparing it to SV (as calculated previously) allows for the determination of the volume of blood that regurgitates back into the left atrium (LA) during systole (LV inflow − LV outflow volume), known as the regurgitant volume. This will be discussed further in future chapters.
- Another application of this principle is to quantify a right to left shunt. This is done by comparing pulmonary flow (Qp) to systemic flow (Qs), where the Qp/Qs ratio is considered elevated if >1.5. Qs is determined by the previous SV calculation, and Qp is similarly calculated by multiplying the area of the RVOT by the RVOT systolic VTI.

$$Qp/Qs = (RVOT\ area) \times (RVOT\ VTI)/(LVOT\ area) \times (LVOT\ VTI)$$

  - *RVOT diameter and VTI are usually best obtained in the parasternal short-axis (PSAX) view at the level of the AoV. Alternatively, the proximal pulmonary artery (PA) diameter and PW VTI at the PA may be used.*

- **Key Points:**
  1. *LVOT diameter is usually best measured in the PLAX view in early to mid systole using a magnified view.*
  2. *SV = (LVOT VTI) × (LVOT area)*
  3. *Qp/Q$_S$ = (RVOT area) × (RVOT VTI)/(LVOT area) × (LVOT VTI)*
  4. *RVOT diameter and VTI are usually best obtained in the PSAX view at the level of the AoV.*

Bernoulli Principle and Estimation of Pressure in Cardiac Chambers

• The Bernoulli principle is a derivation of the Law of Conservation of Energy. Applied to echocardiography, if blood flows across a valve or orifice is viewed as fluid flowing through a cylinder of varying diameters, the energy of the fluid must be conserved at all points in the cylinder.
• The main biologically relevant variables in this system are pressure and velocity of blood; other components such as flow acceleration, viscous friction, and gravitational energy are omitted for simplification.
• Pressure energy$_1$ (P_1) + kinetic energy$_1$ = pressure energy$_2$ (P_2) + kinetic energy$_2$
• Kinetic energy of blood is calculated by the following formula:

$$\tfrac{1}{2}\rho \times V^2$$

where ρ is the mass density of blood and $\tfrac{1}{2}\rho$ is roughly 4

$$P_1 + 4 \times V_1^2 = P_2 + 4 \times V_2^2, \text{ or}$$
$$P_1 - P_2 \ (\Delta P) = 4 \times V_1^2 - 4 \times V_2^2$$

• The velocity proximal to a fixed orifice (V_2) is usually much lower than the peak velocity across it; thus V_2 does not contribute significantly and can usually be ignored.
• Using the simplified Bernoulli equation (ΔP[mm Hg] $= 4 \times V^2$), we can estimate the pressure gradient across an orifice between two cardiac chambers. If the pressure in one chamber is known (or estimated), then the pressure in the adjacent chamber can be calculated by determining the pressure difference between the two chambers.
• The most common application of this principle is the estimation of pulmonary artery systolic pressure (PASP). In the absence of RVOT obstruction or pulmonic valve stenosis, PASP equals RV systolic pressure (RVSP). Peak tricuspid regurgitation (TR) velocity reflects the difference between RVSP and RA pressure:

$$4 \times (\textbf{peak TR velocity})^2 = \textbf{RVSP} - \textbf{RA pressure}$$
$$\textbf{RVSP} = 4 \times (\textbf{peak TR velocity})^2 + \textbf{RA pressure}$$

• RA pressure is estimated clinically by measuring jugular venous pressure (JVP) or by echocardiography by measuring the inferior vena cava (IVC) diameter (see Chapter 5).

Continuity Principle

• The continuity principle is an extension of the Law of Conservation of Mass. In incompressible fluid dynamics, the flow rate varies according to the cross-sectional area so the volume (mass) is preserved. Simply stated in echocardiography, the volume of blood going in must equal that going out (Fig. 1-8).
• As explained previously, the product of VTI and the cross-sectional area where the VTI is measured can measure volume.
• Therefore by **continuity principle (or continuity equation)**:

$$(\textbf{A1}) \times (\textbf{VTI1}) = (\textbf{A2}) \times (\textbf{VTI2})$$

• The continuity equation is commonly applied to the measurement of aortic valve area (AVA) in patients with aortic valve stenosis (AS). Flow velocity will be greatest at the narrowest portion (the stenotic AoV in the case of AS) and can be determined by CW Doppler. Therefore, AVA can be calculated by measuring LVOT diameter, PW Doppler at LVOT, and CW Doppler across the AoV, as follows:

$$(\text{AVA}) \times (\text{AV VTI from AoV CW}) = (\text{LVOT area}) \times (\text{VTI from PW at LVOT}),$$

or

$$\textbf{AVA} = (\textbf{LVOT area}) \times (\textbf{LVOT VTI})/(\textbf{AoV VTI})$$

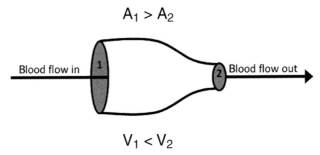

$$A_1 > A_2$$

Blood flow in 1

2 Blood flow out

$$V_1 < V_2$$

Figure 1-8. Diagram illustrating the continuity principle, which states that the product of the cross-sectional area and velocity time integral are the same for blood entering and leaving the heart.

• **Key Points:**
  1. *Simplified Bernoulli equation:* $\Delta P(mm\ Hg) = 4 \times V^2$
  2. *RVSP = 4 × (peak TR velocity)^2 + RA pressure*
  3. *AVA = (LVOT area) × (LVOT VTI)/(AoV VTI)*

Table 1-2 summarizes the application of Doppler echocardiography to measure cardiac hemodynamic indices.

TABLE 1-2	Assessing Cardiac Hemodynamic Indices by Echocardiography	
Hemodynamic	**Parameters needed**	**Calculation**
SV	LVOT VTI, LVOT diameter	$SV = \pi \times (LVOT\ diameter/2)^2 \times (LVOT\ VTI)$
CO	LVOT VTI, LVOT diameter, HR	$CO = \pi \times (LVOT\ diameter/2)^2 \times (LVOT\ VTI) \times HR$
RA pressure/ CVP	IVC diameter	IVC ≤2.1 cm with >50% respiratory variation = 3 mm Hg IVC > 2.1 cm with >50% respiratory variation = 8 mm Hg IVC > 2.1 cm with <50% respiratory variation = 15 mm Hg
PASP	TR jet, IVC diameter	$4 \times (peak\ TR\ jet)^2$ + estimated RAP
PCWP	E/e' (see Chapter 4)	• ≤8 = normal PCWP • ≥15 = elevated PCWP

CO, cardiac output; CVP, central venous pressure; HR, heart rate; IVC, inferior vena cava; LVOT, left ventricular outflow tract; PASP, pulmonary artery systolic pressure; PCWP, pulmonary capillary wedge pressure; RA, right atrium; RAP, right atrial pressure; SV, stroke volume; TR, tricuspid regurgitation; VTI, velocity time integral.

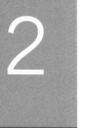

2

The Comprehensive Transthoracic Echocardiographic Examination

David S. Raymer

GETTING STARTED

A quality echocardiogram study starts with the setup (Fig. 2-1).

Patient Positioning

The low-powered ultrasound beam cannot image the entire heart clearly in its natural position behind the sternum.

Helpful Tips:
- Use the left lateral decubitus position to shift the heart laterally.
- Place a wedge or pillow to support the patient on his/her left side.
- Raise the left arm above the head to spread the intercostal spaces.

Patient comfort is key!

Sonographer Positioning

Get comfortable to prevent frequent breaks or a hastily performed examination. The examination can be performed from either side of the patient.

Helpful Tips:
- The examination table height should allow the sonographer's elbow to rest comfortably with a slight arm bend.
- Position the patient so the examination can be performed without leaning.

Handling The Transducer

Helpful Tips:
- The transducer should rest between thumb and index and middle fingers (much like throwing a dart).
- Move the fingers to the tip of the transducer.
- Stabilize the transducer against the patient's chest using the little finger.
- Note the position of the transducer notch (N) to orientate the cardiac views.

Machine Setup

Move the machine beyond the head of the bed; the sonographer should sit at the level of the patient's chest. Make sure to record the following information for each examination:

Patient identification	**Full name**
	Date of birth
	Identification number
Vitals	**Height/weight** (used for indexing measurements)
	Blood pressure (evaluating hemodynamic significance)

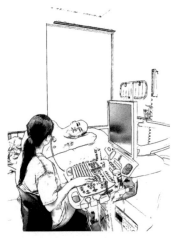

Figure 2-1. Echocardiogram setup.

Additional Imaging Considerations	
Acoustic Windows The optimal acoustic window allows acquisition of bright and clear images. Poor image quality will affect the accuracy of two-dimensional (2D) measurements and Doppler quality.	• **Keep the transducer movements small.**
Respiration Heart position changes with respiration.	• Acquire most **parasternal** and **apical** views at held **end-expiration**. • Acquire the **apical two-chamber** (A2C) and **subcostal** views at held **end-inspiration**.
Transducer Pressure Firm pressure is necessary for good transducer contact. However, applying too much pressure, especially on sensitive bony surfaces, will cause the patient pain!	• When imaging through areas of increased subcutaneous tissue (e.g., adipose tissue or under breasts), **applying increased pressure** often improves the image quality. • Slightly reduce pressure, once a good quality image is found. • Release the transducer pressure when switching intercostal spaces.
Ultrasound Gel Definition: a medium used to conduct sound waves between the patient and the ultrasound transducer	• Use plenty of gel! • Reapply when the gel on the patient spreads to a thin layer.

ADJUSTING THE IMAGE

Two-dimensional Gain

The intracardiac blood pool should be as dark as possible without losing definition of the cardiac structures (Fig. 2-2).

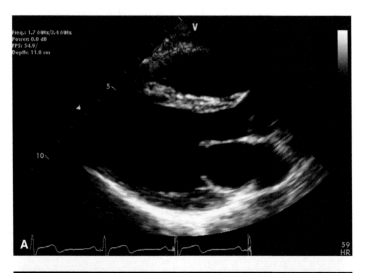

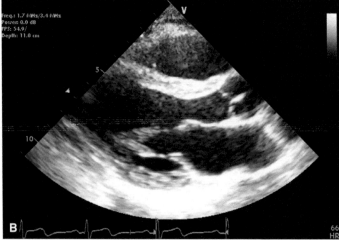

Figure 2-2. A: Optimum gain. **B:** Overgained.

IMAGE DEPTH

The depth should be set to extend approximately 1–2 cm beyond the cardiac boundary most distant from the transducer to ensure that none of the structures are cut off (Fig. 2-3). Sometimes it is necessary to change the depth to visualize pathology posterior to the heart, such as a pleural effusion.

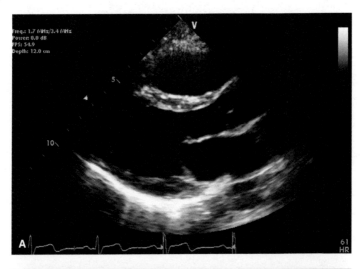

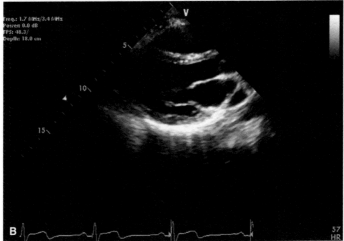

Figure 2-3. A: Optimum depth. **B:** Too deep.

Note: Some laboratories use standard default depths to facilitate comparison of serial examinations. In this case, acquire images at the default depth as well as at the appropriate depth.

Color Doppler

Adjust the color Doppler sampling region to include only the structures of interest so as to avoid decreases in temporal resolution and color quality. Keep the default Nyquist limit at 50–60 cm/sec (Fig. 2-4).

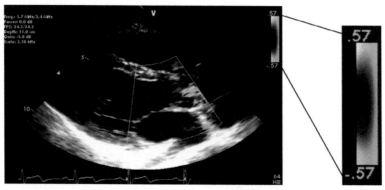

Figure 2-4. Color Doppler sampling region with Nyquist limit (*inset*).

Color Gain

Color gain can be calibrated by moving the color box into the extracardiac space and increasing Doppler gain until there is visible noise. Slowly decrease gain until the noise first disappears.

Frequency

Start imaging with the transducer set at 1.7/3.4 MHz (transmitted/received; second harmonic imaging) (Fig. 2-5). Select a higher (for near-field imaging) or lower (for deeper penetration) frequency to optimize the image quality.

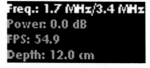

Freq.: 1.7 MHz/3.4 MHz
Power: 0.0 dB
FPS: 54.9
Depth: 12.0 cm

Figure 2-5. Transducer setting.

Focus

Try adjusting the ultrasound focus if an unclear image or artifact is encountered (Fig. 2-6).

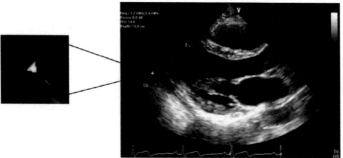

Figure 2-6. The focus of the ultrasound beam is shown by the *arrow* (*inset*).

Pulsed-wave Doppler Sample Volume Sizes

Inflow/outflow: 3–4 mm
Venous flow: 5–7 mm
Tissue or annular velocities: 5–7 mm

An inappropriate sample size may contaminate the Doppler acquisition and nullify spectral Doppler's greatest advantage of range specificity.

Spectral Gain

The background should be dark and the signal bright to ensure it is not under-gained. Overgained images may result in overestimation of blood flow velocities. Measurements should be taken of the modal velocities (bright envelope) and not the spectral broadening ("feathering of the signal") especially seen in overgained or poor quality Doppler (Fig. 2-7).

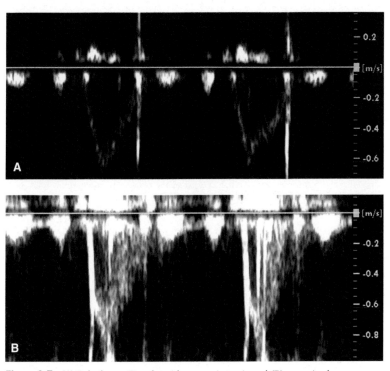

Figure 2-7. (**A**) Pulsed-wave Doppler with appropriate gain and (**B**) overgained.

Sweep Speed

Generally set sweep speed at 50 mm/sec for M-mode and spectral Doppler with normal heart rates. Set the sweep speed at 100 mm/sec to get measurements at a high temporal resolution (Fig. 2-8).

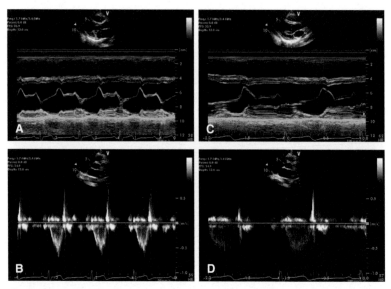

Figure 2-8. Parasternal long-axis view with M-mode through the mitral valve leaflets and parasternal short-axis view with spectral Doppler of the right ventricular outflow tract, with sweep speed at 50 mm/sec **(A,B)** and 100 mm/sec **(C,D)**.

PARASTERNAL LONG-AXIS VIEW (PLAX)

See Figure 2-9.

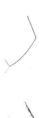

Obtaining the Image

- At the third or fourth intercostal space, point the notch toward the patient's right shoulder.
- Keep the transducer close to but not on the sternum.
- Move the transducer superiorly (high PLAX) to measure aortic root dimensions.

2D Examination

Structures

- *Chambers*: left atrium (LA), left ventricle (LV), left ventricular outflow tract (LVOT), right ventricular outflow tract (RVOT), aorta (Ao), descending aorta
- *Valves*: mitral valve (MV), aortic valve (AoV)

Key Features

- Coaptation of the anterior and posterior MV leaflets.
- Coaptation of the AoV leaflets; right coronary cusp closest to the RVOT with either the non-cusp or left cusp opposite it.
- LV cavity maximized (imaging between papillary muscles).

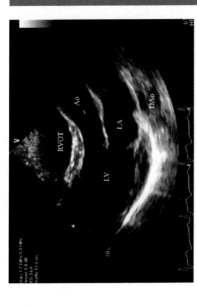

Figure 2-9. Parasternal long-axis view. Ao, aorta; DAo, descending aorta; LA, left atrium; LV, left ventricle; N, transducer notch; RVOT, right ventricular outflow tract.

Doppler Examination

Color Doppler

- MV and AoV: Color box should include the interventricular septum (IVS), AoV, and MV.
- This view is especially useful for identifying eccentric regurgitant jets and ventricular septal defects (VSDs), and for assessing aortic regurgitation (AR) severity.

M-Mode Examination

Chambers

- Midventricle to include the anteroseptum and inferolateral walls

Valves

- MV and AoV structure and leaflet motion

RIGHT VENTRICULAR INFLOW TRACT

See Figure 2-10.

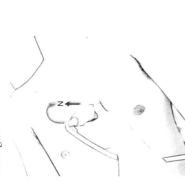

Obtaining The Image
- From the PLAX view, tilt the transducer tail toward the left shoulder.
- The imaging plane will slowly move anteriorly until the tricuspid valve (TV) is in view.

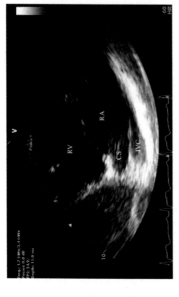

Figure 2-10. Right ventricular inflow tract view. CS, coronary sinus; IVC, inferior vena cava; N, transducer notch; RA, right atrium; RV, right ventricle.

2D Examination

Structures
- *Chambers:* right atrium (RA), right ventricle (RV), inferior vena cava (IVC), coronary sinus (CS)
- *Valves:* TV

Key Features
- The only view in which the posterior TV leaflet is seen
- Coaptation of the TV leaflets

Doppler Examination

Color Doppler
- TV: Color box should include the RA, TV, and RV.

Spectral Doppler
- Continuous wave (CW): Place the cursor through the vena contracta of the TV regurgitant jet (or the valve leaflet coaptation point if the vena contracta is not visualized).

Troubleshooting

The transducer tilt for this view is often directed toward a rib. Open the acoustic window by:
- Sliding the transducer laterally away from the RV
- Moving to a lower intercostal space if the image continues to be difficult to obtain

PARASTERNAL SHORT AXIS (PSAX) VIEW

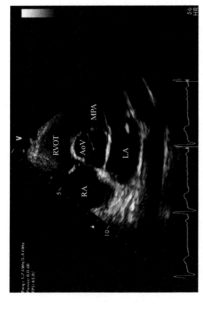

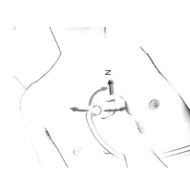

Figure 2-11. Parasternal short-axis view. AoV, aortic valve; LA, left atrium; MPA, main pulmonary artery; N, transducer notch; RA, right atrium; RVOT, right ventricular outflow tract.

Obtaining The Image

- From the PLAX view, rotate the transducer clockwise 90° (red arrow).
- Tilt the transducer tail slightly toward the patient's right shoulder for more apical views and away from the right shoulder for basal views (blue arrows).

2D Examination (AoV Level)

See Figure 2-11.

Structures

- *Chambers:* LA, RA, RV/RVOT, main pulmonary artery (MPA)
- *Valves:* AoV, TV, pulmonic valve (PV)

Key Features

- The three leaflets of the AoV with a circular aortic root

Doppler Examination (AoV Level)

Color Doppler

- AoV: Size color box to include the AoV.
- PV: Color box should include the RVOT, PV, and MPA.
- TV: Color box should include the RA, TV, and interatrial septum.

Spectral Doppler

- PW: PV (place sample volume in the RVOT, 1 cm proximal to PV).
- CW: Place cursor through the vena contracta of the TV or PV regurgitant jet, or the valve leaflet coaptation point.

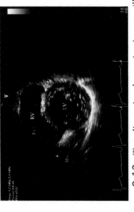

Figure 2-12. Two-dimensional examination, mitral valve (MV) level. LV, left ventricle; RV, right ventricle.

2D Examination (MV Level)

See Figure 2-12.

Structures
- *Chambers:* LV, RV
- *Valves:* MV

Key Features
- Anterior and posterior MV leaflets with the coaptation point at the center of the ventricle

Tip: If the valve appears to open medially, rotate the transducer clockwise for a more complete view; if it opens laterally, rotate counterclockwise.

Doppler Examination (MV Level)

Color Doppler
- MV: Color box should include the MV.

Spectral Doppler
- Generally not useful in this view

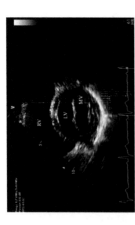

Figure 2-13. Two-dimensional examination, papillary muscle level. LV, left ventricle; RV, right ventricle.

2D Examination (Papillary Muscle Level)

See Figure 2-13.

Structures
- *Chambers:* LV, RV

Key Features
- Circular shape of the LV
- Anterolateral and posteromedial papillary muscles

Doppler Examination (Papillary Muscle Level)

Color and spectral Doppler are not generally useful in this view.

Troubleshooting (PSAX)
Rib artifacts are common and can be minimized by sliding the transducer away from the rib shadowing the ventricle.

APICAL FOUR-CHAMBER (A4C) VIEW

See Figure 2-14.

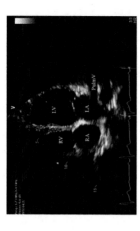
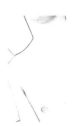
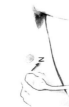

2D Examination

Structures
- Chambers: LA, RA, LV (inferoseptal and anterolateral walls), RV, pulmonary vein (PulmV)
- Valves: MV, TV

Key Features
- Entire length of the LV is visualized.
- LV endocardium is well-defined in all segments.
- Coaptation of the MV and TV (septal and anterior) leaflets
- RV free wall and TV annulus motion

Obtaining The Image
- This view is generally found near the point of maximum impulse.
- Angle the transducer tail away from the patient's right shoulder.

Doppler Examination

Color Doppler
- MV: Color box should include LA, MV, LV inflow tract.
- TV: Color box should include RA, TV, RV, IVS.

Spectral Doppler
- PW: MV (place sample volume at leaflet tips; for volumetric calculations, place sample at mitral annulus level), PulmV
- CW: Place cursor through the vena contracta of regurgitant jet or MV and TV leaflet coaptation point.
- TD: Septal and lateral MV annuli, lateral TV annulus

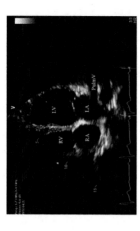

Figure 2-14. Apical four-chamber view. LA, left atrium; LV, left ventricle; N, transducer notch; PulmV, pulmonary vein; RA, right atrium; RV, right ventricle.

Troubleshooting

Common Problems
- If ventricles visualized, but not the atria, tilt the transducer up or down.
- If MV/TV coaptation or LV/RV is cut-off, rotate transducer clockwise or counterclockwise.
- If apex not centered, move transducer medially or laterally.

Note: The location of the optimal acoustic window also varies depending on how much the patient is rolled onto his/her left side (i.e., if the patient is supine, the apical window will be more medial).

APICAL FIVE-CHAMBER (A5C) VIEW
See Figure 2-15.

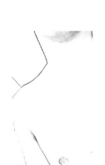

Obtaining The Image

- From the A4C view, tilt the transducer tail toward the patient's left hip (red arrow).

Note: The AoV plane lies only a few degrees anterior to the A4C plane.

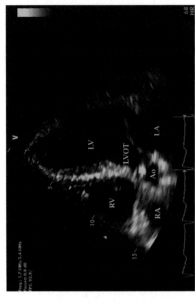

Figure 2-15. Apical five-chamber view. Ao, aorta; LA, left atrium; LV, left ventricle; LVOT, left ventricular outflow tract; N, transducer notch; RA, right atrium; RV, right ventricle.

2D Examination

Structures
- *Chambers:* LA, RA, LV, LVOT, RV, Ao
- *Valves:* MV, TV, AoV

Key Features
- Similar to A4C with additional visualization of the LVOT, AoV, and Ao root

Doppler Examination

Color Doppler
- Color box should include the AoV.

Spectral Doppler
- PW: LVOT (place the sample volume ~1 cm proximal to the AoV).
- CW: Place cursor through the vena contracta of the AoV regurgitant jet or the valve leaflet coaptation point to evaluate aortic stenosis (AS).

APICAL TWO-CHAMBER VIEW

See Figure 2-16.

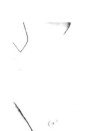

Obtaining The Image

- From the A4C view, rotate the transducer roughly 30° counterclockwise (red arrow).

Note: Be careful not to foreshorten the LV by moving the transducer medially.

2D Examination

Structures

- *Chambers:* LA, LV (anterior and inferior walls)
- *Valves:* MV

Key Features

- Entire length of the LV with well-defined endocardial segments
- Coaptation of the MV leaflets
- Left atrial appendage (LAA) and CS occasionally visualized

Doppler Examination

Color Doppler

- MV: Color box should include the LA, MV, and LV inflow.

Spectral Doppler

- PW: Generally, place the sample volume at MV leaflet tips; for volumetric calculations, place the sample volume at the mitral annulus level.
- CW: MV leaflet coaptation point

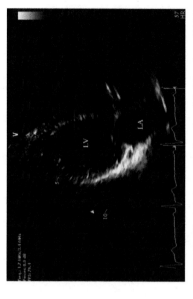

Figure 2-16. Apical two-chamber view. LA, left atrium; LV, left ventricle; N, notch.

Troubleshooting

This view is difficult to obtain because of two common problems:

- The transducer slips as the equipment is rotated
- The transducer is not at the apex

Tip: Anchor the transducer with one hand and rotate it with the other.

APICAL PARASTERNAL LONG-AXIS (APLAX) VIEW

See Figure 2-17.

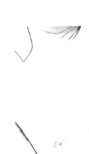

Obtaining The Image

- From the A2C view, rotate the transducer roughly 30° counterclockwise (red arrow).

Tip: Be careful not to fore-shorten the LV by moving the transducer medially.

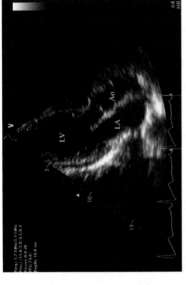

Figure 2-17. Apical parasternal long-axis view. Ao, aorta; LA, left atrium; LV, left ventricle; N, transducer notch.

2D Examination

Structures

- *Chambers:* LA, LV (anteroseptal and inferolateral walls), Ao.
- *Valves:* MV, AoV.

Key Features

- Coaptation of the MV and AoV leaflets.

Doppler Examination

Color Doppler

- MV and AoV: Color box should include the IVS, AoV, and MV.

Spectral Doppler

- PW: LVOT, MV inflow
- CW: MV for regurgitation and AoV for AS

SUBCOSTAL CORONAL VIEW

See Figure 2-18.

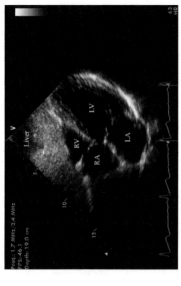

Obtaining The Image

- With the patient lying supine, apply firm pressure at a 45° angle two finger-widths below the xiphoid process.
- Aim the transducer up toward the patient's left shoulder.

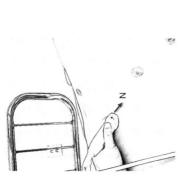

Freq: 1.7 MHz; 3.4 MHz
FPS: 46.1
Depth: 19.0 cm

Figure 2-18. Subcostal coronal view. LA, left atrium; LV, left ventricle; N, transducer notch; RA, right atrium; RV, right ventricle.

2D Examination

Structures
- *Chambers:* LA, RA, LV, RV
- *Valves:* MV, TV

Key Features
- LV function
- Pericardial effusion and tamponade physiology if effusion present
- Look for interatrial septal defects.

Doppler Examination

Color Doppler
- MV: Color box should include the LA and MV.
- TV: Color box should include the RA and TV.
- Interatrial septum

Spectral Doppler
- CW: Through TV coaptation or vena contracta of regurgitant jet

Troubleshooting

- Utilize the liver's low acoustic impedance by imaging slightly to the right of the xiphoid process.
- Image at end-inspiration.
- Relax the abdominal muscles by bending the patient's knees.
- Decrease the transducer frequency to increase the depth of ultrasound penetration.

27

SUBCOSTAL SAGITTAL VIEW

See Figure 2-19.

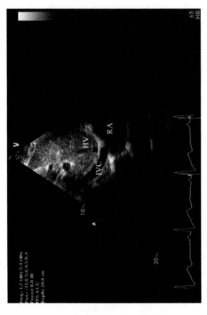

Figure 2-19. Subcostal sagittal view. HV, hepatic vein; IVC, inferior vena cava; N, transducer notch; RA, right atrium.

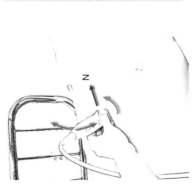

Obtaining The Image

- Angle the transducer per-pendicular to the patient.
- From the coronal view, rotate the transducer counterclockwise until the notch is toward the patient's head.
- A slight tilt of the transducer tail to the patient's left brings the IVC into view; tilting to the patient's right brings the abdominal Ao into view.

2D Examination

Structures

- Chambers: RA, IVC, hepatic vein (HV), Descending aorta (DAo) (not shown).

Key Features

- IVC size and change with respiration (may require "sniff" maneuver if there is no significant change in size with normal breathing).

Doppler Examination

Color Doppler

- IVC and hepatic vein
- DAo for turbulent flow

Spectral Doppler

- PW: Hepatic vein and DAo

SUPRASTERNAL NOTCH (SSN) VIEW

See Figure 2-20.

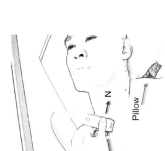

Obtaining The Image
- Move the pillow under the shoulder blades, extending the patient's neck.
- The transducer is placed above the suprasternal notch.
- The transducer notch points to the patient's head, with the transducer tail also angled slightly in this direction.

2D Examination

Structures
- *Chambers:* LA, aortic arch, brachiocephalic artery (BCA), left common carotid artery (LCA), left subclavian artery (LSC), right pulmonary artery (RPA).

Key Features
- Look for anatomic abnormalities to suggest an aortic dissection, aortic coarctation, or patent ductus arteriosis.

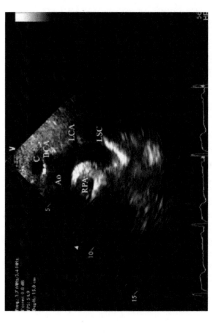

Figure 2-20. Suprasternal notch view. Ao, aorta; BCA: brachiocephalic artery; C, brachiocephalic vein; LCA, left common carotid artery; LSC, left subclavian artery; N, transducer notch; RPA, right pulmonary artery.

Doppler Examination

Color Doppler
- Arch vessels: Color box should include all of the arch vessels.

Spectral Doppler
- PW sampling of the proximal DAo (holodiastolic flow reversal seen in moderate to severe AR) or any areas of turbulence.
- CW of AoV for aortic valve jet.

Tips For Technically Difficult Studies

Patients with Hyperinflated Lungs
The heart lies lower in the thoracic cavity in patients with longstanding pulmonary disease.

* Lower-than-normal parasternal windows should be attempted. It is not uncommon to obtain the best parasternal orientation from the subcostal view.
* Have the patient lie flat.
* Transducer orientation is the same, and all axis views are often attainable.

Obesity
* Reduce transducer frequency for deeper penetration.
* Increase transducer pressure slightly for better tissue compression.
* Optimize width and depth.
* Decrease frame rates.

3

The Role of Contrast in Echocardiography

Majesh Makan

KEY POINTS FOR CONTRAST OPTIMIZATION

- Mechanical index (MI) <0.5
- Optimize time gain compensation and overall gain settings
- Minimize near-field gain
- Generally have focus point at the base of the heart
- Optimize probe position for nonforeshortened views
- Doppler enhancement measuring the modal/darkest envelope
- Correct timing and dose of contrast require good communication between sonographer and nurse

INDICATIONS

- Reduced image quality with ≥2 wall segments not visualized
- Increase the accuracy of ventricular volume measurement
- Stress testing for enhanced endocardial edge detection
- Doppler signal enhancement
- Evaluation for left ventricular (LV) thrombus, LV aneurysm
- Intracardiac masses

CONTRAINDICATIONS

- Pregnant or lactating women
- Patients who have known allergic reaction to perflutren (octafluoropropane gas)
- Right-to-left, bidirectional, or transient right-to-left cardiac shunts
- Sensitivity to blood, blood products, or albumin (Optison only)

GENERAL PRINCIPLES

Using contrast while performing an echocardiogram can play a vital role and provide additional information in the patient's diagnosis and management. Contrast consists of microbubbles that when mixed with red blood cells in the cardiac chambers increase the scatter of the ultrasonic signal, therefore enhancing the blood–tissue interface. Optison is a perfluoropropane-filled shell derived from human serum albumin, whereas Definity is a perfluoropropane lipid-coated microbubble that has to be agitated before use. The FDA has approved contrast for LV opacification and enhancement of endocardial border definition.

Contrast should be given to a patient in the following circumstances:

- **Reduced image quality:** When two or more wall segments cannot be visualized in any one view
- **Doppler signal enhancement:** For valvular stenosis and regurgitation
  - The best Doppler signal is obtained at the beginning of contrast administration. This helps avoid "blooming" artifact and overestimation of the Doppler signal.
  - Measure only the modal envelope (Fig. 3-1).
- **To rule out LV apical pathology:** LV thrombus, aneurysm, pseudoaneurysm, apical hypertrophy, noncompaction (Fig. 3-2)
- **To assess regional wall motion abnormalities**
- **In exercise/pharmacologic stress testing**
  - Ensures visualization of all myocardial segments
- **To increase accuracy of ejection fraction and LV volume calculations** (Fig. 3-3)
- **In ICU and ER settings**
  - ICU patients are usually technically difficult to image because of mechanical ventilation equipment, chest tubes, and bandages, as well as the presence of lung disease, and inability to reposition these patients.
  - Most patients are imaged supine rather than in the left lateral position.
  - When patients present in the ER with chest pain, using contrast is helpful to provide complete analysis of all myocardial segments for regional wall motion abnormalities.
- **To identify intracardiac masses**
  - Thrombus does not enhance and is outlined as a "black" mass with contrast enhancement of the cardiac chambers.
  - Tumors within the cardiac chambers can similarly be outlined by contrast.
  - The use of contrast increases the sensitivity of detection of intracardiac masses and also helps in differentiating these from normal structures (e.g., LV trabeculation) (Fig. 3-4).

- **Key Points:**
  1. *Move focus point transiently from the base of the heart to the apex to evaluate the LV apex for pathology.*
  2. *Although IV contrast may help with endocardial definition, it does not reduce image foreshortening secondary to nonoptimal probe or patient positioning. Try to optimize the image prior to contrast administration.*

PREPARING DEFINITY (LANTHEUS MEDICAL IMAGING) CONTRAST

- Definity has to be agitated in the vial mixer. Do not use unless it has completed the cycle. It is a clear liquid that turns milky after activation.
- Draw 1.5 mL of Definity with a vented spike and dilute in 8.5 mL of saline.
- Turn MI down <0.5 to achieve maximum LV opacification.
- Change gain settings to optimize endocardial border detection.
- Inject saline flush *slowly*; otherwise this will cause apical contrast attenuation.

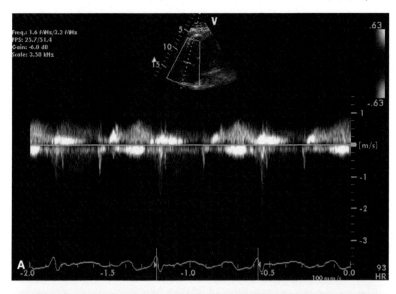

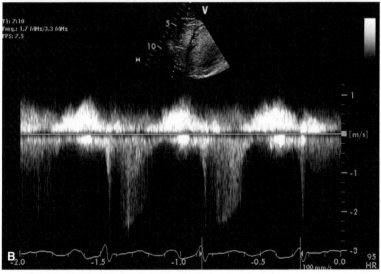

Figure 3-1. A: No measurable envelope is seen on spectral Doppler in patient with trace tricuspid regurgitation (TR). **B:** After contrast enhancement, a clear TR Doppler envelope can be accurately measured.

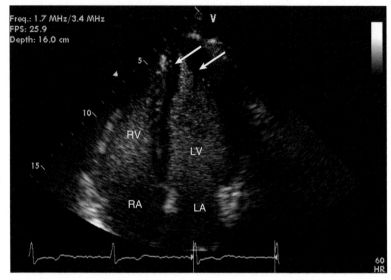

Figure 3-2. Contrast-enhanced apical four-chamber view during diastole showing focal increase in myocardial thickness at the apex (*arrows*), giving a "spadelike" appearance to the left ventricle (LV) cavity. LA, left atrium; RA, right atrium; RV, right ventricle.

- Follow with a 1 mL *slow* flush.
- Repeat as needed. Increase or decrease injection rate based on image quality.

PREPARING OPTISON (GE HEALTHCARE) CONTRAST

- Draw 3 mL of Optison with a vented spike and dilute in 5 mL of saline.
- Suspend the solution until milky by rolling between the palms of your hands.
- Lower MI to 0.3–0.4.
- Inject 1–2 mL of Optison solution followed by a *slow* saline flush.
- Change gain settings to optimize endocardial border detection.
- Repeat as needed. Increase or decrease injection rate based on image quality.

PITFALLS

High Mechanical Index
- This disrupts and destroys the contrast microbubbles.
- This is seen as a dark swirling artifact, especially close to where the ultrasound beam is focused.
- To fix, decrease MI and reinject contrast slowly.

Attenuation
- This is caused by injecting contrast too fast or pushing too much.
- This is seen as a bright "pool" of contrast in the apex that casts a shadow over the rest of the heart.

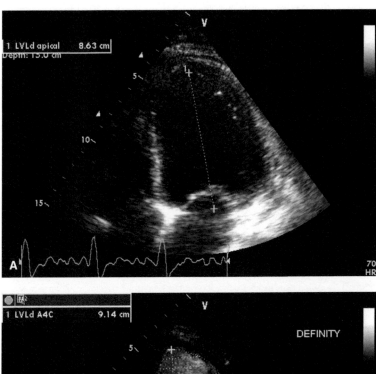

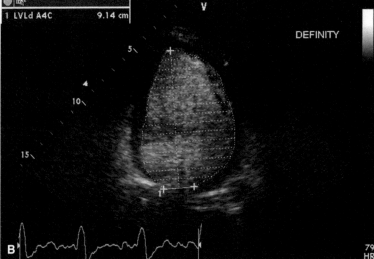

Figure 3-3. The difference in accuracy in measuring left ventricular volume and long-axis dimensions between **(A)** unenhanced end-diastolic apical four-chamber view and **(B)** contrast-enhanced end-diastolic apical four-chamber view.

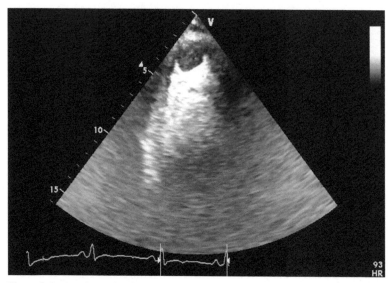

Figure 3-4. Apical two-chamber view with contrast delineating a "black" ovoid mass attached to an akinetic left ventricular apex consistent with thrombus.

- To fix, either wait for some of the contrast to transit through the heart or move the focus point to the apex and turn the MI up to destroy some of the bubbles. Then turn the MI back down and return the focus point to the base of the heart (Fig. 3-5).

LV Underfilled with Contrast
- This is especially seen affecting the apex or in patients with dilated LV (Fig. 3-6).
- This is seen as "swirling" of contrast as it mixes with unopacified blood in the LV.
- To fix, inject more contrast, then flush with a faster flush. This will help push the contrast to the apex.

AGITATED BACTERIOSTATIC SALINE CONTRAST

Reasons to Perform an Agitated Saline Contrast
- With patients who have unexplained right heart enlargement.
- In patients with suspected transient ischemic attack (TIA) or cerebral vascular accident (CVA) (<55 years of age).
- To evaluate for patent foramen ovale (PFO)/atrial septal defect (ASD).
- In the presence of atrial septal aneurysm.
- To enhance tricuspid regurgitation (TR) jet for pulmonary artery (PA) systolic pressure measurement (not as accurate as using commercially available contrasts because of spectral broadening).

Contraindications
- Known ASD/ventricular septal defect (VSD)
- Pregnancy

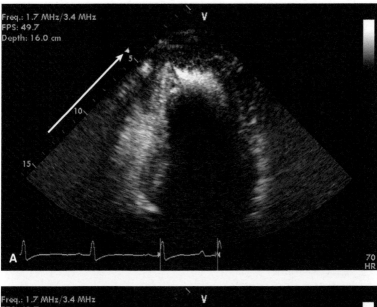

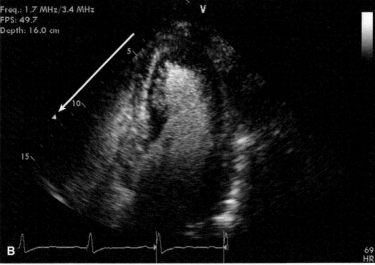

Figure 3-5. (**A**) Pooling of the contrast in the left ventricular (LV) apex causing attenuation of the basal to mid-LV cavity in this apical four-chamber view. The focus (▷) is transiently shifted to the apex to "destroy" excess bubbles and allow the proximal chamber to be visualized. The focus can then be readjusted back to the normal position at the base of the heart (**B**).

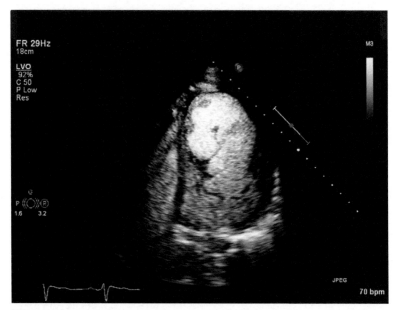

Figure 3-6. Swirling unenhanced blood is seen in a dilated left ventricle secondary to inadequate amount of contrast injected.

PREPARING AGITATED BACTERIOSTATIC SALINE CONTRAST

If patients have both contrast and agitated saline contrast ordered, the saline contrast should be given for the evaluation of shunt before contrast is used!

- Draw 8 mL bacteriostatic saline into a 10 mL syringe, connect to a three-way stop-cock, and connect an empty 10 mL syringe to the other port.
- Leave 1 mL of air in the saline syringe, but ensure that there is no air in the IV line or stop-cock.
- Agitate the solution (with stop-cock in closed position to patient) by rapidly transferring the volume of one syringe to the other, back and forth several times until the solution is foamy.
- Inject the agitated saline.
- Repeat injection with patient performing Valsalva maneuver.
- Capture 8–10 beat loops of both normal and Valsalva injections (long capture is important to evaluate for extracardiac shunts).

INJECTION OF AGITATED SALINE

- This is typically performed for detection of cardiac shunts.
- Saline "bubbles" are generally too large to pass through the pulmonary circulation and opacify the left heart, unless a right-to-left shunt bypassing the pulmonary capillary bed is present.
- Shunts are defined as intracardiac at the level of the atria (PFO, ASD) or extracardiac (pulmonary or hepatic arterial-venous malformations).

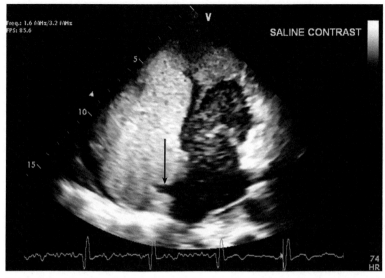

Figure 3-7. Apical four-chamber view with injected saline bubble study showing "negative contrast" (*arrow*) in right atrium secondary to left-to-right shunt.

- Left-to-right shunts may be seen as "negative" contrast in the right atrium (RA), where nonopacified blood from the left atrium (LA) is outlined by the injected agitated saline in the RA (Fig. 3-7).
- If persistent left superior vena cava (PLSVC) is suspected, the bubble study should be performed from an IV placed in the left arm and opacification should be observed from a parasternal long-axis (PLAX) view. The coronary sinus will opacify before the right ventricle (RV) if PLSVC is present (Fig. 3-8).

- **Key Points:**
  1. *Intracardiac shunt: Quick, dense opacification of LV (<3 to 4 beats); opacification is intensified or occurs only with Valsalva (PFO). If shunt is significant, RV enlargement may be present (ASD).*
  2. *Extracardiac shunt: Delayed opacification (>5 to 6 beats); opacification slowly builds in intensity in the LV with each successive beat as the bubbles slowly circulate to the LV. Site of bubble entry into the LA is from the pulmonary veins.*
  3. *"Pseudocontrast" (faint, diffuse bubbles), may be seen transiently (1 to 2 beats) in the LA and LV, unrelated to injection of agitated saline, secondary to the release of "stagnant" blood in the pulmonary veins after Valsalva, causing spontaneous echo contrast. This can be confirmed by repeating Valsalva without agitated saline injection to reproduce the "pseudocontrast" effect.*
  4. *False-negative agitated saline studies may be related to the inability to transiently increase RA pressure above LA pressure (e.g., inadequate Valsalva, severe LV diastolic dysfunction) or antecubital vein injection of agitated saline being directed away from the interatrial septum, especially in the presence of a prominent eustachian valve.*

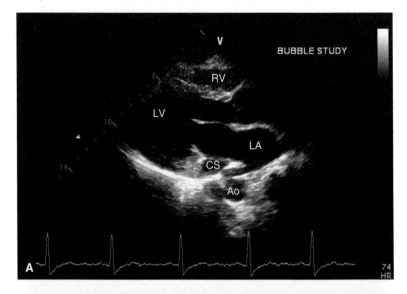

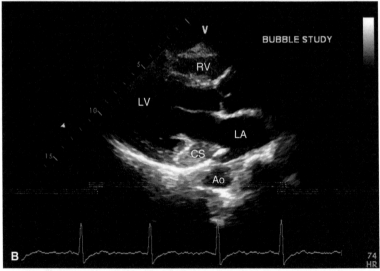

Figure 3-8. Patient with persistent left superior vena cava with bubble study performed from IV in left arm. **A:** Parasternal long-axis (PLAX) view prior to injection showing a dilated coronary sinus (CS). **B:** Early after injection of agitated saline, PLAX showing opacification of the CS before the right ventricle (RV). **C:** Later after injection of agitated saline, PLAX showing opacification of both CS and RV. Ao, aorta; LA, left atrium; LV, left ventricle.

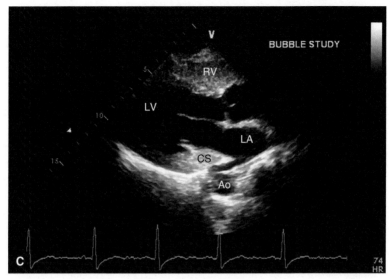

Figure 3-8. (*Continued*)

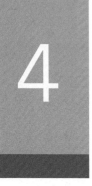

4

Quantification of Left Ventricular Systolic and Diastolic Function

Praveen K. Rao and Christopher L. Holley

HIGH-YIELD CONCEPTS

- *Normal left ventricle (LV) size:* Parasternal long-axis (PLAX) diameter ≤4.5 (± 0.36) cm ♀, 5.0 (± 0.41) cm ♂; apical four-chamber (A4C) end-diastolic volume indexed to body surface area (BSA) ≤45 (± 8) mL/m^2 ♀, ≤54 (± 10) mL/m^2 ♂
- *Normal LV systolic function:* Ejection fraction (EF) ≥54% ♀; ≥52% ♂
- *Normal LV mass, indexed to BSA:* <89 mL/m^2 ♀, <103 mL/m^2 ♂
- *Normal left atrium (LA) size, indexed to BSA:* <35 mL/m^2
- *Normal diastolic function* is quickly assessed by tissue Doppler imaging (TDI) of the mitral annulus; e' lateral ≥10 cm/sec or medial ≥7 cm/sec

---

KEY VIEWS

- *PLAX:* Two-dimensional (2D) (linear) measurements of LV, LA, and aortic root (AR)
- *Parasternal short axis (PSAX):* Assessment of LV mass
- *A4C:* Tracings for LV and LA volumes; Doppler assessment of mitral inflow (MIF) and annular velocities

---

INTRODUCTION

Accurate quantitative assessment of the LV is an essential aspect of echocardiography. Calculating systolic and diastolic function impacts prognosis and treatment of many cardiac diseases. At the time of interpretation, indexed measurements (to BSA or height) should be used in reports, as "normal" measurements vary significantly by gender and body size.

Tips for Optimizing Image Quality

- Adjust image acquisition settings as detailed in Chapter 1. Optimizing patient positioning and acquiring images at held end-expiration may also improve image quality.
- Use contrast (see Chapter 3) when appropriate to visualize the endocardium (i.e., unable to assess ≥ two myocardial segments).

Tips for Interpreting Studies

- *Qualitative* size and function estimates should be avoided except as a "reality check" for measured values.
- Use *multiple views* for assessment.

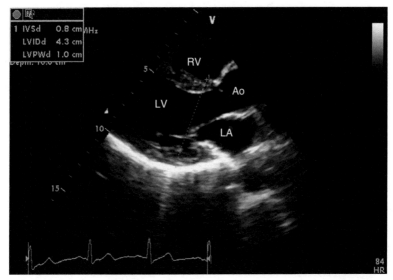

Figure 4-1. Parasternal long-axis view with linear left ventricular measurements performed at the level of the mitral valve leaflet tips. Ao, aorta; LA, left atrium; LV, left ventricle; RV, right ventricle.

- Beware of *off-axis* views as they may distort the comparative size of chambers and not allow use of standardized normal ranges.

> - **Key Point:** *Use of contrast does not increase accuracy of chamber measurements if the apical images are foreshortened. Optimize probe and patient positioning before injection of contrast and reduction of machine mechanical index.*

LV DIMENSIONS

Plax

- At a minimum, make simple linear measurements and compare to (nonindexed) upper limits of normal (Fig. 4-1 and Table 4-1).

TABLE 4-1	Linear Dimensions			
	LVIDd (cm)	SWT or PWT (cm)	RWT (cm)	LA volume index (mL/m^2)
Normal	4.5 ± 0.36 ♀, 5.0 ± 0.41 ♂	1	0.42	16–34

LA, left atrial; LVIDd, left ventricular internal diameter at end-diastole; PWT, posterior wall thickness; RWT, relative wall thickness; SWT, septal wall thickness.
Adapted from Lang RM, Badano LP, Mor-Avi V, et al. Recommendations for chamber quantification by echocardiography in adults: an update from the American Society of Echocardiography and the European Association of Cardiovascular Imaging. *J Am Soc Echocardiogr.* 2015;28:1–39.

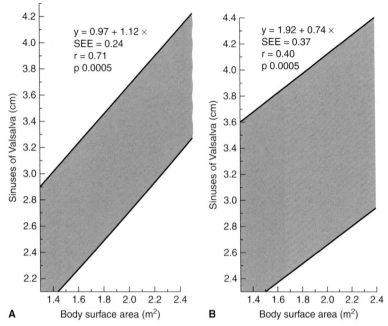

Figure 4-2. Ninety-five percent normal confidence intervals for aortic root dimension at the sinuses of Valsalva indexed to body surface area for adults <40 years of age (**A**) and those ≥40 years (**B**). From Roman MJ, Devereux RB, Kramer-Fox R, et al. Two-dimensional echocardiographic aortic root dimensions in normal children and adults. *Am J Cardiol*. 1989;64:507–512, with permission from Elsevier.

- Left ventricular internal diameter (LVID) ("minor axis," left ventricular internal diameter at end-diastole [LVIDd] and LVIDs, measured at mitral valve [MV] leaflet tips in end-diastole and end-systole, respectively).
- Septal and inferolateral wall thicknesses (measured at MV leaflet tips in end-diastole).
- Aortic root diameter at the sinuses, sinotubular junction, and proximal ascending aorta (Fig. 4-2).
- LA size more accurately measured as a volume in A4C rather than linear dimensions in PLAX view.
- M-mode measurements may be used, although beware of errors related to beam angle (Fig. 4-3).

Apical Views—A4C and Apical Two Chamber (A2C)

The minimum assessment should include LA volume assessment and measurement of LV volume in systole and diastole for left ventricular ejection fraction (LVEF) (Table 4-2).

- The LA is measured at end-systole tracing from the MV annulus and excluding the pulmonary veins (PVs) and LA appendage.

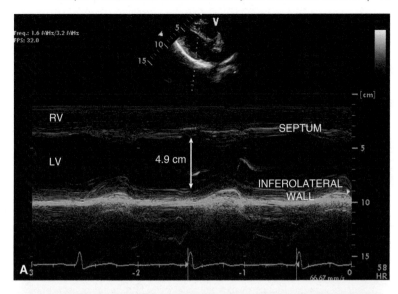

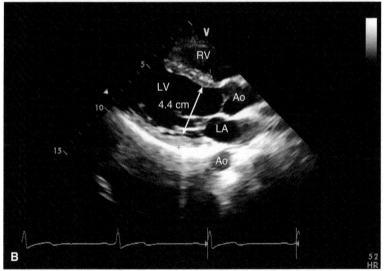

Figure 4-3. (**A**) M-mode oblique to long axis of the left ventricle (LV) in the parasternal long-axis view leading to overestimation of the LV end-diastolic internal diameter compared to two-dimensional measurement (**B**) in the same patient. Ao, aorta; LA, left atrium; RV, right ventricle.

TABLE 4-2	Volumes and Mass		
	LV diastolic volume indexed to BSA (mL/m^2)	LV systolic volume indexed to BSA (mL/m^2)	LV mass by 2D method indexed to BSA (g/m^2)
Normal	45 ± 8 ♀ 54 ± 10 ♂	16 ± 4 ♀ 21 ± 5 ♂	44–88 ♀ 50–102 ♂

BSA, body surface area; LV, left ventricular; 2D, two dimensional.
Adapted from Lang RM, Badano LP, Mor-Avi V, et al. Recommendations for chamber quantification by echocardiography in adults: an update from the American Society of Echocardiography and the European Association of Cardiovascular Imaging. *J Am Soc Echocardiogr.* 2015;28:1–39.

- The LV volume tracing should exclude the papillary muscles and trabeculations. Ensure that a *nonforeshortened* view is used (apex should move inward rather than toward the annulus).
- The LV long-axis length at end-diastole is also used in the calculation of LV mass and is another method to ensure that images are not foreshortened.

Three-dimensional Echocardiography (3DE)

- In patients with good image quality, the accuracy of 3DE in the assessment of LV volume and mass is comparable to cardiac magnetic resonance imaging.
- 3DE images can be reconstructed offline from a set of 2D cross-sections, or obtained real time using a matrix-array transducer.
- 3DE is not subject to plane positioning errors that can lead to chamber foreshortening that can be seen in 2D imaging.

- Key Points:
  1. *PLAX: Measures LVIDd, left ventricular internal diameter at end-systole (LVISd), septal wall thickness (SWT), and posterior wall thickness (PWT), all made at the level of the mitral leaflet tips.*
  2. *M-mode generally overestimates LV internal dimensions.*
  3. *3D image quality depends on good 2D images.*

LV SYSTOLIC FUNCTION

- The preferred method is the modified Simpson's biplane estimate (summation of elliptical discs along LV long axis; formula not shown but available in standard analysis packages) (Table 4-3). If there are no regional wall motion abnormalities, a single plane estimate may be used instead.

TABLE 4-3	LV Functional Assessment	
	LVEF (%)	2D-peak global longitudinal strain (mean,%)
Normal	52–74	≤–18.6[*]

LV, left ventricle; LVEF, left ventricular ejection fraction; 2D, two dimensional.
*Negative sign denotes shortening; that is, more negative numbers = increased shortening.

- *Biplane method:* Use A4C and A2C views to trace LV volumes for end-systole and end-diastole.
- *Single plane method:* Use A4C or A2C view to trace LV volumes for end-systole and end-diastole (Fig. 4-4).

$$EF = (EDV - ESV)/EDV$$

- LVEF is not only influenced by intrinsic myocardial function *but also LV geometry.* For example, patients with concentric left ventricular hypertrophy (LVH) may have a normal or even increased LVEF but significant intrinsic myocardial dysfunction. This is because LVEF relies on inward endocardial displacement that is independently affected by relative wall thickness (RWT). LV strain measurements can uncover intrinsic myocardial dysfunction *independent of LV geometry.* Systolic strain describes how the myocardium deforms by comparing the original myocardial length (L_o) at end-diastole to its final length (L_f) at end-systole ($L_f - L_o$).
- 2D LV strain tracks the intrinsic inhomogeneities or "speckles" in the myocardium to measure these changes. From the three apical views, a global or mean peak systolic strain can be calculated as an indicator of global LV systolic function (see Fig. 4-4, C). Global and regional strain imaging has become a powerful echocardiographic tool. It is more sensitive than assessment for regional wall motion abnormalities or tissue Doppler imaging for the detection of early cases of myocardial ischemia. Strain imaging and speckle tracking can also aid in the assessment of electromechanical dyssynchrony and optimization of cardiac resynchronization therapy.

- **Key Points:**
    1. *EF = (EDV − ESV)/EDV*
    2. *LV strain is more sensitive than assessment of regional wall motion abnormalities in detecting cases of early myocardial ischemia.*

LV MASS

2D and 3D Methods Are Preferred over M-mode (Fig. 4-5A,B).

- Area-length (use SAX epicardial/endocardial areas to determine myocardial thickness, plus LV long axis from A4C) assumes the LV shape is a prolate ellipse.
- Truncated ellipsoid method (need the above, *plus* A4C MV annular width) is used when significant distortion to LV shape is present.
- Calculations are automated on most machines.

Linear Method: Uses LVIDd, SWT, PWT from PLAX view

- LV mass = $0.8 \times (1.04 [(LVIDd + PWT + SWT)^3 - (LVID)^3]) + 0.6$ g
- Characterization of hypertrophy based on RWT from PLAX in conjunction with calculated LV mass (indexed to BSA) (Table 4-4).
- RWT indexes wall thickness to long-axis dimension of ventricle:

$$RWT = 2 \times PWT/LVIDd$$

- **Key Points:**
    1. *LV mass = $0.8 \times (1.04 [(LVIDd + PWT + SWT)^3 - (LVID)^3]) + 0.6$ g*
    2. *RWT = $2 \times PWT/LVIDd$*

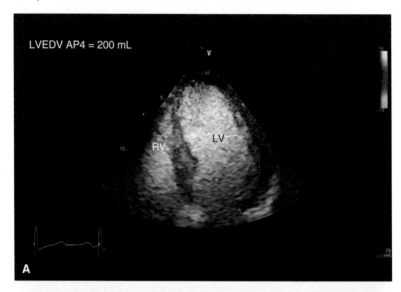

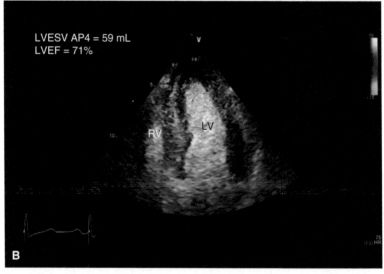

Figure 4-4. Quantifying left ventricular systolic function in a patient with left ventricular hypertrophy by calculating left ventricular ejection fraction (LVEF) using the single plane modified Simpson's method **(A,B)** and global 2D longitudinal peak strain (GLPS) **(C)**. Note despite normal LVEF (71%) there is a marked reduction in GLPS (−14%). APLAX, apical parasternal long axis; A4C, apical four chamber; A2C, apical two chamber; LV, left ventricle; LVEDV, left ventricular end-diastolic volume; LVESV, left ventricular end-systolic volume; RV, right ventricle.

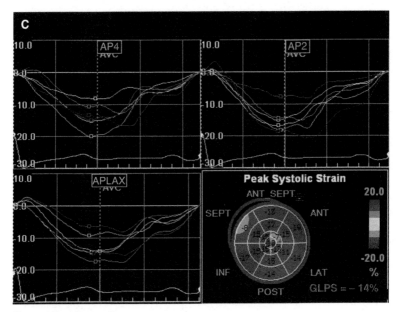

Figure 4-4. (*Continued*)

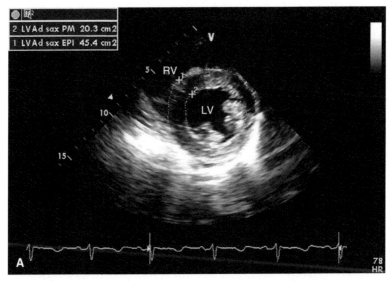

Figure 4-5. Calculation of left ventricular (LV) mass using the area-length method. **A:** Parasternal short axis at the mid-LV level with tracing of endocardium (excluding papillary muscles) and epicardium. (*continued*)

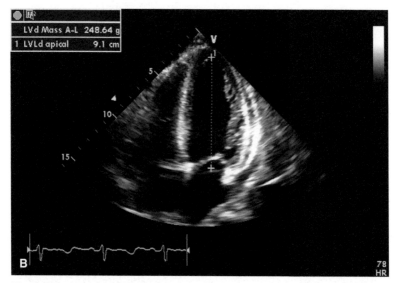

Figure 4-5. (*Continued*) **B:** Apical four-chamber view with LV long-axis measurement at end-diastole from mitral annulus to LV apex. RV, right ventricle.

DIASTOLIC FUNCTION ASSESSMENT

See Table 4-5 and Figure 4-6.

Doppler echocardiography, unlike invasive manometer-based methods, indirectly measures LV diastolic function through changes that occur in the pressure gradients between the LA and LV.

Mitral Inflow Pulsed-Wave (PW) Doppler: E and A Waves
- A4C view, PW Doppler at MV leaflet tips
- Key parameters:
  - E = peak early mitral inflow velocity

TABLE 4-4	Relationships Between LV Mass and RWT (cm)	
	LVMI ≤95 ♀, 115 ♂	**LVMI >95 ♀, 115 ♂**
RWT ≤0.42	Normal	Eccentric hypertrophy
RWT >0.42	Concentric remodeling	Concentric hypertrophy

LVMI, left ventricular mass indexed to body surface area (g/m²); RWT, relative wall thickness.
Adapted from Lang RM, Bierig M, Devereux RB, et al. Recommendations for chamber quantification: a report from the American Society of Echocardiography's Guidelines and Standards Committee and the Chamber Quantification Writing Group, developed in conjunction with the European Association of Echocardiography, a branch of the European Society of Cardiology. *J Am Soc Echocardiogr.* 2005;18: 1440–1463.

TABLE 4.5	Doppler Parameters and LV Diastolic Function			
Classification	**Normal**	**Grade I**	**Grade II**	**Grade III**
LV relaxation	Normal	Impaired	Impaired	Impaired
LAP	Normal	Low or normal	Elevated	Elevated
Average E/e' ratio	<10	<10	10–14	>14
Peak TR velocity (m/sec)	<2.8	<2.8	>2.8	>2.8
LA volume index	Normal	Normal or increased	Increased	Increased

LV: left ventricular; LAP: left atrial pressure; TR: tricuspid regurgitant; LA: left atrial. Nagueh SF, Smiseth OA, Appleton CP et al. Recommendations for the evaluation of left ventricular diastolic function by echocardiography: An update from the American Society of Echocardiography and the European Association of Cardiovascular Imaging. *J Am Soc Echocardiogr* 2016;29:277–314.

- A = peak late mitral inflow velocity
- DT = deceleration time (time from E to baseline)
- IVRT = isovolumic relaxation time (time between aortic valve closure and MV opening)
- Normally filling occurs predominantly early in diastole because of rapid LV relaxation that "sucks" blood from the LA; that is, E > A.
- Impairment of myocardial relaxation leads to a reliance on filling during late diastole; that is, E < A.
- In more severe stages of diastolic dysfunction, as LA pressure rises in response to ineffective filling, this ratio may "normalize." LA blood is then "pushed" into the LV; that is, E > A (pseudonormal) or E >> A (restrictive).
- Aging itself leads to gradual diastolic impairment, such that E = A by around age 65 (E/A = 1), with E < A by age 70.
  - In patients with atrial fibrillation (AF), the usual criteria for classifying diastolic filling patterns cannot be used due to a lack of an mitral inflow "A" wave. Peak velocity and DT of the mitral E wave vary with the irregular cardiac cycles.
    - E/E' of the septum can be used for the assessment of pulmonary capillary wedge pressure in patients with AF.
    - The duration and initial DT of PV diastolic flow may also be useful in determining LV filling pressures.
- The strain phase of Valsalva may be used to unmask underlying impaired myocardial relaxation in patients with a "pseudonormal pattern" by transiently reducing LA filling pressure. Similarly, this may be seen in "reversible" restrictive filling patterns. The use of this technique has been limited by the variability in patient effort to effect a reduction in LA pressure.
- IVRT and DT lengthen with impaired myocardial relaxation as the rate of LV pressure decline is reduced in early diastole, therefore reducing the transmitral filling gradient (loss of "suction"). In more severe diastolic dysfunction, IVRT and DT will shorten, secondary to a marked rise in LA driving pressure and reduced LV compliance (increase in "pushing").

	MIF (Mitral Inflow)	Valsalva	PV (Pulm. Vein)	Septal TDI	Key Features
Young NML	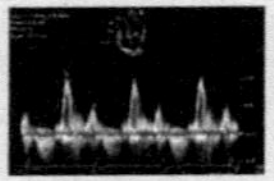	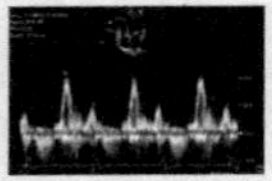	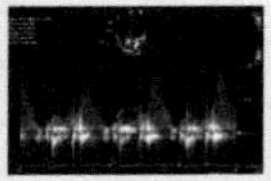	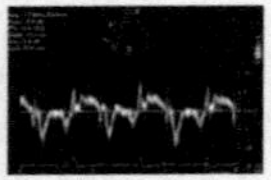	MIF pattern similar to restrictive where PV shows S < D; however, TDI is normal revealing rapid early filling related to vigorous LV suction.
NML	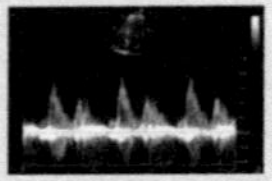	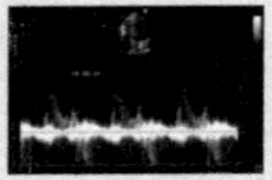	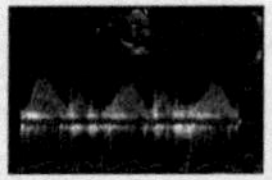	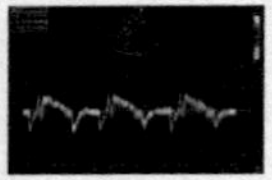	If TDI is normal, it is likely diastolic function is normal. Note that with Valsalva both E and A reduce proportionally.
Impaired	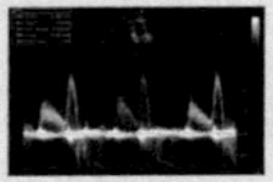	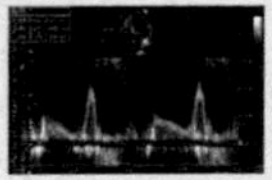	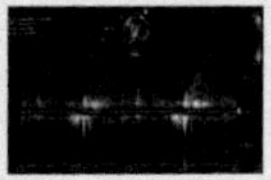	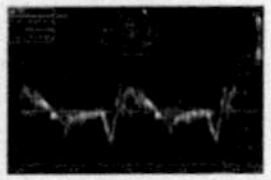	E < A ratio, increased DT, reduced TDI. S > D and E/e' not increased suggesting normal LA pressure.
Pseudonormal	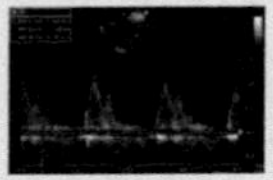	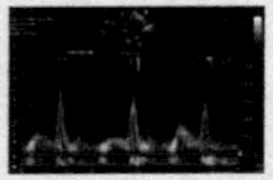	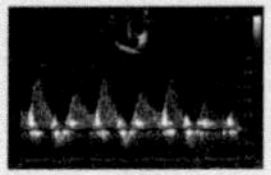	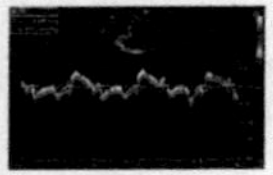	Valsalva unmasks E < A by transiently reducing LA pressure. S < D with increased E/e' suggesting increased LA pressure.
Restrictive	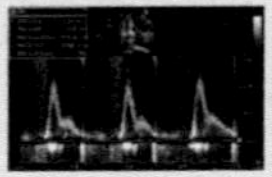	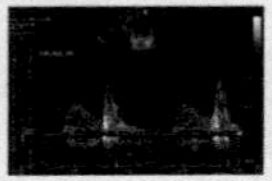	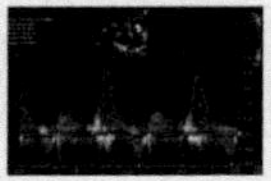	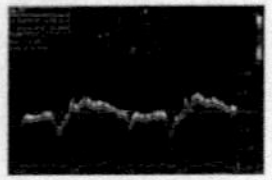	Tall E (MIF) and D (Pulm. Vein) waves with short DT secondary to increased LA pressure and reduced LV compliance. Valsalva unmasks E < A.
Fixed Restrictive	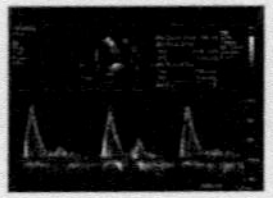	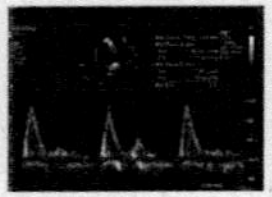	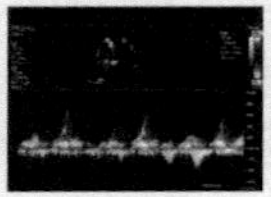	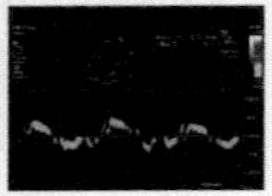	High LA pressure not affected by Valsalva.

Figure 4-6. Use of diastolic (D) function indices to categorize stage of diastolic dysfunction. DT, deceleration time; E/A, ratio of peak early mitral inflow velocity to peak late mitral inflow velocity; E/e', ratio of peak early mitral inflow velocity to early diastolic mitral annular velocity; LA, left atrial; LV, left ventricular; NML, normal; S, systolic; TDI, tissue Doppler imaging.

- **Key Points:**
  1. *Vigorous LV "suction" suggests normal diastolic function with active LV relaxation and a compliant ventricle drawing blood from the LA under low filling pressures. The need to "push" blood into the LV suggests significant diastolic dysfunction as now filling pressures are elevated so as to move blood into a noncompliant LV. This is seen with pseudonormal and restrictive Doppler patterns and portends increased morbidity for patients with heart failure.*
  2. *It may be difficult to determine diastolic function using mitral inflow pattern alone because (a) fusion of the E and A waves may not allow analysis, and (b) it cannot differentiate between normal or "pseudonormal" or restrictive patterns. Therefore, mitral inflow should be used in combination with tissue Doppler, as well as other indices of diastolic function.*

Tissue Doppler of the Mitral Annulus

Tissue Doppler is the most sensitive and reliable echocardiographic index of diastolic function, as long as there are no localized influences affecting annular motion. Rely on this parameter more than any other.

- A4C view, PW Doppler sample volume on septal or lateral MV annulus.
- e′ = tissue Doppler velocity of mitral annulus; normal septal ≥8 cm/sec, lateral ≥10 cm/sec (age dependent; younger patients = potentially higher values).
- Low frequency, high amplitude signal; recorded velocities much lower than blood flow velocities.
  - Lateral annulus velocity > septal annulus (exceptions: any regional influences on annular motion, e.g., constrictive pericarditis).
  - Less affected by preload than MIF.
- E/e′ correlates with LV filling pressures.
  - Increased LV filling pressures denoted by an average of septal and lateral E/e′ >14.
  - If only the lateral or septal E/e′ is available, then lateral E/e′ ratio >13 or septal E/e′ >15 is considered abnormal.
  - When available, age specific cut off values should be utilized.
  - In general, those with septal e′ <7 cm/sec, lateral e′ <10 cm/sec, average E/e′ ratio >14, LA volume index >34 ml/m², and peak TR velocity >2.8 m/sec are considered to have abnormal diastolic function.
  - Change in E/A ratio with Valsalva ≥0.5, pulmonary S < D wave peak velocities, pulmonary atrial reversal (aR) duration exceeds mitral A duration ≥30 msec (see later) are also considered abnormal.

Pulmonary Vein (PV): S/D (Systolic to Diastolic Filling Ratio)

A4C view, PW Doppler at atrial "back wall" (right superior PV)

- Normal: Triphasic (S1, S2, D) or biphasic with fusion of S waves. Also seen is brief aR at atrial contraction. S1 signifies atrial relaxation and is decreased in AF; S2 signifies propagation of flow through the pulmonary circulation and is decreased by elevated left atrial pressure and mitral regurgitation. Timing of the atrial D wave corresponds to the mitral E wave and reflects LV relaxation. The normal adult pattern is S > D with brief aR.
- Abnormal filling pressures: As mean LA pressure rises, filling during ventricular systole diminishes and the atrium fills primarily during early ventricular diastole (S < D). With reduced LV compliance, there is an increase in left ventricular end-diastolic

pressure and aR duration (≥30 msec longer than mitral A wave duration) and amplitude (>35 cm/sec) (i.e., blood refluxes back into PVs upon atrial contraction with increasing LV filling pressures).

• **Key Points:**
1. *The right superior PV is located near the interatrial septum and is best aligned for parallel Doppler interrogation. Slight anterior angulation of the probe (almost to an apical five chamber) offers best visualization of the vein. This is vital to obtain a good quality Doppler profile.*
2. *Despite Doppler echocardiography being the main modality for evaluating diastolic function, always place these measurements in the context of the 2D images; for example, diastolic function is unlikely to be normal if there is significant LVH, cardiomyopathy, or LA enlargement. Use 2D imaging to corroborate Doppler findings of increased LA pressure and also to identify reasons that Doppler indices may be discrepant and not reflective of LV diastolic function, such as significant mitral annular calcification or adherent pericardium limiting mitral annular motion.*

Diastolic Function Assessment in Special Populations

1. Hypertrophic Cardiomyopathy
   a. Look for E/e' >14, LA volume index >34 mL/m², pulmonary vein atrial reversal velocity (Ar-A duration ≥30 msec), and peak TR jet velocity >2.8 m/sec.
   b. If more than half of these variables met, LA pressure is elevated.
2. Restrictive Cardiomyopathy
   a. In those with grade 3 diastolic dysfunction, E/A ratio >2.5, DT <150 msec, IVRT <50 msec, and markedly reduced e' velocities.
   b. In those with constrictive pericarditis, septal e' is usually higher than lateral e' (annulus reversus) and thus the E/e' ratio should not be used to assess filling pressures.
3. Valvular Heart Disease
   a. Mitral stenosis: Look for a short IVRT <60 msec. Also if the mitral A wave is >1.5 m/sec at end diastole, LA pressure is elevated. E/e' ratio is not very useful here.
   b. Mitral regurgitation: E/e' evaluation in the setting of moderate or severe MR may not be very useful if the EF is normal. In those with depressed LVEF and severe MR, E/e' can be used to predict LV filling pressures.
4. Mitral Annular Calcification: LV filling pressures are difficult to estimate from E/e' in these patients.
5. Heart Transplantation
   a. A restrictive pattern is a common finding in heart transplant patients with normal diastolic function since donor hearts are usually from younger patients.
   b. No single diastolic parameter has yet to be proven to be highly predictive of graft rejection.
6. Atrial Fibrillation
   a. Septal E/e' ≥11, short IVRT are indicative of increased LV filling pressures.

5

Right Ventricular Function and Pulmonary Hemodynamics

Deana Mikhalkova and Nishath Quader

ANATOMY AND PHYSIOLOGY OF THE RIGHT VENTRICLE

- The RV is fundamentally different from the LV in both structure and function such that methods typically used to assess the LV do **not** work for the RV.
- The RV is a thin-walled pyramidal structure that "wraps around" the LV and it appears triangular when viewed in cross section. Shape of the RV is also influenced by the interventricular septum.
- The RV can be described in terms of three components: 1) the inlet, with the TV, chordae tendineae, and papillary muscles; 2) the trabeculated apical myocardium; and 3) the infundibulum, or conus, which is the smooth myocardial outflow region and pulmonic valve.
  - Additional structures unique to the RV: crista supraventricularis, prominent trabeculations, moderator band.

- Three prominent muscular bands are present in the RV: the parietal band, the septomarginal band, and the moderator band.
- The RV is connected in series with the LV and thus has the same stroke volume. In contrast to the LV, the RV is highly compliant and energetically efficient; designed to pump blood into the low-impedence, highly distensible pulmonary vascular system.
  - The RV is less capable of maintaining stroke volume in the setting of acute increases in afterload.
- In an adult, the volume of the RV is larger than the volume of the LV, whereas RV mass is about one sixth that of the LV.
- The RV contracts by three separate mechanisms: inward movement of the free wall to the interventricular septum (i.e., "bellows" motion, allowing for a large volume shift with little transverse motion), contraction of longitudinal fibers, and traction on the free wall as a result of LV contraction.
  - This method of contraction is fundamentally different than that of the LV. The main driving force of the LV comes from a layer of circumferential constrictor fibers that act to reduce ventricular diameter.
  - The RV lacks these fibers and thus must rely more heavily on longitudinal shortening than does the LV.
  - In addition, although the RV does undergo torsion, this does not contribute substantially to RV contraction.
- RV systolic function is a reflection of contractility, afterload, and preload. RV performance is also influenced by heart rhythm, synchrony of ventricular contraction, and ventricular interdependence.
- The RV and the LV are interdependent with common encircling muscle fibers, a shared interventricular septum, and the pericardium. Ventricular interdependence refers to the concept that the size, shape, and compliance of one ventricle affects the size, shape, and pressure-volume relationship of the other ventricle. Ventricular interdependence is most apparent with changes in loading conditions such as seen with respiration or sudden postural changes.

TWO-DIMENSIONAL ECHOCARDIOGRAPHIC ASSESSMENT OF RIGHT VENTRICULAR SIZE

- The RV is a complex three-dimensional (3D) shape, and unlike the LV is difficult to model with a single two-dimensional (2D) echocardiographic view. Therefore, **multiple** views should be assessed before determining that RV enlargement is present.

Qualitative RV Size
- A standard A4C view is best to assess RV size compared with that of the LV.
- Mildly enlarged: RV is enlarged but < LV
- Moderately enlarged: RV ≈ LV
- Severely enlarged: RV > LV; apex of heart comprised of RV

Quantitative RV Size
- RV dimension is estimated at end-diastole from an RV-focused A4C view with the goal of demonstrating the maximum diameter of the RV without foreshortening (Fig. 5-1).
  - This is best accomplished by ensuring the crux and apex of the heart are in view.

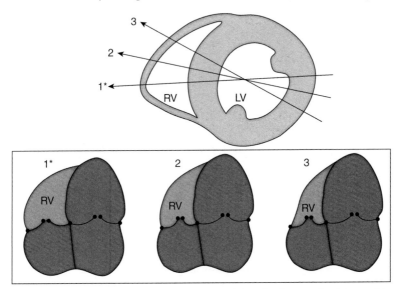

Figure 5-1. Diagram showing the recommened apical four-chamber view for right ventricle (RV) assessment. The size of the RV changes with slight angulation of the transducer. RV as assessed by 1* is the correct plane for RV assessment. LV, left ventricle. From Rudski LG, Lai WW, Afilalo J, et al. Guidelines for echocardiographic assessment of the right heart in adults. *J Am Soc Echocardiogr.* 2010;23:685–713.

- diameter in diastole >4.2 cm, >3.5 cm at the mid level, and longitudinal dimension >8.6 cm indicates RV dilation (Fig. 5-2).
- As RV enlarges, it assumes more of a spherical shape and can impair LV output (Fig. 5-3).

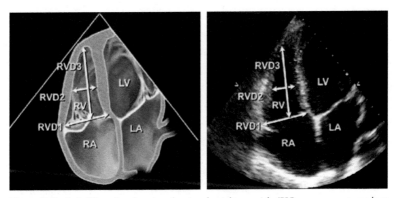

Figure 5-2. Apical four-chamber view showing the right ventricle (RV) measurements made at the base and mid-cavity along with the longitudinal dimension. LA, left atrium; LV, left ventricle; RA, right atrium. From Rudski LG, Lai WW, Afilalo J, et al. Guidelines for echocardiographic assessment of the right heart in adults. *J Am Soc Echocardiogr.* 2010;23:685–713.

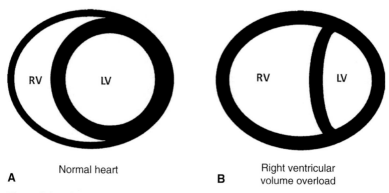

A Normal heart   **B** Right ventricular volume overload

Figure 5-3. Changes in normal left ventricle (LV) and right ventricle (RV) shape **(A)** with RV volume overload **(B)**.

Quantitative RVOT Size

- Measured in the PSAX view with focus on the RVOT and pulmonic valve
- RVOT at the level of the pulmonic valve insertion is the distal diameter; measured at end-diastole
- PLAX RVOT proximal diameter >3.3 cm indicated enlargement
- PSAX RVOT distal diameter >2.7 cm indicated enlargement

Quantitative RV Thickness

- RV wall thickness measured at peak of R wave on electrocardiogram (ECG) at the level of TV chordae in subcostal view (normal ≤5 mm) (Fig. 5-4).
- RVH may suggest RV pressure overload in the absence of other pathologies.
- *It is critical that qualitative assessment of RV size be made in standard transducer locations. If the transducer is placed too medially in the A4C view, the RV will always appear larger.*

- **Key Points:**
  1. *RV basal diameter >4.2 cm, RVOT PSAX distal diameter >2.7 cm, RVOT PLAX proximal diameter >3.3 cm indicates RV enlargement.*
  2. *RV subcostal wall thickness >0.5 cm indicates increased RV wall thickness.*

ASSESSMENT OF RIGHT VENTRICULAR FUNCTION

Two-dimensional Assessment

- Fractional area change (FAC) is calculated by tracing the RV area, including apex and lateral wall, in systole and diastole.
- Trabeculations should be excluded while tracing the area.
- FAC <35% indicates RV systolic dysfunction.

M-mode

- As RV systolic function primarily relies on longitudinal myocardial shortening, measurement of tricuspid annular plane systolic excursion (**TAPSE**) can be used.

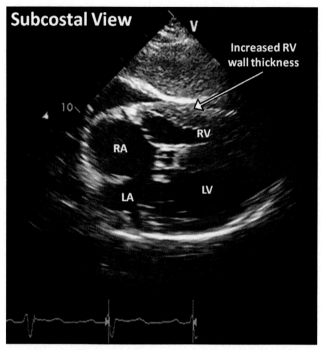

Figure 5-4. A subcostal image showing clear delineation of the borders of the hypertrophied right ventricle (RV) wall. For accurate measurement, a zoomed two-dimensional view or M-mode should be acquired. LA, left atrium; LV, left ventricle; RA, right atrium.

- In the A4C view, an M-mode cursor is oriented to the junction of the TV plane with the RV free wall. TAPSE is the difference in the displacement of the RV base during diastole and systole. **Abnormal excursion is <1.6 cm** (low sensitivity but high specificity) (Fig. 5-5).

Doppler Assessment

- Right index of myocardial performance (RIMP) provides an index of global RV function; it is also known as myocardial performance index (MPI) or Tei index. It is a measure of both systolic and diastolic function. RIMP is a ratio of isovolumic time (contraction and relaxation) to ventricular ejection time (ET). RIMP >0.40 by pulsed Doppler and >0.55 by tissue Doppler indicates RV dysfunction.
  - 2D Doppler: TR jet duration (continuous-wave [CW] Doppler) and RVOT jet duration (pulsed-wave [PW] Doppler) are recorded. The duration of TR is holosystolic and includes both isovolumic relaxation and contraction. RVOT ET only includes active ejection. Thus, the difference between the TR jet duration and RVOT jet duration is the isovolumic periods.
  - MPI = (isovolumic contraction time [IVCT] + isovolumic relaxation time [IVRT])/ ET
  - However, IVCT + IVRT = TR time – RVOT ET

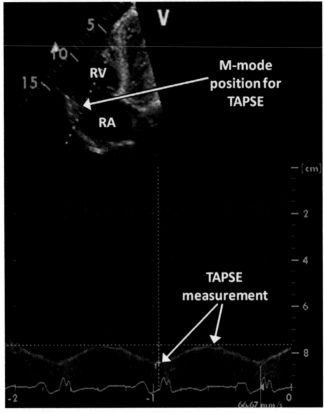

Figure 5-5. Using M-mode positioned from the right ventricle (RV) apex through the RV free wall and tricuspid annulus intersection to measure tricuspid annular plane systolic excursion (TAPSE). RA, right atrium.

- Thus, **MPI also is given as: (TR time – RVOT ET)/RVOT ET** (Fig. 5-6)
- Tissue Doppler: IVCT, IVRT, and ET are measured from tissue Doppler velocity of the lateral tricuspid annulus (TA). This technique avoids errors related to heart rate variability.
- RIMP is falsely low with elevated RA pressures, which decrease the IVRT.
- S′ is a measure of RV systolic function and is measured by tissue Doppler at the lateral TA. S′ <10 cm/sec indicates RV dysfunction (Fig. 5-7).

RV Diastolic Function

- PW Doppler of the tricuspid inflow, tissue Doppler of the lateral TA, PW Doppler of hepatic veins, and IVC should be measured.
- Impaired relaxation: E/A ratio <0.8; pseudonormal filling: E/A ratio of 0.8 to 2.1 with an E/e′ ratio of >6 including a diastolic flow predominance in the hepatic veins; restrictive filling: E/A ratio >2.1 with a deceleration time <120 msec.

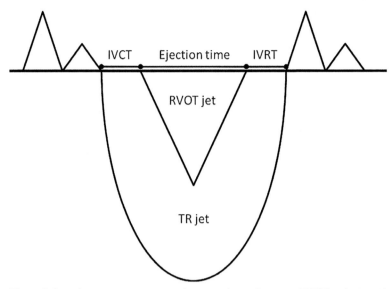

Figure 5-6. A drawing superimposing right ventricular outflow tract (RVOT) and tricuspid regurgitant (TR) Doppler jets to demonstrate the intervals measured for calculation of RV myocardial performance index. IVCT, isovolumic contraction time; IVRT, isovolumic relaxation time.

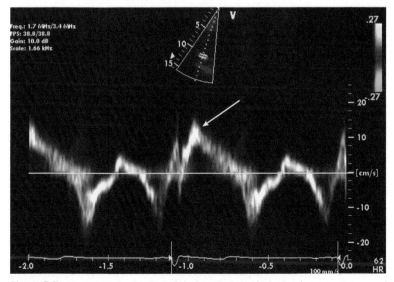

Figure 5-7. Tissue Doppler imaging of the lateral tricuspid annulus demonstrating normal systolic peak velocity ~11.5 cm/sec (*arrow*).

• **Key Points:**
Indicators of RV dysfunction
1. *FAC <35%*
2. *TAPSE <1.6 cm*
3. *S' velocity <10 cm/sec*
4. *RIMP >0.4 by PW Doppler and >0.55 by tissue Doppler*

RIGHT VENTRICULAR PATHOLOGY

RV Volume Overload

- Typically seen as a result of **L → R shunt** (atrial septal defect, anomalous pulmonary venous return, arteriovenous malformation) or severe pulmonary insufficiency (Fig. 5-8).
- In the short-axis view, the LV assumes a more D-shaped cavity as the ventricular septum flattens and loses its circular shape.
  - Isolated volume overload results in most marked shift of the ventricular septum at end-diastole.
  - Analysis of septal motion is best performed in the absence of significant conduction delays, particularly left bundle branch block or in post cardiac surgery patients.
- Classic findings are a dilated RV with **diastolic interventricular septal flattening** (see Fig. 5-8).
- Signs of concomitant **increased right heart pressure** may also be seen.

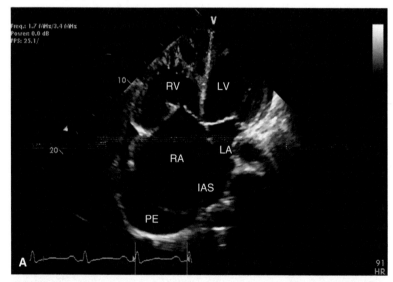

Figure 5-8. Patient with arteriovenous malformations and marked right ventricle (RV) volume overload. **A:** Apical four-chamber view with massive right atrium (RA) and RV dilation and bowing of interatrial septum (IAS) to the left atrium (LA). Small, medium posterior pericardial effusion (PE) seen. (*continued*)

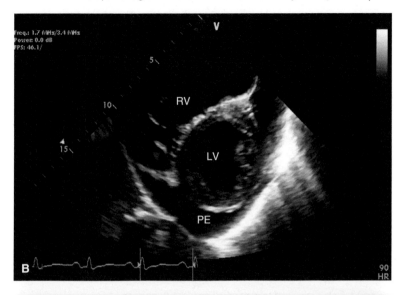

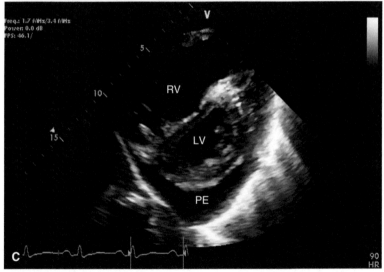

Figure 5-8. (*Continued*) **B:** Parasternal short-axis view in systole with paradoxical interventricular septal motion. **C:** Parasternal short-axis view in diastole with diastolic septal flattening. (*continued*)

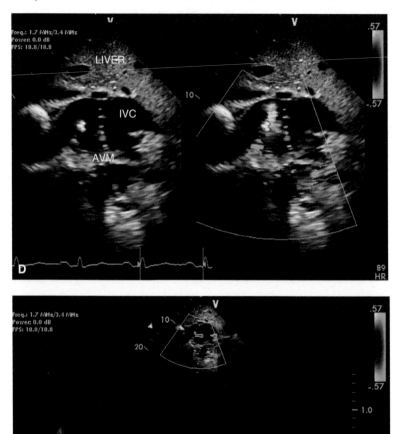

Figure 5-8. (*Continued*) **D:** Side-by-side subcostal view of the dilated inferior vena cava (IVC) with color Doppler showing communication and a larger area of flow from the posterior lumbar artery. **E:** Spectral Doppler of the shunt shows a continuous dense envelope. AVM, arteriovenous malformation; LV, left ventricle.

RV Pressure Overload

- Pressure overload distorts the normal circular short-axis geometry of the LV by shifting the septum leftward away from the center of the RV and toward the LV, resulting in flattening of the ventricular septum and a D-shaped short-axis LV cavity profile, predominantly during systole.
- Pressure overload results from **high pulmonary artery pressures, pulmonary stenosis, or when the RV is the systemic ventricle in congenital heart disease**.
- Acute increases in pulmonary artery (PA) pressures, as seen in acute pulmonary embolism, can cause RV failure, as the RV cannot adapt quickly to changes in afterload.
- With chronically elevated PA pressures, the RV hypertrophies, spherically remodels, and can maintain systolic function at higher pressures than seen in the acute setting.
- RV pressures can be estimated using the TR jet and the RV outflow pattern. In the absence of a gradient across the pulmonary valve (i.e., pulmonary stenosis), **RV pressure estimates PA pressure**.
  - Qualitative signs of high PA pressures: **dilated pulmonary arteries, RVH** (in cases of chronic elevation in PA pressures), **systolic interventricular septal flattening** (i.e., "D-shaped" LV; best seen in PSAX at level of papillary muscles and indicates marked increase in RV pressure to near systemic levels), **high velocity TR jet, short RVOT AT** (<90 msec), **shortened RVOT velocity time integral, mid-systolic closure of pulmonic valve flow**

- **Key Points:**
  1. *"60:60 sign"—In the setting of an acute pulmonary embolism, the RVOT AT may be shortened (<60 msec), secondary to local fluid hemodynamic changes, and does not accurately reflect mean pulmonary artery pressure (MPAP). This phenomenon is confirmed by a low velocity TR jet, reflecting only a modest increase in peak pulmonary artery systolic pressure (PASP) (<60 mm Hg gradient).*
  2. *McConnell's sign—In addition to changes in pulmonary hemodynamics, acute pulmonary embolism can produce regional RV wall motion abnormalities, with severe hypokinesis of the RV basal to mid free wall and hyperdynamic apical contraction.*

RV Infarction

- If the ECG is concerning for acute inferior myocardial infarction, obtain a careful assessment of RV function by echocardiography.
- Typical findings would be **hypokinesis/akinesis of the inferior LV wall in addition to the RV**. Quantitative evidence of RV dysfunction—high RV MPI, abnormal TAPSE
- Clinically, these patients are **preload-dependent:** Volume depletion and nitroglycerin can precipitate profound hypotension.

Arrhythmogenic Right Ventricular Dysplasia

- Arrhythmogenic right ventricular dysplasia (ARVD) is a rare congenital disorder involving focal or diffuse replacement of RV myocardium with adipose tissue.
- This clinically manifests as syncope or sudden cardiac death resulting from ventricular tachycardia originating from these abnormal areas of infiltration.
- Echocardiographic findings are **RV enlargement, free wall thinning, focal aneurysms, and systolic dysfunction**.
  - Aneurysms are most frequently seen in the RV basal inferior, apical, and anterior outflow walls.

PULMONARY HEMODYNAMICS

- **PASP and pulmonary artery end-diastolic pressure (PAEDP) can be estimated using the modified Bernoulli equation,** which calculates the pressure difference between two chambers of the heart using the velocity of a jet between them:

$$\Delta P \text{ (measured in mm Hg)} = 4 \times V^2 \text{ (measured in m/sec)}$$

- To estimate RV systolic pressure (which estimates PASP in the absence of a gradient across the RVOT/pulmonary valve, try to obtain the TR jet in multiple views: PLAX/RV inflow, PSAX at level of aortic valve (AoV), A4C, and subcostal views. Use the highest velocity TR jet where the Doppler envelope is *complete, measuring the modal peak velocity (darkest part of jet).*
  - RV systolic pressure – RA pressure = $4 \times$ (peak velocity of TR jet)^2
  - **PASP = $4 \times$ (peak velocity of TR jet)^2 + mean RA pressure**
- PAEDP can be estimated using the PR jet (obtainable in the PSAX at the level of the AoV). The end velocity of the PR jet represents the end-diastolic gradient between the PA and the RV (Fig. 5-9).

PAEDP = $4 \times$ (end velocity of PR jet)^2 + RA pressure

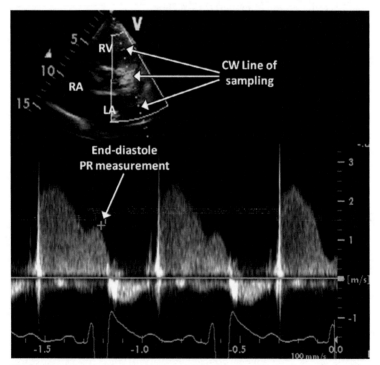

Figure 5-9. Continuous-wave (CW) Doppler across the pulmonic valve demonstrating estimation of the pulmonary end-diastolic pressure from the end-diastolic velocity of the pulmonic regurgitation (PR) jet. LA, left atrium; RA, right atrium; RV, right ventricle.

- **MPAP can be estimated using the following formulae:**

$$MPAP = 1/3(PASP) + 2/3(PAEDP)$$

$$MPAP\ 90 - (0.62 \times AT)\ \text{(Fig. 5-10)}$$

$$MPAP = 4 \times (\text{peak velocity of PR jet})^2 + RA\ \text{pressure}$$

- In cases of very elevated PA pressures, a midsystolic notch can be seen in the RVOT outflow Doppler jet, resulting from early transient closure of the PV.
- The following equation has been shown to noninvasively estimate pulmonary vascular resistance (PVR):

$$PVR = [(TRV)/VTI_{RVOT}] \times 10 + 0.16$$

where TRV, TR velocity; VTI_{rvot}, RVOT VTI

- **Key Points:**
  1. *When measuring Doppler acquired gradients, ensure that the cardiac rhythm is regular. If the rhythm is irregular, average measurements from at least 5–10 cardiac cycles.*
  2. *In the setting of severe TR, the Doppler envelope is often low velocity and early peaking because of high RA pressure. In this circumstance it is difficult to estimate PASP.*

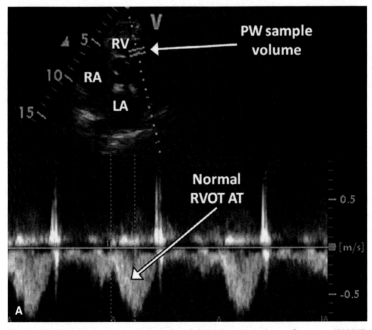

Figure 5-10. Pulsed-wave (PW) Doppler of the right ventricular outflow tract (RVOT) with correct positioning of the sample volume so that only the closing click is recorded. Measurement of the RVOT acceleration time (AT) from onset to peak velocity allows estimation of mean pulmonary artery pressure (MPAP). **A:** Normal RVOT AT. (*continued*)

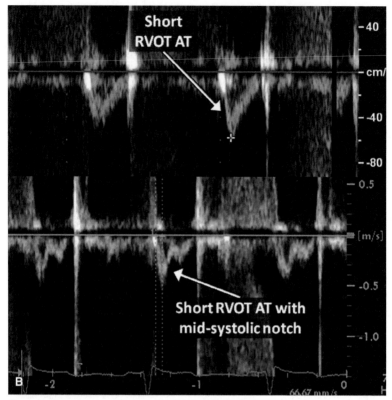

Figure 5-10. (*Continued*) **B:** Short RVOT AT and mid-systolic notching suggesting elevation of MPAP. LA, left atrium; RA, right atrium; RV, right ventricle.

RIGHT ATRIAL ASSESSMENT

RA Size Assessment

- Measured in the A4C view at end-diastole: Tracing of the RA is performed from the plane of the TA along the interatrial septum, superior, and anterolateral wall of the RA.
- The RA major dimension is the distance from the superior wall to the TA. The minor dimension is the distance from the interatrial septum to the anterolateral wall.
- RA area >18 cm^2, RA length (major dimension) >53 mm, and RA diameter (minor dimension) >44 mm measured in end-diastole indicate RA enlargement.

Estimating Mean RA Pressure

- RA pressure is estimated by the size and compressibility of the IVC. Diameter of the IVC is measured in the subcostal view just proximal to the entrance of the hepatic veins during quiet respiration and after "sniff" maneuver. M-mode can be placed on the IVC for more accurate quantification (Fig. 5-11).

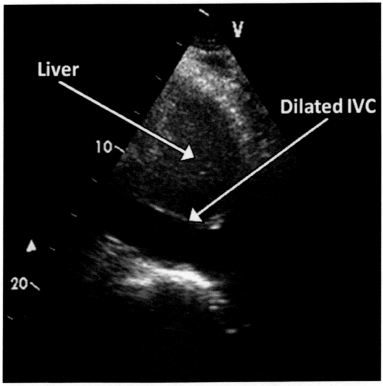

Figure 5-11. Subcostal image showing dilated inferior vena cava (IVC). Measurement of the IVC diameter should be taken close to the right atrium and IVC junction.

- **IVC diameter ≤2.1 cm and collapse >50% with sniff—normal RA pressure of 3 mm Hg (range 0–5 mm Hg)**
- **IVC diameter >2.1 cm and collapse <50% with sniff—high RA pressure of 15 mm Hg (range 10–20 mm Hg)**
- **In scenarios where IVC diameter and collapse do not fit these two criteria, RA pressure is intermediate value of 8 mm Hg (range 5–10 mm Hg).**
- In normal young athletes, the IVC may be dilated with normal RA pressures.
- Ventilated patients may have dilated and noncollapsible IVC; therefore, it should not be used to estimate RA pressure in those cases.
- Hepatic Doppler can be used to corroborate IVC findings. Systolic flow is greater than diastolic flow when mean RA pressure is normal. In the absence of severe TR, blunting of systolic flow suggests elevated mean RA pressure (Fig. 5-12).

- **Key Points:** *In assessing IVC diameter, ensure that the reduction in caliber, suggesting normal RA pressure, is due to changes with respiration rather than translational movement secondary to probe or patient motion.*

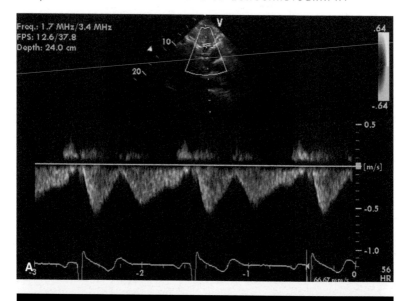

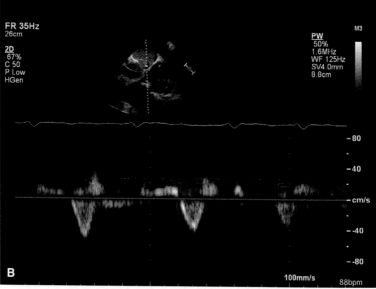

Figure 5-12. A: Normal hepatic Doppler showing systolic dominant flow in patient with normal right atrial (RA) pressure. **B:** Abnormal hepatic Doppler showing systolic blunting and diastolic dominant flow in patient with elevated RA pressure and severe pulmonary hypertension.

DISCREPANCY BETWEEN DOPPLER AND CARDIAC CATHETERIZATION

There are several explanations as to why a Doppler-derived estimation of right-sided pressures may be inconsistent with invasive pressure measurements.

- If the transducer is **not parallel** to the flow of the TR jet, the peak velocity of the jet will be reduced and lead to an underestimation of the PASP.
- In TR Doppler envelopes where spectral broadening is present, not measuring the modal velocity may result in overestimation of PASP. Note any error in velocity measurement is "**squared**" using the modified Bernoulli equation.
- Incorrectly estimating mean RA pressure from the **IVC** can lead to underestimation or overestimation of pulmonary pressures.
- Inability to accurately estimate mean RA pressure in the setting of severe TR.
- Accidently capturing the mitral regurgitant (MR) jet instead of the TR jet can lead to a gross overestimation of PA pressures. In cases where pulmonary pressures are near systemic pressures, it is imperative to ensure that the TR and not the MR jet Doppler envelope is measured. The jet of TR will always be **longer** in duration than the MR (as a result of longer IVRT and IVCT) and will demonstrate respiratory variation.

Using multiple methods to confirm findings will improve accuracy and consistency in reporting pulmonary pressures. With the exception of acute pulmonary embolism, a high-velocity TR jet should be accompanied by a short RVOT AT. Additional findings to support a diagnosis of pulmonary hypertension should also be found (e.g., RVH or RV enlargement, "D-shaped" LV, PA enlargement, IVC and coronary sinus dilation, blunted systolic hepatic flow, interatrial septum bowed toward left atrium).

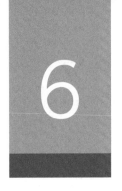

6

Stress Testing for Ischemia and Viability

Pedro M. Calderón-Artero and Daniel H. Cooper

HIGH-YIELD CONCEPTS

- Echocardiographic stress testing is a sensitive and specific modality for detecting the presence of stress-induced ischemia in appropriately selected patients.
- Ischemia manifests as regional wall motion abnormalities and changes in **myocardial thickening** during stress.
- Exercise echocardiography yields additional prognostic information and is preferred over pharmacologic stress testing.
- Causes of **false-negative** results include: failure to reach target heart rate, delayed peak stress image acquisition, single-vessel disease (especially involving the circumflex artery), and antianginal/β-blocker use before testing.
- Causes of **false-positive** results include: hypertensive response to exercise, left ventricular hypertrophy (LVH), coronary spasm, and paradoxical septal motion secondary to conduction abnormality (e.g., left bundle branch block [LBBB], pacing).
- To avoid these pitfalls, recognize the importance of achieving an adequate level of stress (>85% maximally predicted heart rate [MPHR]), timely image acquisition (<60 seconds for exercise echo protocols), and **confirming wall motion abnormalities in multiple views**.
- Dobutamine stress echocardiography can be utilized to confirm myocardial viability by noting the presence of a **biphasic response** to increasing rates of dobutamine infusion.

GENERAL PRINCIPLES

- The use of stress echocardiography for detection of ischemia is based on the principles outlined by the ischemic cascade (Fig. 6-1).
- Impaired myocardial perfusion stemming from coronary artery disease (CAD) leads to a progression of manifestations during exercise or pharmacologic stress that ultimately results in regional or global wall motion or thickening abnormalities.
- The goal is to determine whether ischemia is present or, if there are baseline wall motion abnormalities and reduced left ventricular ejection fraction (LVEF), if there is viable myocardium and left ventricle (LV) contractile reserve.
- Obtaining an adequate level of stress is vital to maintaining the modality's sensitivity for detecting CAD.
  - Achieving 85% of the MPHR (220 – age) improves sensitivity greatly.
  - However, if changes consistent with ischemia are detected at lower (submaximal) levels of stress, this improves specificity of the result.

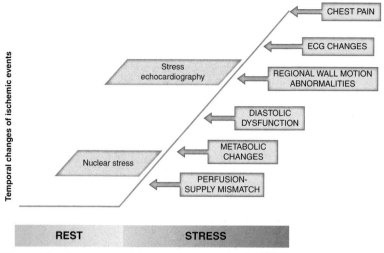

Figure 6-1. Ischemic cascade showing at what stage stress echocardiography and nuclear stress detect changes. ECG, electrocardiogram. (Adapted from Schinkel AFL, Bax JJ, Geleijnse ML, et al. Noninvasive evaluation of ischaemic heart disease: myocardial perfusion imaging or stress echocardiography? *Eur Heart J.* 2003;24:789–800, by permission of Oxford University Press.)

- Continuous patient monitoring by medical staff is required, including frequent symptom inquires, continuous ECG, and intermittent blood pressure (BP) measurement.
  - Crash carts, stocked with resuscitation equipment and medications, should be available.

ANATOMY

- Stress echocardiography typically focuses on images obtained in the apical (four- and two-chamber [A4C and A2C], and long-axis) and parasternal (short- and long-axis [PSAX and PLAX]) views, allowing for observation of all myocardial segments.
- Knowledge of the **typical distribution of coronary artery blood flow** to the various myocardial segments is vital. It allows:
  - Confirmation in multiple views of suspected lesions, especially when image quality in one view is suboptimal
  - Correlation of findings to specific location(s) of coronary artery stenosis (Fig. 6-2)
    ○ **Left anterior descending (LAD):** anterior, anteroseptum, apex, +/– inferoapical (wrap-around LAD)
    ○ **Circumflex:** anterolateral, inferolateral
    ○ **Right coronary artery:** inferior, inferoseptal (basal, mid), +/– inferolateral (depending on dominance)
    ○ **Distal versus proximal:** A proximal LAD lesion; for example, will result in basal to distal wall motion abnormalities of the anteroseptum (septal perforators), anterior wall, anterolateral wall; whereas distal LAD disease will affect only the apex.

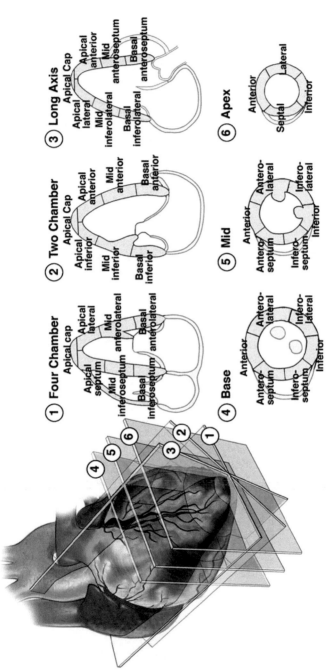

Figure 6-2. The standard echocardiographic views demonstrating the 17-segment model color coded for typical coronary artery distribution. (Reprinted from Lang RM, Bierig M, Devereux RB, et al. Recommendations for chamber quantification: a report from the American Society of Echocardiography's Guidelines and Standards Committee and the Chamber Quantification Writing Group, developed in conjunction with the European Association of Echocardiography, a branch of the European Society of Cardiology. *J Am Soc Echocardiogr.* 2005;18:1440–63, with permission from Elsevier.)

EXERCISE STRESS ECHOCARDIOGRAPHY

- In general, all exercise stress protocols involve staged increases in workload to increase myocardial oxygen demand. This is accomplished by treadmill or stationary bicycle exercise.
  - The Bruce protocol (most common) involves exercise on a treadmill where **grade and speed increases** every **3 minutes**.
  - Patient exercises until target heart rate is achieved, significant symptoms develop, or marked ECG changes are noted.
  - Maximal metabolic equivalents <5 suggest poor prognosis if <65 years old.

Absolute Contraindications

- Acute myocardial infarction (MI)
- High-risk unstable angina
- Uncontrolled ventricular tachycardia (VT) or supraventricular tachycardia (SVT)
- Severe arterial hypertension; systolic blood pressure (SBP) >200 mm Hg and/or diastolic blood pressure (DBP) >110 mm Hg
- Symptomatic severe aortic stenosis (AS)
- Uncontrolled, symptomatic congestive heart failure
- Acute pulmonary embolism (PE) or pulmonary infarct
- Acute myocarditis or pericarditis
- Acute aortic dissection

Relative Contraindications

- Left main coronary stenosis
- Moderate stenotic valvular disease
- Electrolyte abnormalities
- Tachy- or bradyarrhythmias
- Hypertrophic cardiomyopathy or other forms of outflow obstruction
- Mental or physical impairment inhibiting exercise
- High-degree atrioventricular block

Absolute Indications to Terminate Exercise Testing

- Drop in SBP >10 mm Hg from baseline despite increase in workload, if accompanied by other evidence of ischemia
- Moderate to severe angina
- Increasing central nervous system symptoms (ataxia, near-syncope)
- Signs of poor perfusion (cyanosis, pallor)
- Technical difficulties in monitoring BP/ECG
- Patient's request
- Sustained VT
- ST elevation ≥1 mm in leads without Q waves (other than V1 or aVR)

Relative Indications to Terminate Exercise Testing

- Drop in SBP >10 mm Hg from baseline despite increase in workload, without other evidence of ischemia
- ECG changes such as marked ST drop (>2 mm, horizontal or downsloping) or marked axis shift

- Other arrhythmias (multifocal nonsustained VT, SVT, high-degree heart block, bradyarrhythmia)
- Fatigue, shortness of breath, wheezing, leg cramps, claudication
- Increasing chest pain
- Hypertensive response (SBP >220 mm Hg and/or DBP >115 mm Hg)

DOBUTAMINE STRESS ECHOCARDIOGRAPHY

- Pharmacologic stress is indicated in patients unable to exercise. Dobutamine is the most commonly utilized pharmacologic stress agent.
  - Dobutamine, like exercise, increases myocardial oxygen demand by augmenting contractility (positive inotropy), increasing heart rate (positive chronotropy), and elevating BP.
- Images are obtained at rest and at increasing doses of dobutamine infusion.
  - Typically, four to five 3-minute stages are utilized: 5, 10, 20, 30, 40 μg/kg/min.
  - Atropine (0.2–0.4 mg every 2 minutes to a maximum of 2 mg) is commonly used to help achieve target heart rates, especially if patients have resting bradycardia or in the setting of β-blockade.
  - Use of this medication also reduces the occurrence of the Bezold–Jarisch reflex (profound vagal response) that may occur, especially in the elderly (small LV cavity) and in patients with hypovolemia.
- Other supplementary maneuvers such as isometric hand grip are used to achieve peak heart rate.
- Side effects
  - Anxiety, nausea, headache, and palpitations from isolated premature beats are not uncommon.
  - Estimated risk for sustained ventricular arrhythmias or MI is ~1/2000.

INTERPRETATION

Baseline Transthoracic Echocardiography

- Particular attention should be given to **other possible causes of the symptoms** that prompted the ischemic evaluation. This is assessed from a baseline transthoracic echocardiography (TTE) performed prior to stress testing.
  - Specifically, new depressed LV function with regional wall motion abnormalities, pericardial tamponade, evidence of PE, severe AS, and aortic dissection should be excluded.
- In the absence of acute coronary syndrome, prior MI, or cardiomyopathy, wall motion and thickening should be normal on resting images in patients presenting with chest pain, even in the setting of significant CAD.
- However, be aware that regional wall motion abnormalities may be related to non-CAD causes. For example, "pseudodyskinesis" describes diastolic flattening of the inferior wall related to localized compression by the diaphragm. This is overcome during systole when the inferior wall becomes rounded giving the appearance of dyskinesis despite normal wall thickening. Pathologic causes of LV regional wall motion abnormalities include infiltrative disease (e.g., sarcoidosis), conduction abnormalities (e.g., LBBB), postcardiac surgical changes (paradoxical septal motion, myocardial patch repair), right heart abnormalities (e.g., volume or pressure overload), and stress-induced cardiomyopathy.

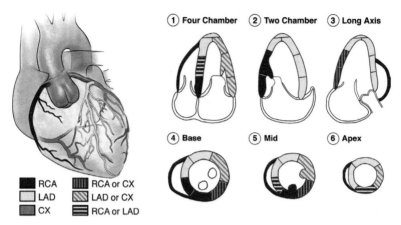

Figure 6-3. Segmental analysis of left ventricle walls based on schematic views, in a parasternal short- and long-axis orientation, at three different levels. The "apex segments" are usually visualized from apical two-, three-, and four-chamber views. The apical cap can only be appreciated on some contrast studies. CX, circumflex; LAD, left anterior descending; RCA, right coronary artery. (Reprinted from Lang RM, Bierig M, Devereux RB, et al. Recommendations for chamber quantification: a report from the American Society of Echocardiography's Guidelines and Standards Committee and the Chamber Quantification Writing Group, developed in conjunction with the European Association of Echocardiography, a branch of the European Society of Cardiology. *J Am Soc Echocardiogr.* 2005;18:1440–63, with permission from Elsevier.)

Peak Stress Transthoracic Echocardiography

- Rapid image acquisition, **within 1 minute** after exercise discontinuation, improves sensitivity. Blunting of wall motion abnormalities can, however, persist for ~3–5 minutes depending on severity of ischemia elicited.
- Hyperdynamic ventricular response, increase in endocardial excursion (>5 mm), uniform **thickening** during systole, and **increase in LVEF** with associated decrease in end-systolic volume (with exception of recumbent bicycle protocol) constitute a normal stress echocardiogram response.
- A comprehensive stress echocardiogram report should include exercise capacity, heart rate response, rhythm and BP changes, along with wall motion abnormalities.
- Compare rest and stress **global and regional LV function in all available views** (PSAX and PLAX, A4C, A2C, and apical long axis).
  - Wall thickening and movement is assessed in all myocardial segments (Fig. 6-3; see also Fig. 6-2).
  - Each of the 17 myocardial segments is graded by a five-point scale: (1) normal; (2) hypokinetic, <30% wall thickening; (3) akinetic, <10% wall thickening; (4) dyskinetic, systolic outward movement; and (5) aneurysmal, outwardly displaced segment in systole and diastole.
  - A wall motion score index (WMSI) can be calculated to quantify the extent of regional wall motion abnormalities.
  - WMSI = sum of wall motion scores/number of segments visualized (e.g., normal = 1).
  - The LV cavity should appropriately decrease in size with peak stress.

- Abnormal segments should be confirmed in **multiple views** to improve specificity.
  - For example, hypokinesis of the anteroseptal wall seen on the PLAX view should be confirmed on the PSAX view. In addition, confirm if other myocardial segments subtended by the same coronary artery are affected.
- **Recovery images** should be obtained to confirm resolution in patients with stress-induced wall motion abnormalities prior to discharge from the laboratory.

False Results

- *False negatives*
  - Submaximal stress (<85% MPHR) is the most common cause.
  - Late image acquisition (>60 seconds) after peak exercise can result in a false negative.
  - Single-vessel disease is more likely to be missed than multivessel because of the reduced extent of wall motion abnormalities seen.
  - Circumflex stenosis in particular is more commonly missed because of the relatively small myocardial territory involved.
  - Marked LVH and small LV cavity increase the possibility of missing wall motion abnormality.
  - β-Blocker/antianginal use can also yield a false-negative result.
- *False positives*
  - Ischemia in the absence of epicardial CAD
    - Hypertensive response to stress
    - LVH
    - Microvascular disease (e.g., diabetes)
    - Coronary spasm (especially seen with dobutamine)
  - Nonischemic causes of stress-induced wall motion abnormalities
    - Nonischemic cardiomyopathy
    - Long-standing hypertension
    - Paradoxical septal motion (e.g., LBBB)

PROGNOSIS

- Negative predictive value
  - Event-free survival (MI or death) at 3 years is ~99% if exercise stress echocardiogram is negative.
  - Patients with a negative pharmacologic stress echocardiogram tend to have a slightly higher event rate, presumably secondary to the inability to exercise, selecting for a "sicker" patient population.
- Cardiac risk increases incrementally with abnormal findings on a stress echocardiogram. In general, the following factors suggest a worse prognosis:
  - Ischemia at low thresholds (exercise or pharmacologic)
  - Extensive (four to five myocardial segments) ischemia
  - Failure to reduce LV or worse, an increase in cavity size at peak exercise

OTHER CONSIDERATIONS

- *Stress echocardiography versus myocardial perfusion imaging*
  - In general, stress echocardiography offers better specificity and slightly reduced sensitivity than myocardial perfusion imaging. This reduction in sensitivity is mostly related to single-vessel (especially circumflex artery) disease.

- Accounting for slight differences in sensitivity and specificity, both modalities offer similar accuracy and prognostic implications overall for patients presenting with symptoms and an intermediate risk of CAD.
- Given the importance of achieving target heart rate, β-blockers should typically be held the day of the procedure.
  - However, for patients with known CAD, some physicians prefer to continue medical therapy to help gauge adequacy of treatment.
- Given the importance of endocardial border definition, echocardiographic contrast should be considered in patients with poorly defined myocardial segments.
- Modified protocols are available for elderly patients who may have impaired proprioception and may not be able to quickly adapt to increasing treadmill speed and incline.
- For patients with moderate to severely depressed EF or multivessel disease, or for those at high risk for arrhythmia, a low-dose dobutamine protocol (starting at 2.5 μg/kg/min) along with a gradual uptitration can be sometimes used with attentive monitoring.
- Dobutamine stress testing should be terminated when a patient reaches 85% MPHR, or when a patient exhibits new wall motion abnormalities, significant arrhythmias, hypotension, severe hypertension, or when intolerable symptoms occur.
- Short-acting β-blockers (e.g., esmolol) are used to reserve the effects of dobutamine.

STRESS TESTING FOR MYOCARDIAL VIABILITY

General Principles
- The role of stress echocardiography in detecting myocardial viability involves the demonstration of myocardial contractile reserve.
- Myocardial thickening is impaired when 20% or more of the wall is affected by ischemia or infarction.
- Therefore despite resting regional akinesis, a large proportion of myocardium may be viable and, when stimulated, will allow for normal myocardial thickening.
- "Hibernating" myocardium describes akinesis secondary to chronic ischemia with the important prognostic implication that coronary revascularization will restore normal myocardial function.
- Akinetic segments that are thinned and fibrotic (echogenic) at rest are less likely to be viable.
- Response of akinetic segments to increasing dobutamine infusion allows differentiation of viable myocardium from myocardial scar.

Protocol
- Initial infusion typically begins at 2.5 μg/kg/min with staged increases in dose to 5, 10, and 20 μg/kg/min.
- 40 μg/kg/min can be utilized if improvement is sustained at 20–30 μg/kg/min.
- TTE images are obtained at rest and at each stage of dobutamine infusion.
- The test should be terminated if there is absence of functional improvement or worsening of function during infusion.
- **Medical staff awareness of arrhythmia risk and careful monitoring for arrhythmias should be a particular focus during these studies.**
- By definition, these patients have some degree of scar-based structural heart disease that may serve as substrate for reentrant ventricular arrhythmias, particularly during dobutamine infusion.

TABLE 6-1	Characteristic Echocardiographic Responses to Dobutamine Infusion to Determine the Etiology of Regional Akinesis			
Patient	Low-dose dobutamine	Peak-dose dobutamine	Viable myocardium	Critical coronary stenosis
Myocardial scar/ infarction	No increase	No increase	No	Yes
Hibernating myocardium	Increase	Decrease	Yes	Yes
Nonischemic cardiomyopathy	Increase	Increase	Yes	No

Interpretation

- *Rest images*
  - Baseline wall thickness and motion abnormalities should be noted in each segment.
  - Bright, thinned-out (<0.6 cm) segments are consistent with nonviable scar that would not respond to revascularization.
  - Evidence of comorbid valvular heart disease should be carefully evaluated as it may change surgical risk and approach.
- *Stress images*
  - Evidence of functional improvement in affected segments with stress should be gauged.
  - Viability is defined as the improvement by one grade or more (i.e., akinetic → hypokinetic, normal, or hyperkinetic) in two or more myocardial segments.
  - Potential responses of affected segments to dobutamine infusion are shown in Table 6-1.
  - Dobutamine stress echocardiography for viability is most reliable (specific) when a "biphasic response" is noted (i.e., improved myocardial thickening at low-dose dobutamine that worsens at high-dose dobutamine infusion).
  - Worsening LV dysfunction with dobutamine infusion suggests nonviable myocardium (poor prognosis), and the test should be stopped.

Other Considerations

- **β-blockade can limit the ability to detect viable segments.** If limited viability is detected on β-blockers, then consideration should be given to repeating the test without β-blockade.

7

Ischemic Heart Disease and Complications of Myocardial Infarction

Olusegun Olusesi and Michael Yeung

HIGH-YIELD CONCEPTS

- Echocardiography is useful in the evaluation of acute chest pain because it allows for assessment of wall motion to rule out myocardial ischemia (MI) and evaluate other causes of chest pain such as aortic dissection and pulmonary embolism.
- Quick calculation of stroke volume (SV) may provide additional information in the unstable patient as follows, where CSA = cross sectional area, VTI = velocity time integral, and LVOT = left ventricular outflow tract:

$$SV = CSA_{LVOT} \times VTI_{LVOT}$$

- Color flow (CW) Doppler and agitated saline are helpful in the localization of ventricular septal defects (VSD) or ventricular free wall rupture.
- The posteromedial papillary muscle is often affected in acute ischemic mitral regurgitation (IMR), given its single coronary supply from the posterior descending artery.
- Assessment of the etiology and severity of acute MR may require transesophageal echocardiography (TEE) evaluation.
- A neck diameter to maximal aneurysmal diameter ratio of <0.5 suggests pseudoaneurysm (PsA).

EVALUATION OF CHEST PAIN SYNDROME IN THE ACUTE SETTING

- In the acute setting, the rapid detection of new wall motion abnormalities as well as mechanical complications is crucial. The ischemic cascade has been described in Chapter 6. Echocardiography plays an integral part in the evaluation of chest pain syndrome as it can detect wall motion abnormalities even before electrocardiogram (ECG) changes occur. In addition, the screening of other critical causes of chest pain such as aortic dissection, pulmonary embolism, and pericarditis makes echocardiography an essential diagnostic tool.
- Infarct can be differentiated from regions of ischemia by areas of akinetic, thinned-out myocardium. Hypokinesis usually refers to lack of endocardial wall thickening during systole. Other nonischemic causes of wall motion abnormalities include a conduction abnormality such as a left bundle branch block (LBBB), right ventricular (RV) pacing, RV pressure/volume overload, and recent cardiac surgery. These etiologies of wall motion abnormalities have to be differentiated from ischemic wall motion abnormalities.

- If the patient has a history of infarct, assessment of a prior echocardiogram is helpful for comparison of regional and overall LV function.
- Contrast agents have greatly improved the echocardiographic diagnostic accuracy of MI in the acute setting by enhancing the detection of regional wall motion abnormalities as well as endocardial thickening.

- **Key Points:**
  1. *Echocardiography can detect wall motion abnormalities even before ECG changes occur.*
  2. *Ischemic causes of wall motion abnormalities must be differentiated from nonischemic causes such as LBBB, RV pacing, RV pressure/volume overload, and recent cardiac surgery.*
  3. *Review prior echocardiograms to compare and assess wall motion abnormalities.*

MECHANICAL COMPLICATIONS OF ACUTE MYOCARDIAL INFARCTION

- Recurrent chest pain after MI should prompt suspicion and evaluation of recurrent ischemia, post-MI pericarditis, pericardial effusion, aortic dissection, or LV rupture.
- Cardiogenic shock after MI can be due to RV dysfunction, LV dysfunction, acute MR caused by papillary muscle rupture (PMR), or tamponade resulting from LV rupture. Right-sided dysfunction can be differentiated clinically from left-sided dysfunction by the presence of marked neck vein distension, peripheral edema, and the conspicuous absence of pulmonary edema.
- A new holosystolic murmur after MI suggests either (1) ischemic MR caused by papillary muscle dysfunction/rupture or (2) ischemic VSD.

LEFT VENTRICULAR DYSFUNCTION AND CARDIOGENIC SHOCK

- Echocardiography provides important quantitative information regarding chamber size, ventricular systolic and diastolic function, valvular hemodynamics, and pericardial involvement.
- SV is an important indirect measurement that can assist in the evaluation of the patient's hemodynamic status as follows, where CO = cardiac output and HR = heart rate:

$$CO = SV \times HR$$

- SV can be estimated by measuring the CSA and VTI of the LVOT by pulsed-wave (PW) Doppler:

$$SV = CSA_{LVOT} \times VTI_{LVOT}$$

- Early mitral blood flow (E) and annular (e′) velocities have been correlated with pulmonary capillary wedge pressure (PCWP). **A septal E/e′ ≥15 corresponds to a PCWP >20 mm Hg.**

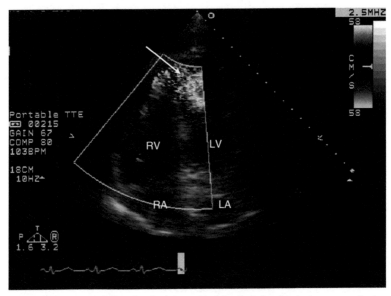

Figure 7-1. An apical four-chamber view with color Doppler showing a communication between the left and right ventricles in this apical ventricular septal defect (*arrow*). LA, left atrium; LV, left ventricle; RA, right atrium; RV, right ventricle.

VENTRICULAR SEPTAL DEFECT

- VSD markedly increases risk of mortality and occurs within the first 3–6 days after a MI.
- Risk factors include age (>65 years), hypertension, female gender, first infarction, and single-vessel coronary disease. Its classic presentation is recurrent chest pain and hypotension several days after MI, along with the presence of a new harsh pansystolic murmur and thrill in about 50% of patients.
- The left anterior descending and right coronary arteries are most commonly implicated in the development of VSD. Anatomically, the left anterior descending artery supplies the apical portion of the ventricular septum and the right coronary artery gives rise to the posterior septal perforators that supply the basal inferoseptal wall (Figs. 7-1 and 7-2).
- VSDs may be simple or complex; the latter is often associated with multiple areas as well as different dissection planes that track along the myocardium in a serpiginous fashion.
- The use of CW Doppler is essential to identify the location of the left-to-right shunt. Off-axis views may be needed to better localize the rupture.
- The two most common locations are **inferoseptal** and **anteroapical walls**.
- Additional evaluation for worsening pulmonary hypertension and left and right ventricular function is important for prognosis.
- Percutaneous closure is feasible in simple, apical VSDs.

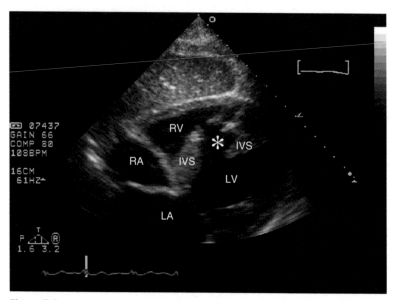

Figure 7-2. A subcostal view showing a complex, serpiginous ventricular septal defect (*) in the interventricular septum (IVS). LA, left atrium; LV, left ventricle; RA, right atrium; RV, right ventricle.

> • **Key Point:** *Any localized areas of color disturbance or turbulence near the interventricular septum (IVS) should be thoroughly investigated with off-axis imaging and spectral Doppler.*

LEFT VENTRICULAR FREE WALL RUPTURE

• Cardiac free wall rupture is often a catastrophic event. Approximately 40% of LV free wall ruptures occur in the first day and 85% within the first week of the MI. High clinical suspicion by a rapidly deteriorating hemodynamic status after MI should prompt evaluation for myocardial rupture, often in the anterior location.

• Predisposing factors include female gender, elderly (>65 years old), single coronary disease (often total occlusion), anterior location, and transmural MI. Unsuccessful reperfusion and the delayed use of thrombolytics have also been associated with a higher incidence of free wall ruptures.

• Effusions are common in the setting of MI (up to 25% in acute setting). However, an expanding pericardial effusion with considerable wall thinning along the infarct region should raise suspicion of a LV wall rupture. In addition, fibrinous echodensities in the pericardial space may be related to the presence of blood. CW Doppler increases the diagnostic yield and may help localize the site of myocardial tear (Figs. 7-3 and 7-4).

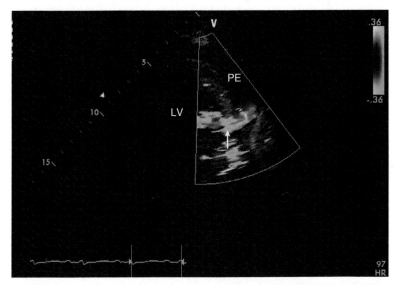

Figure 7-3. Apical four-chamber with color flow Doppler. Color Doppler is instrumental in delineating the region of free wall rupture, which in this case is in the anterolateral wall (*arrow*). Notice the prominent pericardial effusion (PE) present. LV, left ventricle.

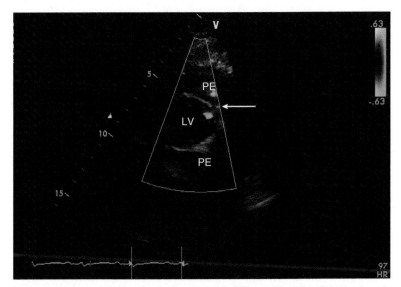

Figure 7-4. Short-axis view with color flow Doppler of left ventricle (LV) wall rupture (*arrow*). PE, pericardial effusion.

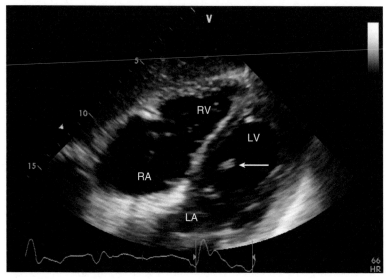

Figure 7-5. Modified subcostal view. A patient presenting with an inferior myocardial infarction and unexplained hypotension. An ovoid mass attached to the mitral valve chordae tendinae (*arrow*) is part of the posterior medial papillary muscle that has ruptured. LA, left atrium; LV, left ventricle; RA, right atrium; RV, right ventricle.

PAPILLARY MUSCLE RUPTURE AND ISCHEMIC MITRAL REGURGITATION

- IMR may complicate MI, classically presenting in the acute setting as sudden onset of hypotension and pulmonary edema.
- Adjacent MI, infarction, and remodeling surrounding the valve lead to IMR as a result of leaflet tethering.
- One of the complications of acute MI is PMR. The posterior papillary muscle is most commonly affected, because of a single arterial supply (right coronary or left circumflex artery, depending on dominance). In contrast, the anterolateral papillary muscle shares a dual supply from the left anterior descending and left circumflex arteries (Figs. 7-5 and 7-6).
- In the setting of acute MI and MR, special attention should be paid not only to the severity of the MR but also to the presence of abnormal leaflet motion (prolapse or flail). Acute IMR is suspected when the MR jet is eccentric and brief in duration (because of rapid rise in LA pressure). A hyperdynamic LV post MI may suggest a PMR. **The mitral E velocity is typically high**.
- Highly eccentric MR may be difficult to appreciate qualitatively or quantitatively by standard echocardiographic methods and TEE may be helpful.
- IMR is also exquisitely sensitive to afterload. Occasionally, at relatively low systolic blood pressures such as under conscious sedation, IMR may only appear mild on TEE.
- Provocative maneuvers such as administration of phenylephrine may be required to elucidate the true volume overload as a result of IMR.

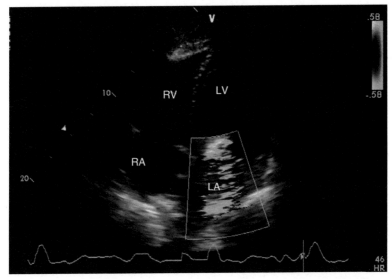

Figure 7-6. Same patient as Figure 7-5 with severe mitral regurgitation by color Doppler secondary to papillary muscle rupture seen in this apical four-chamber view. LV, left ventricle; RA, right atrium; RV, right ventricle.

- Mortality associated with IMR is greater than with nonischemic causes of MR and this is reflected in lower reference values used to define severe IMR (effective regurgitant orifice area [EROA] ≥20 mm^2, regurgitant volume ≥30 mL).

- **Key Points:**
  1. *Severity of IMR may be visually underestimated because of eccentricity of jet and high LA pressure influencing jet size.*
  2. *A hyperdynamic LV in the setting of severe MR and acute MI may indicate a PMR.*
  3. *IMR is very sensitive to afterload.*
  4. *In IMR, an EROA ≥20 mm^2, regurgitant volume ≥30 mL is associated with increased mortality. These values are used to define severe IMR.*

PERICARDIAL EFFUSION

- Small, uncomplicated pericardial effusions are common in transmural infarction and are usually transient in nature. These effusions result from inflammation of the epicardial wall and rarely result in tamponade.
- Large pericardial effusions after MI should raise the suspicion of ventricular free wall rupture, especially if the effusion appears to be hemorrhagic with thrombus or fibrinous material present in the pericardial space.
- Dressler's syndrome is a clinical entity that occurs 6 weeks to 3 months after MI. It is due to pericardial inflammation leading to reproducible chest pain and diffuse ST segment elevations on ECG. This inflammatory process results in

increased permeability of the pericardium and subsequent accumulation of pericardial fluid.

> • **Key Point:** *The subcostal view is usually best to visualize the full extent of a pericardial effusion, especially if loculations and hematoma are present.*

ACUTE DYNAMIC LEFT VENTRICULAR OUTFLOW TRACT OBSTRUCTION

- Acute dynamic LVOT obstruction is primarily seen in elderly females who present with an anterior MI. They often have a history of long-standing hypertension with subsequent localized basal septal hypertrophy and small LV cavities. The obstruction develops as a result of the compensatory hyperdynamic function of the anteroseptal and lateral walls. This in turn leads to systolic anterior motion (SAM) of the mitral valve with corresponding LVOT obstruction and mitral valve (MV) regurgitation.
- Likewise, acute dynamic LVOT may be present in ICU patients on inotropic therapy who are volume depleted.
- This entity has also been reported in patients with Takotsubo or stress-induced cardiomyopathy.

> • **Key Point:** *Suspect acute dynamic LVOT obstruction in a patient with worsened hemodynamic status after initiation of inotropic therapy with no other obvious cause.*

LEFT VENTRICULAR PSEUDOANEURYSM

- LV PsA is the result of a rupture along the ventricular free wall with hemorrhage into the pericardial space that is self-contained by an organizing clot or thrombus. It occurs most often after MI but may also occur secondary to trauma or cardiac surgery.
- A small, narrow neck connects the ventricular cavity with the walled-off pericardial space.
- Pseudoaneurysms can be differentiated from true aneurysms by the following features:
  - The neck diameter to maximal aneurysmal diameter ratio is **<0.5.**
  - Color and spectral Doppler show **bidirectional** flow through the narrowed neck.
  - Spontaneous echo contrast (stasis of blood) and **thrombus** can be seen in the pericardial space.
- Pseudoaneurysms occur most commonly in the inferior/inferolateral walls (Fig. 7-7), and less frequently in the apical walls (Fig. 7-8).
- Recognition of a PsA is critical because of a high risk of rupture and death.

TAKOTSUBO SYNDROME

- Takotsubo syndrome is also referred to as stress-induced cardiomyopathy or apical ballooning syndrome.
- Classic presentation is that of a postmenopausal woman who has just experienced a psychological or physically **stressful event.**

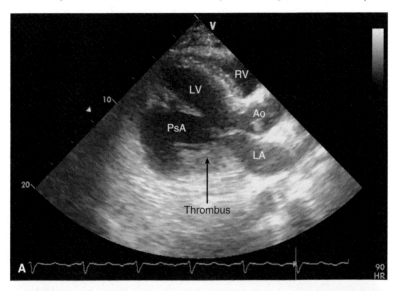

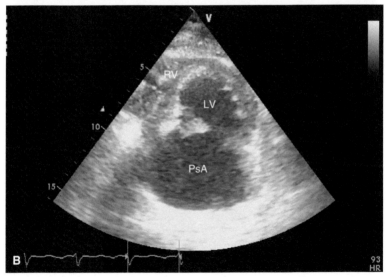

Figure 7-7. Pasternal long-axis (**A**) and short-axis (**B**) views showing a large basal inferolateral pseudoaneurysm (PsA). Note thrombus within the PsA. Ao, aorta; LA, left atrium; LV, left ventricle; RV, right ventricle.

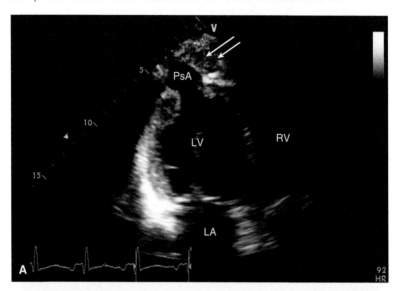

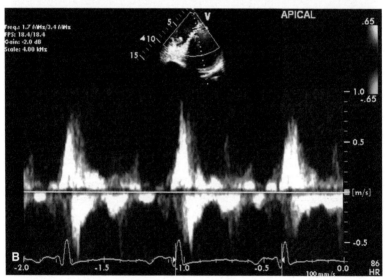

Figure 7-8. A: An apical pseudoaneurysm (PsA) seen on an "off-axis" apical long-axis image. Note the narrow neck and thrombus in the pericardial space (*arrows*). **B:** Spectral Doppler shows flow back and forward into the PsA.

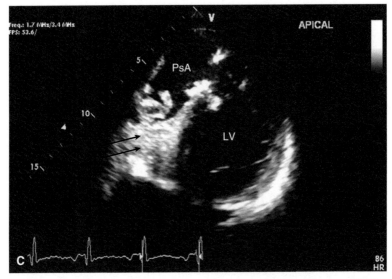

Figure 7-8. (*Continued*) **C:** Off-axis apical two-chamber view shows the full extent of the PsA and thrombus (*arrows*). LA, left atrium; LV, left ventricle; RV, right ventricle.

- Often mimicking a true MI, this entity often presents with **ST-segment elevation** as well as mildly elevated **biomarkers** for infarction. However, cardiac catheterization reveals **absence of obstructive coronary disease or coronary disease that is disproportional to** the patient's presentation.
- Although there are variants, the classic echocardiographic feature is **apical ballooning with a hypercontractile base,** giving an appearance similar to a Japanese octopus trap (Takotsubo).
- Treatment is analogous to that of patients with heart failure and often resolves within days to months (see subsequent chapters for examples of this entity).

CHRONIC COMPLICATIONS OF ACUTE MYOCARDIAL INFARCTION

Left Ventricular Aneurysm and Thrombus

- LV aneurysm is usually the result of a transmural infarction, causing thinning and remodeling of the ventricular wall.
- LV aneurysm occurs most frequently in the **apical** region, but can occur anywhere.
- Complications of aneurysms include LV thrombus formation and ventricular arrhythmias.
- In general, thrombi are dark and heterogeneous masses on echocardiography, but may be bright if extensive fibrosis has taken place. They are almost always related to an akinetic or aneurysmal wall and may be laminar or pedunculated (the latter are more prone to embolism).
- Contrast echocardiography has significantly increased detection of thrombi and also helps differentiate these masses from normal structures such as trabeculations.

> • **Key Point:** *A foreshortened apical view is the most common reason normal myocardial trabeculations may be mistaken for thrombus. This especially occurs when the heart is enlarged and the apex is aneurysmal, causing trabeculations to appear prominent. Conversely, thrombus may be missed when the view is foreshortened. Use of a more lateral probe position and contrast for LV opacification will allow better visualization of the "true" LV apex and reduce these errors.*

RIGHT VENTRICULAR DYSFUNCTION

- RV infarction occurs in the setting of inferior wall MI; patients usually present with hypotension.
- On echocardiography, a dilated and hypokinetic RV is seen. A dilated inferior vena cava with lack of respiratory variability and bowing of the interatrial septum toward the LA may also be seen due to elevated right atrial (RA) pressure.
- The apical RV may contract normally as a result of interaction with the LV and unaffected blood supply from the left anterior descending artery.
- Tricuspid regurgitation (TR) resulting from annular dilation is usually present.
- Other characteristics of right-sided volume overload secondary to severe TR include flattening of the IVS during diastole, best seen on the parasternal short-axis view.
- In a patient with inferior MI presenting with sudden onset hypoxemia, suspect a patent foramen ovale and the sudden development of right-to-left shunt caused by elevated right-sided pressures from RV infarction. This can be detected by color Doppler, injection of agitated saline, or TEE.

8 Cardiomyopathies

Mirnela Byku, Praveen K. Rao, and
Christopher L. Holley

HIGH-YIELD CONCEPTS

- *Dilated cardiomyopathy (DCM)* is accompanied by both increased left ventricular (LV) mass *and* volume, depressed ejection fraction (EF), diastolic dysfunction, and more commonly central mitral regurgitation.
- *Restrictive cardiomyopathy (RCM)* involves restrictive filling and should prompt a search for underlying causes such as amyloid or other infiltrative diseases.
- *Arrhythmogenic right ventricular dysplasia (ARVD)* echocardiographic findings include RV akinesis, dyskinesis, or RV aneurysm.
- *Takotsubo* cardiomyopathy is transient LV dysfunction with apical hypokinesis and basal hyperkinesis; *it requires angiography to exclude significant coronary artery disease (CAD)*.
- *Noncompaction* is a disorder characterized by echocardiographic findings of abnormal LV trabeculation and cardiomyopathy.
- Echocardiography can help evaluate for *transplant rejection and coronary vasculopathy*.

KEY VIEWS

- *DCM:* Parasternal long-axis (PLAX) and apical four-chamber (A4C) views to show increased LV cavity diameter and volume; A4C Doppler to demonstrate diastolic dysfunction and look for MR
- *RCM:* A4C to assess restrictive filling by transmitral pulsed-wave (PW) Doppler and low mitral annular tissue Doppler velocities
- *ARVD:* PLAX or parasternal short-axis (PSAX) view to demonstrate RVOT enlargement; off-axis A4C to evaluate RV function and search for structural abnormalities
- *Takotsubo:* PLAX and A4C to show apical ballooning and hypercontractile basal segments
- *Noncompaction:* Apical and PSAX views *with contrast enhancement* to demonstrate abnormal LV trabeculation

The five most commonly recognized categories of cardiomyopathy are:

- Hypertrophic cardiomyopathy (HCM), including obstructive forms
- DCM
- ARVD
- RCM
- Other (including takotsubo and noncompaction cardiomyopathy)

DILATED CARDIOMYOPATHY

DCM is defined as LV dilation and LV systolic dysfunction in the absence of significant CAD.

Background

- Approximately 25% of cases are familial.
- Remaining cases are inflammatory/toxic/metabolic, with the breakdown as follows:
  - Myocarditis (infectious, toxic, immune-mediated)
  - Drugs/alcohol
  - Endocrine (e.g., thyroid)
  - Nutritional (e.g., thiamine/beriberi)
  - Tachycardia-mediated
  - Postpartum cardiomyopathy

Echocardiographic Findings

- DCM often affects all four cardiac chambers: Lateral probe position for image acquisition is important to provide nonforeshortened images because of cardiac enlargement.
- LV mass is uniformly increased.
- LV is dilated (Figs. 8-1, *A* and *B;* see also Table 8-1 for normal LV chamber values).
  - Increased sphericity (ratio of long/short LV axes; in these cases approaching 1.0 [normal = 1.5])
  - MR is common as the mitral annulus dilates and papillary muscles are apically displaced leading to incomplete mitral valve (MV) coaptation; this is often termed "functional MR" (see Fig. 8-1, *C*).
- Impaired LV systolic function
  - Stroke volume may be preserved despite reduced EF, since LV diastolic volume is increased.
- Impaired diastolic filling
  - Look for elevated E/e' as evidence of elevated mean left atrial (LA) pressure.

- **Key Points:**
  1. *DCM usually affects all cardiac chambers.*
  2. *LV is dilated along with an increased LV mass.*
  3. *DCM may be accompanied by MR as a result of displacement of the papillary muscles.*

TABLE 8-1	Chamber Dimensions		
	LVIDd	**LV diastolic volume**	**LV systolic volume**
♀	4.5 ± 0.36 cm	76 ± 15 mL	28 ± 7 mL
♂	5.0 ± 0.41 cm	106 ± 22 mL	41 ± 10 mL

Adapted from Lang RM, Badano LP, Mor-Avi V, et al. Recommendations for cardiac chamber quantification by echocardiography in adults: an update from the American Society of Echocardiography and the European Association of Cardiovascular Imaging. *J Am Soc Echocardiogr.* 2015;28:1–38.
LV, left ventricular; LVIDd, left ventricular internal diameter in diastole.

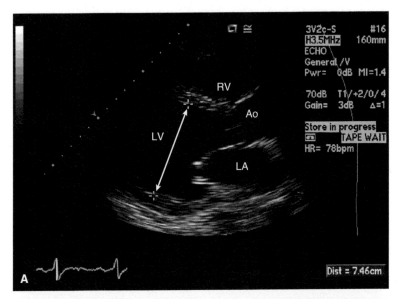

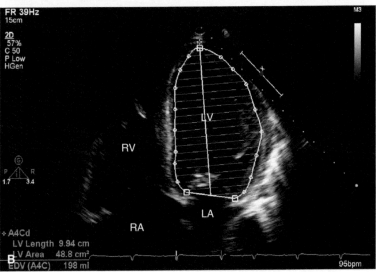

Figure 8-1. A: Marked left ventricular dilation, with left ventricular internal diameter in diastole of 7.46 cm. **B:** Another patient with significant dilated cardiomyopathy and LV diastolic volume of 198 mL. See Table 8-1 for normal values. (*continued*)

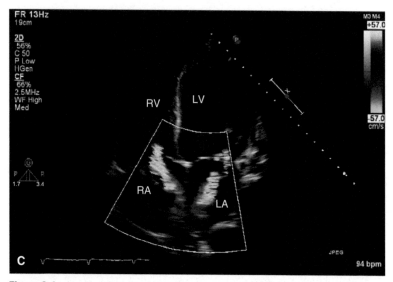

Figure 8-1. (*Continued*) **C:** Functional mitral regurgitation and tricuspid regurgitation secondary to mitral and tricuspid annular dilation. Ao, aorta; LA, left atrium; LV, left ventricle; RA, right atrium; RV, right ventricle.

RESTRICTIVE CARDIOMYOPATHY

Background

RCM is characterized by a LV that is normal sized or slightly enlarged; LV relaxation can be present if LV is severely impaired. RCM can be seen in infiltrative diseases (such as amyloid).

- Familial causes: Familial amyloidosis (e.g., transthyretin abnormality), hemochromatosis, glycogen storage disease, Fabry's (X-linked recessive lysosomal storage disease), and cardiac troponin mutations
- Nonfamilial causes: Primary amyloidosis (AL), endomyocardial fibrosis (including hypereosinophilic syndrome, carcinoid, radiation, chemotherapy [e.g., anthracyclines], scleroderma

Echocardiographic Findings

- Restrictive diastolic filling, biatrial enlargement, normal systolic function
- Restrictive mitral filling because of noncompliant LV
  - E >100 cm/sec, E/A >2, DT ≤160 msec, septal e′ <7 cm/sec, lateral e′ <10 cm/sec, average E/e′ ratio >14.
- RCM is also characterized by markedly reduced tissue Doppler myocardial velocities, and hepatic Doppler flow reversals are most marked during *inspiration*.
- Myocardium may have an abnormal echogenic, sparkling appearance suggestive of infiltrative disease.
- "Binary" appearance of LV myocardium in Fabry's disease with bright endocardium and myocardium with "clearing" of intervening subendocardium related to

the compartmentalization and accumulation of glycosphingolipids in certain layers of the wall

- Cardiac involvement in hypereosinophilic syndrome involves eosinophilic infiltration of the myocardium causing necrosis and obliteration of the ventricular apex with thrombus. Endomyocardial fibrosis leads eventually to RCM (Fig. 8-2).

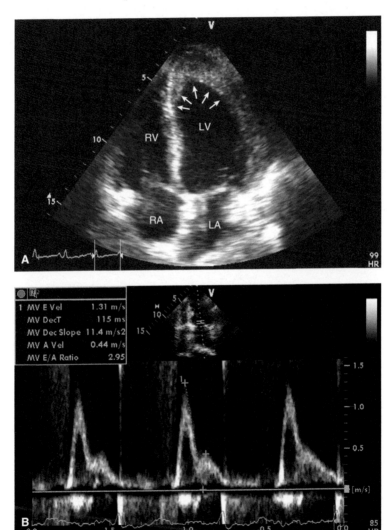

Figure 8-2. A: Apical four-chamber view showing a thrombus obliterating the left ventricular (LV) apex (*arrows*) in a patient with hypereosinophilic syndrome. No regional wall motion abnormalities were seen. **B:** Restrictive mitral inflow Doppler with E/A ratio ≥2 and E wave deceleration time <160 msec. LA, left atrium; RA, right atrium; RV, right ventricle.

• **Key Point:** *LV apical thrombus typically occurs in an area of akinesis or aneurysm formation. Hypereosinophilic syndrome is an example where thrombus can form without the presence of regional wall motion abnormalities.*

ARRHYTHMOGENIC RIGHT VENTRICULAR DYSPLASIA

Background

• ARVD is a genetic disorder affecting cardiac desmosomes. It primarily involves the right ventricle with fibrofatty replacement of the RV myocardium and associated arrhythmias.

Echocardiographic Findings

• Major criteria by two-dimensional (2D) echocardiography (Fig. 8-3)
  • RV akinesis, dyskinesis, or RV aneurysm and one of the following:
    ○ PLAX RVOT ≥32 mm
    ○ PSAX RVOT ≥36 mm
    ○ Fractional area change ≤33%
• Minor criteria by 2D echocardiography
  • Regional RV akinesis or dyskinesis and one of the following:
    ○ PLAX RVOT ≥29 to <32 mm
    ○ PSAX RVOT ≥32 to <36 mm
    ○ Fractional area change >33% to ≤40%

TAKOTSUBO CARDIOMYOPATHY

No Consensus Criteria, But Modified Mayo Clinic Criteria Often Used

• Takotsubo cardiomyopathy is characterized by transient hypokinesis, akinesis, or dyskinesis of mid to distal LV with apical involvement, in the setting of acute chest pain after physical or emotional stress (Fig. 8-4).
• Electrocardiographic abnormalities and modest troponin elevation mimic acute coronary syndrome.
• No angiographic evidence of obstructive coronary disease or acute plaque rupture is typically present.
• There is no evidence of myocarditis or pheochromocytoma.

Background

• Typical patient is postmenopausal woman with severe emotional (e.g., death of a spouse) or physical stress (e.g., surgery, severe pain, intracranial bleeding).
• Presents as acute chest pain and/or left heart failure that is reversible.
• This specific cardiomyopathy resolves over time.

Echocardiographic Findings

• ECHOCARDIOGRAPHY CANNOT DEFINITIVELY DIAGNOSE STRESS-INDUCED CARDIOMYOPATHY! *CAD must be excluded by angiography.*
• Takotsubo refers to the appearance of transient LV apical ballooning.
  • Hypocontractile apical segments: involving more than one coronary territory
  • Hypercontractile basal segments
• Takotsubo may affect both LV and RV.

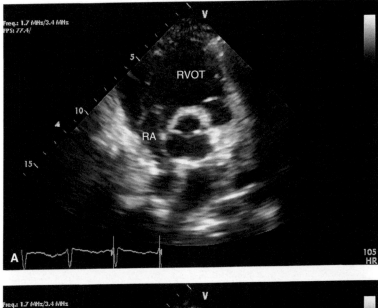

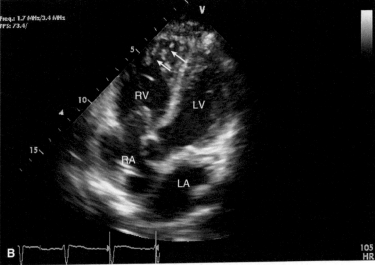

Figure 8-3. Patient with arrhythmogenic right ventricular dysplasia. **A:** Parasternal short-axis view with marked right ventricular outflow tract (RVOT) enlargement. **B:** Off-axis apical four-chamber view demonstrates hypertrabeculation of the right ventricle (RV) (*arrows*). LA, left atrium; LV, left ventricle; RA, right atrium.

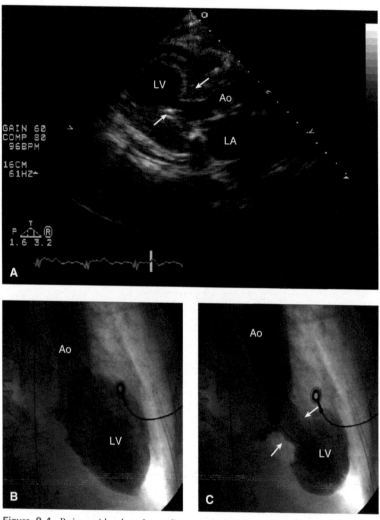

Figure 8-4. Patient with takotsubo cardiomyopathy. **(A)** Parasternal long-axis view during systole with marked basal hypercontractility and apical ballooning. Left ventriculograms from the same patient in diastole **(B)** and systole **(C).** The patient presented with pulmonary edema and cardiogenic shock in the setting of anterolateral ST elevation on electrocardiography. Peak serum troponin was 9 mcg/dL. Ao, aorta; LA, left atrium; LV, left ventricle.

- Myocardial involvement is much greater than expected by cardiac enzyme elevation.
- Less commonly "inverted" takotsubo pattern has also been described. This involves basal hypokinesis and apical sparing as well as a "Mid-LV" takotsubo pattern where there is mid-LV hypokinesis with sparing of the apex and basal segments.

- **Key Points:**
  1. *Takotsubo cardiomyopathy is a diagnosis of exclusion after coronary anatomy reveals no flow limiting lesions.*
  2. *This cardiomyopathy usually is reversible.*
  3. *It can also affect the RV.*

ISOLATED NONCOMPACTION OF THE LEFT VENTRICLE

Background
- **Prominent LV trabeculations, deep intertrabecular recesses**
- Frequently familial, with evidence in up to 25% of asymptomatic relatives
  - Thought to be failure of normal LV trabecular compaction during fetal development (weeks 5–8)
- Clinical presentation: High prevalence of heart failure (systolic and diastolic), **thromboembolism,** and arrhythmia (atrial fibrillation and ventricular tachycardia)

Echocardiographic Findings
- LV trabeculation with deep intertrabecular recesses (Fig. 8-5)
  - Primarily at the **apex** and mid-**inferior/lateral** walls
  - CW Doppler demonstrates flow in the trabecular recesses
  - "Two-layered" ventricular wall, with **noncompacted endocardial layer ≥2× the thickness of compacted epicardial layer** (i.e., greater trabeculation than what would be expected in simple LV dilation)

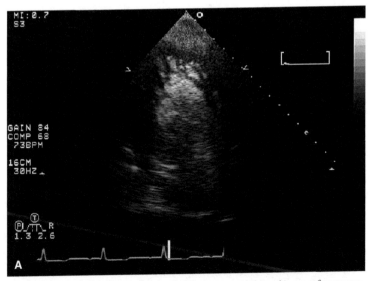

Figure 8-5. Noncompaction. Panels A and B show contrast-enhanced images of a noncompacted left ventricle in the apical four-chamber and apical two-chamber views, respectively. Note the conspicuous trabeculation with deep intertrabecular recesses. (*continued*)

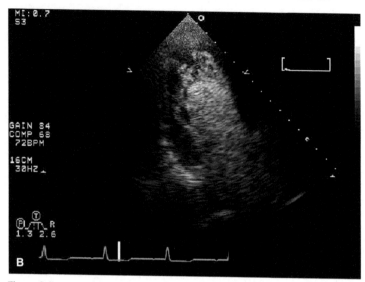

Figure 8-5. (*Continued*)

• **Key Point:** *The use of IV contrast for LV opacification increases sensitivity in detecting trabeculae, trabecular recesses, and thrombi in LV noncompaction.*

POST HEART TRANSPLANT

Background

The prognosis of patients post heart transplant has greatly improved over the past few decades, but allograft rejection, transplant vasculopathy, pericardial diseases, and valvular abnormalities continue to limit survival. Transthoracic echocardiography (TTE) can aid in the diagnosis of these complications.

Echocardiographic Findings

Allograft Rejection

• A healthy allograft should have normal systolic function. Acute changes in LV systolic and diastolic function, even if subtle, can help in the clinical diagnosis of rejection. These findings may be enough to begin aggressive immunosuppressive treatment and lead to an earlier endomyocardial biopsy.

• Endomyocardial biopsy can be performed safely from the jugular approach solely with TTE guidance. An off-axis A4C view can be used to visualize the bioptome, assess for possible perforation, pericardial effusion, or changes to tricuspid regurgitation.

• There is ongoing research into the applications of strain imaging and speckle tracking to aid in the diagnosis of allograft rejection.

Cardiac Allograft Vasculopathy (CAV)

• Stress testing can be used to identify patients at risk for CAV. A normal dobutamine stress echocardiogram can predict an uneventful clinical course and can be used to postpone invasive testing.

Hypertrophic Cardiomyopathy

Sharon Cresci

- *Hypertrophic cardiomyopathy (HCM)* is characterized by left ventricular (LV) hypertrophy in the absence of pressure overload; 60–70% of patients have significant resting or provocable LV outflow obstruction.
- *Hypertrophic obstructive cardiomyopathy (HOCM)* is a variant of HCM with outflow obstruction >30 mm Hg, often with asymmetric septal hypertrophy (ASH), systolic anterior motion (SAM), and eccentric, posteriorly directed mitral regurgitation (MR).
- Apical HCM is a variant of HCM with hypertrophy predominantly in the LV apex with a typical "spade-shaped" configuration of the LV at end-diastole; it accounts for 15–25% of HCM in Japan but is much less prevalent in Western populations.

KEY VIEWS

- Parasternal long axis (PLAX) to show abnormal septal or inferolateral wall thickness
- PLAX (two-dimensional [2D] and M-mode) to look for ASH and SAM; apical four-chamber (A4C) or apical three-chamber (A3C) Doppler to demonstrate and localize left ventricular outflow tract (LVOT) gradient
- A4C and apical two chamber (A2C) to look for apical variant
- Contrast enhancement may be necessary to demonstrate full extent of apical variant of HCM.
- HCM is one of the five most commonly recognized categories of cardiomyopathy.
- HCM is characterized by the presence of increased ventricular wall thickness associated with nondilated ventricular chambers in the absence of another cardiac or systemic disease that itself would be capable of producing the magnitude of hypertrophy evident in a given patient.

BACKGROUND

- Prevalence is around 1:500 adults in the general population; men and women are affected equally.
- HCM is a genetic form of cardiomyopathy caused by more than 1,000 mutations in genes encoding sarcomere and related proteins. Causative gene(s) are inherited in an autosomal dominant pattern with variable penetrance.
- HCM is an important cause of sudden cardiac deaths in young adults.

TABLE 9-1	Guidelines for Echocardiography in Patients with Hypertrophic Cardiomyopathy

Class	Recommendation
I	TTE in the initial evaluation of all patients with suspected HCM
I	TTE as a component of the screening algorithm for family members of patients with HCM unless the family member is genotype negative in a family with known definitive mutations
I	Periodic (12–18 months) TTE screening for children of patients with HCM, starting by age 12 years or earlier if a growth spurt or signs of puberty are evident and/or when there are plans for engaging in intense competitive sports or there is a family history of SCD
I	Repeat TTE for the evaluation of patients with HCM with a change in clinical status or new cardiovascular event.
I	TEE for the intraoperative guidance of surgical myectomy
I	TTE or TEE with intracoronary contrast injection of the candidate's septal perforator(s) for the intraprocedural guidance of alcohol septal ablation
I	TTE to evaluate the effects of surgical myectomy or alcohol septal ablation for obstructive HCM
III	TTE studies should not be performed more frequently than every 12 months in patients with HCM when it is unlikely that any changes have occurred that would have an impact on clinical decision making.
III	Routine TTE and/or contrast echocardiography is not recommended when TTE image is diagnostic of HCM and/or there is no suspicion of fixed obstruction or intrinsic mitral valve pathology.

Adapted from Gersh et al. ACCF/AHA hypertrophic cardiomyopathy guideline. *JACC* 2011;58: e212–e260.
HCM, hypertrophic cardiomyopathy; SCD, sudden cardiac death; TEE, transesophageal echocardiography; TTE, transthoracic echocardiography.

- A *majority* of patients have resting or provocable LV outflow obstruction.
  - 60–70% of patients have LV outflow obstructed at rest *or* with provocation.
- There are specific guidelines for echocardiography in HCM (Table 9-1) and for first-degree family members of patients with HCM (Table 9-2).

Echocardiographic Findings
- LV cavity is crescent-shaped (Fig. 9-1).
- LV systolic function is usually normal to supranormal (also termed hyperdynamic).
  - Left ventricular ejection fraction (LVEF) is often greater than 70%. The reason for this hypercontractile state is unclear.
- LV hypertrophy (increased mass) is typically asymmetric.
  - Wall thickness >1.5 cm, (1.3–1.5 cm is considered borderline), typically in the basal anteroseptum.

TABLE 9-2	Screening Strategies with Echocardiography for Detection of Hypertrophic Cardiomyopathy with Left Ventricular Hypertrophy

Age < 12 years: optional unless
Malignant family history of premature death from HCM or other adverse complications
Patient is a competitive athlete in an intense training program
Onset of symptoms
Other clinical suspicion of early LVH

Age 12 to 18–21: every 12–18 months

Age > 18–21 years: *At onset of symptoms or at least every 5 years; more frequently in families with a malignant clinical course or late onset of HCM*

Adapted from Gersh et al. ACCF/AHA hypertrophic cardiomyopathy guideline. JACC 2011;58: e212–e260.
HCM, hypertrophic cardiomyopathy; LVH, left ventricular hypertrophy.

- **ASH:** ratio of septum to posterior wall of 1.3:1
- No LV dilation
- Decreased early diastolic mitral annular velocities (e′)
  - Abnormal longitudinal peak systolic strain; may be seen in any segment or segments, but often in anteroseptal segments
- *HOCM: HCM with obstructive physiology*
  - LVOT obstruction is **dynamic,** that is, changes with loading conditions
  - **ASH** of the basal anteroseptum (Fig. 9-2, *A*)

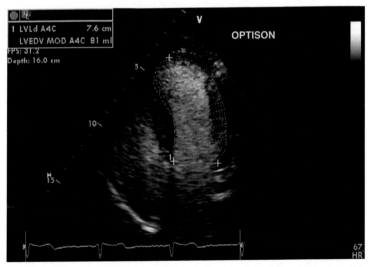

Figure 9-1. Typical crescent-shaped left ventricular cavity in a subject with hypertrophic cardiomyopathy.

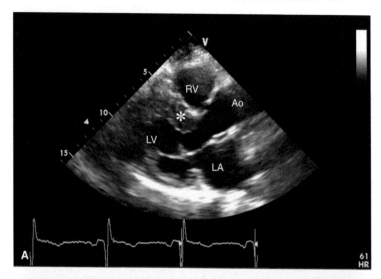

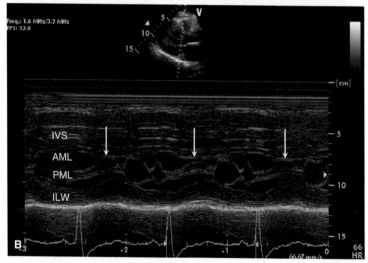

Figure 9-2. A: Typical parasternal long-axis view for hypertrophic obstructive cardiomyopathy, with eccentric hypertrophy of the basal anteroseptum (*). **B:** M-mode from the same view, demonstrating systolic anterior motion of the anterior mitral valve leaflet in systole (*arrows*). AML, anterior mitral leaflet; Ao, aorta; ILW, inferolateral wall thickness; IVS, interventricular septum; LA, left atrium; LV, left ventricle; PML, posterior mitral leaflet; RV, right ventricle.

- **SAM** of the anterior mitral leaflet toward the septum
  - Best seen in PLAX 2D or M-mode (see Fig. 9-2, *B*)
    - May see midsystolic contact of anterior leaflet with the septum in severe obstruction (Fig. 9-3).

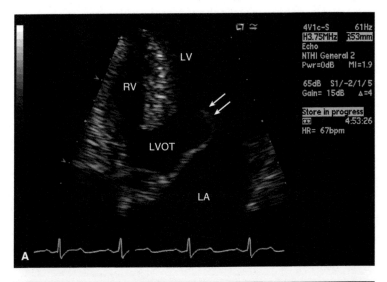

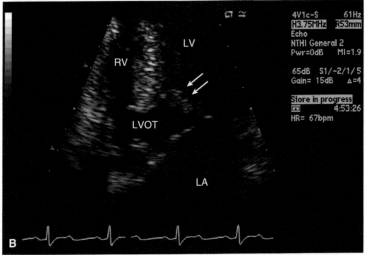

Figure 9-3. Apical four-chamber view of the mitral valve (MV) during early systole (**A**) and mid-systole (**B**) of the same beat, demonstrating systolic anterior motion of the anterior MV leaflet (*arrows*). Note that in midsystole, the MV contacts the septum, suggestive of significant left ventricular outflow tract (LVOT) obstruction. LA, left atrium; LV, left ventricle; RV, right ventricle.

- - LVOT obstruction may lead to midsystolic closure of the aortic valve because of reduced subvalvular pressure (Fig. 9-4, *A*).
- Eccentric, **posteriorly directed MR** jet secondary to SAM causing incomplete leaflet apposition (see Fig. 9-4, *B*)

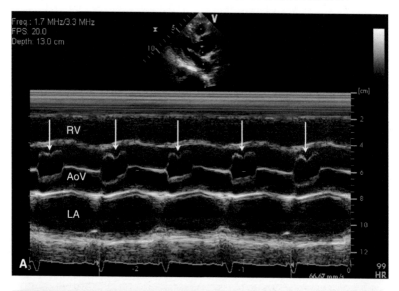

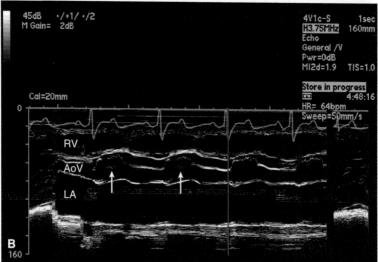

Figure 9-4. A and **B.** Mid-systolic closure of the aortic valve (AoV) (*arrows*), which indicates that left ventricular outflow tract obstruction is present.

- As MR increases as the anterior mitral valve (MV) leaflet is pulled away from the posterior MV leaflet, it also appears mid-to-late peaking and may be confused with the dynamic LVOT gradient (Fig. 9-5).
- A central or anteriorly directed jet should raise concern for intrinsic MV pathology.

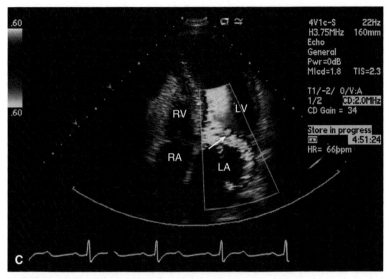

Figure 9-4. (*Continued*) **C.** Mid-systolic mitral regurgitation (*arrow*) with posteriorly directed jet resulting from systolic anterior motion of the mitral valve. LA, left atrium; LV, left ventricle; RA, right atrium; RV, right ventricle.

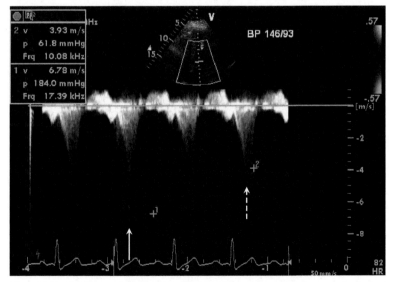

Figure 9-5. Continuous-wave Doppler showing mid- to late-peaking appearance of mitral regurgitation (MR) (*arrow*) in hypertrophic obstructive cardiomyopathy (the MR increases as the anterior mitral valve (MV) leaflet is pulled away from the posterior MV leaflet (also see text). Because of this profile, the MR may be confused with the dynamic left ventricular outflow tract gradient (*dotted arrow*).

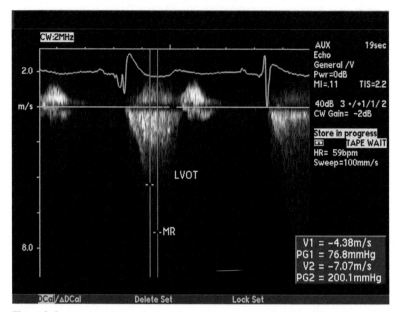

Figure 9-6. Continuous-wave Doppler shows a higher velocity, slightly broader mitral regurgitation jet superimposed on a late-peaking left ventricular outflow tract (LVOT) jet. The patient's systolic blood pressure of 120 mm Hg at the time of the study serves as an additional indicator that the measured gradients were accurate (assuming a left atrial pressure of ~15; see text).

- The MR jet peak velocity and systolic blood pressure (SBP) can be used to estimate and/or verify the LVOT gradient and as an "internal check." In Figure 9-6, continuous-wave (CW) Doppler shows the broader MR jet superimposed on the LVOT jet with measured gradients fitting with measured SBP.

  MR peak gradient = LVSP – LAP
  LVSP = MR peak gradient + LAP
  SBP = LVSP – LVOT gradient
  LVOT gradient = LVSP – SBP

  where LVSP = left ventricular systolic pressure and LASP = left atrial pressure.
- Dynamic LVOT gradient ≥30 mm Hg (velocity ≥2.7 m/sec)
  - M-mode will show midsystolic closure of aortic valve (note that this finding can also be seen with fixed LVOT obstruction [i.e., fixed subaortic obstruction that mimics aortic stenosis [AS]).
  - CW Doppler will show **late-peaking Doppler** envelope ("broad-blade dagger" shape) (Fig. 9-7, *A*). Intracavitary LV gradients resulting from hyperdynamic LV function and small LV cavity are distinguished from LVOT gradients by having a "scythe-shaped" late-peaking gradient (see Fig. 9-7, *B*). These both are in contrast to the early or mid-peaking Doppler envelope of fixed outflow obstruction (e.g., valvular AS, subaortic membrane) (see Fig. 9-7, *C*).
  - Pulsed-wave or high pulse repetition frequency Doppler must be used to identify the location of obstruction, which is often seen as turbulence at the point of the "septal bulge" on color Doppler (Fig. 9-8).

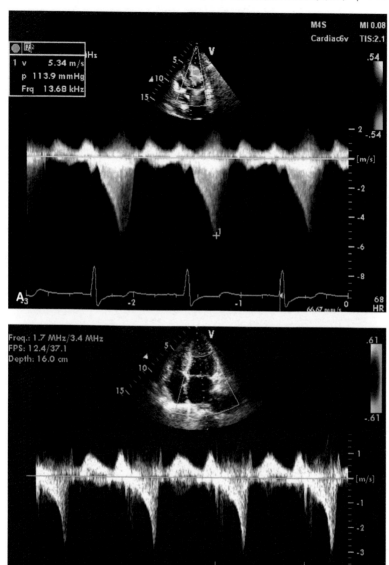

Figure 9-7. Typical left ventricular outflow tract with "broad-blade," late-peaking gradient (**A**), intracavitary "scythe-shaped," late-peaking gradient (**B**), and fixed, mid-peaking aortic stenosis gradient (**C**). (*continued*)

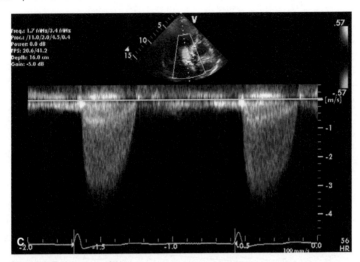

Figure 9-7. (*Continued*)

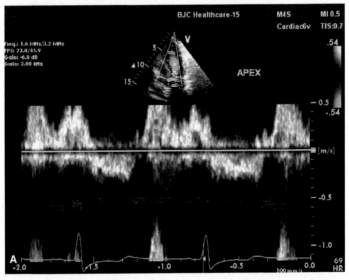

Figure 9-8. Pulsed-wave (PW) Doppler can be used to localize the gradient in subjects with hypertrophic obstructive cardiomyopathy. **A–C:** PW Doppler starting at the apex and moving into the left ventricular outflow tract (LVOT) (showing aliasing at the site of systolic anterior motion [SAM] and demonstrating that the obstruction is in the LVOT (**C**) and not in the apex (**A**) or mid-cavity (**B**). Continuous-wave Doppler (**D**) and broader mitral regurgitation jet (**E**) in the same subject. The subject's systolic blood pressure of 120 mm Hg at the time of the study serves as an additional "internal check" (assuming a left atrial pressure of ~15 mm Hg). **F.** From a different subject, shows how high pulse repetition frequency Doppler can also be used to localize the peak jet velocity (~2.3 m/sec) in the LVOT.

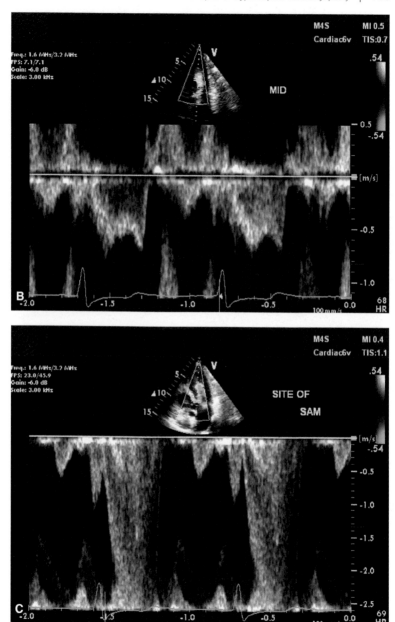

Figure 9-8. (*Continued*)

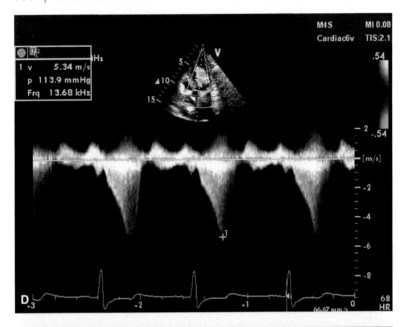

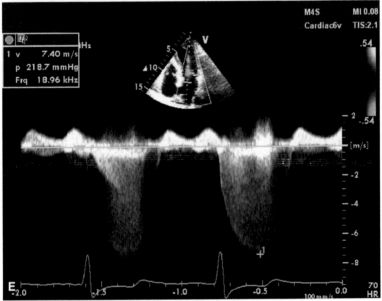

Figure 9-8. (*Continued*)

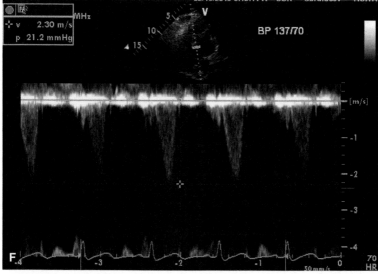

Figure 9-8. (*Continued*)

○ The gradient is influenced by both preload and afterload.
  - The gradient can be provoked/increased during echocardiography by Valsalva maneuver (decreases preload during strain phase), amyl nitrite inhalation (short-acting vasodilator decreasing preload and afterload), exercise (increased contractility), or inotropic medications (increased contractility).
  - The gradient may decrease with vasoconstrictors such as phenylephrine (increased afterload) or large fluid bolus (increased preload).
• If an early- or mid-peaking (parabolic) subvalvular gradient that does not change with dynamic maneuvers is seen, transesophageal echocardiography (TEE) should be used to exclude a subaortic membrane (i.e., fixed subaortic obstruction that mimics AS).

> • **Key Point:** *Evaluation of the Doppler profile and change in peak velocity with hemodynamic maneuvers help differentiate dynamic LVOT obstruction of HOCM from fixed LVOT obstruction seen with, for example, a subaortic membrane. Aortic insufficiency is also more typically seen with a subaortic membrane, whereas eccentric posterior MR is seen with HOCM.*

• *Apical variant of HCM*
  • Accounts for 15–25% of HCM in Japan; much less prevalent in Western populations
  • Electrocardiography typically shows T-wave inversions, especially in precordial leads.
  • Hypertrophy predominantly in LV apex
    ○ Apical hypertrophy
      - Results in the typical "spade shaped" configuration of the LV at end-diastole

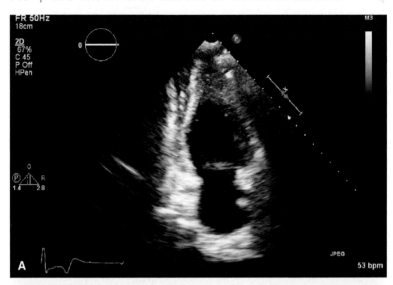

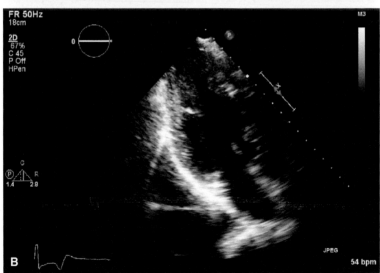

Figure 9-9. Apical two-chamber (**A**) and three-chamber (**B**) views, without contrast enhancement, in a subject with the apical variant of hypertrophic cardiomyopathy.

- Best seen in A2C or A3C view (Fig. 9-9)
- Contrast enhancement may be necessary to demonstrate the full extent of the apical hypertrophy (Fig. 9-10).
- Peak systolic strain pattern is typically abnormal in the apex (Fig. 9-11).
- Typically, there is no LVOT obstruction.

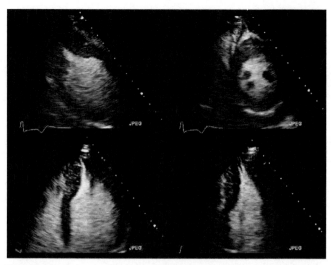

Figure 9-10. Contrast enhancement may be necessary to demonstrate the full extent of the apical hypertrophy. The typical "spade-shaped" configuration of the left ventricle at end-diastole is easily seen in the apical two-chamber view (*bottom right panel*).

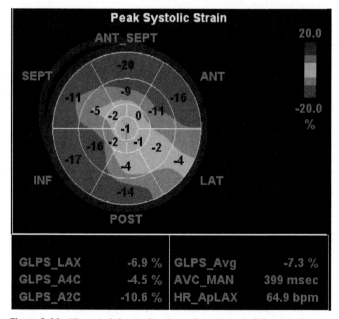

Figure 9-11. The typical abnormal peak systolic strain in the left ventricular apex in a subject with the apical variant of hypertrophic cardiomyopathy. A2C, apical two chamber; A4C, apical four chamber; ANT, anterior; Ap, apical; AVC_MAN, manual measure of aortic valve closure; GLPS, global longitudinal peak systolic strain; HR, heart rate; INF, inferior; LAT, lateral; LAX, long axis; POST, posterior; SEPT, septal.

10 Aortic Valve Disease

Brian R. Lindman and Jacob S. Goldstein

HIGH-YIELD CONCEPTS

- *Left ventricular outflow tract (LVOT) dimension* is a significant source of error when measuring aortic valve area (AVA).
- Make sure the numbers are internally consistent (AVA, gradients, left ventricular ejection fraction [LVEF]).
- Subvalvular obstruction: Evaluate flow through the LVOT.
- *Low-dose dobutamine test* is helpful in patients suspected of having severe aortic stenosis (AS) in the setting of low flow, low gradients.
- *LV size, shape, and function* are helpful in determining acute (normal LV size) versus chronic aortic regurgitation (AR) (dilated LV).

KEY VIEWS

- *Parasternal long-axis (PLAX) view*—initial screening for AS severity (ability of valve to open, calcification) and AR severity (width of jet, LV dimensions); LVOT measurement
- *Parasternal short-axis (PSAX) view*—aortic valve (AoV) morphology
- *Apical three-chamber (A3C) and apical five-chamber (A5C) views*—quantitative assessment of AS and AR: LVOT and AoV gradients, AR pressure half-time (PHT) using Doppler
- *Apical four-chamber (A4C) view*—LV dimensions and LV function for AR chronicity
- *Transesophageal echocardiogram (TEE)*—higher resolution views for valve morphology, planimetry for AVA, AR severity

ANATOMY

- **Leaflets**
  - The normal AoV is trileaflet.
  - A bicuspid valve occurs in 1–2% of the population; the abnormal leaflet number may cause inherent valvular stenosis and regurgitation.
  - Different valve pathologies are shown in Figure 10-1.
- **Annulus**
  - The leaflets form semilunar attachments at the annulus forming a "crown"-like interlocking of ventricular and arterial tissue.
  - They also attach at the sinotubular junction.

| Normal | Rheumatic | Calcific | Bicuspid |

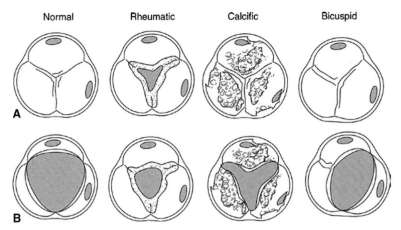

Figure 10-1. Typical appearance of aortic valve in diastole (**row A**) and systole (**row B**) suggestive of underlying etiology. Adapted from C. Otto, *The Practice of Clinical Echocardiography.* 3rd ed. Philadelphia, PA: Saunders Elsevier; 2007.

- **Sinuses of Valsalva**
  - As the proximal aortic root meets the LV outlet, there are three sinuses that bulge out and form the supporting structure for the corresponding AoV leaflets.
  - The sinuses and corresponding valve leaflet (or cusp) are named according to the origin of the coronary arteries; two sinuses give rise to coronary arteries (right and left) while the third, lying immediately adjacent to the mitral valve (MV), does not (non).
- **Sinotubular junction**
  - This is the place where the superior portion of the sinuses narrows and joins the proximal tubular portion of the ascending aorta.

AORTIC STENOSIS

- **Standard echocardiographic assessment of AS**
  - **Severity of AS**
    See Table 10-1.
  - **Two-dimensional (2D) assessment**
    - ○ **Leaflets**
      - *Motion of the valve*
        - AVA can be planimetered in the PSAX view.
        - This is most often only possible in TEE studies using a side-by-side, zoomed, short-axis, 2D image with corresponding color Doppler image to ensure that correct margins are drawn.
          - □ Ensure that the visual estimate of valve orifice area corresponds with other measurements; if, for example, the valve appears to open fairly well but measured gradients are considerably higher than expected, there may be a supravalvular/subvalvular obstruction.

TABLE 10-1	Severity of Aortic Stenosis			
	Aortic sclerosis	Mild	Moderate	Severe
Aortic jet velocity (m/sec)	≤2.5	2.6–2.9	3.0–4.0	>4.0
Mean gradient (mm Hg)	—	<20	20–40	>40
AVA (cm^2)	—	>1.5	1.0–1.5	<1.0
Indexed AVA (cm^2/m^2)	—	>0.85	0.60–0.85	<0.6
Velocity ratio	—	>0.50	0.25-0.50	<0.25

AVA, aortic valve area.
Adapted from Baumgartner H, Hung J, Bermejo J, et al. Echocardiographic assessment of valve stenosis: EAE/ASE recommendations for clinical practice. *J Am Soc Echocardiogr.* 2009;22:1–23, with permission from Elsevier.

□ Conversely, if the valve appears calcified and stenotic, but the recorded gradients are lower than expected, consider the following possibilities: (1) Doppler acquisition is not parallel to flow; (2) there is low flow, low gradient, reduced LVEF AS; or (3) there is low flow, low gradient, preserved LVEF AS (discussed later).
- Eccentric closure, doming, and prolapse of the valve in the PLAX view suggest the presence of a bicuspid valve.
- *Classifications of AoV (based on 2D assessment)*
  - *Bicuspid aortic valves (BAVs)*—This is most commonly a result of fusion of the right and left coronary cusps (~80%) or fusion of the right and noncoronary cusps (~20%).
    □ BAVs have an elliptical orifice during systole; they can easily be mistaken for trileaflet valves during diastole, particularly when a raphe is present.
    □ Leaflet doming is present because of restricted leaflet motion (Fig. 10-2A–D).
    □ Valvular regurgitation is usually highly eccentric and posteriorly directed (see Fig. 10-2E). There may be associated aortic abnormalities (e.g., dilation of aortic root, coarctation).
  - *Rheumatic aortic valve*—Leaflet thickening and fusion affects the **tips** predominantly, causing doming of the valve.
  - *Calcification*—The distribution and amount of calcification is important to note as it suggests an etiology and impacts prognosis. In senile calcific AS, there is calcification of the **body** of the leaflets as well as the supporting aortic root.
- **Subvalvular or supravalvular obstruction**
  - *Subvalvular obstruction*
    - This can be *fixed* (e.g., subaortic membrane) or *dynamic* (e.g., hypertrophic cardiomyopathy with obstruction).
    - A subaortic membrane is often seen best in the ALAX or A5C view and is usually a tunnel-shaped circumferential fibrous ring or a discrete fibrous ridge.
    - There is often concomitant AR secondary to LVOT turbulence affecting the AoV.

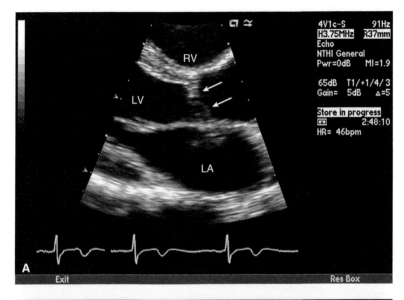

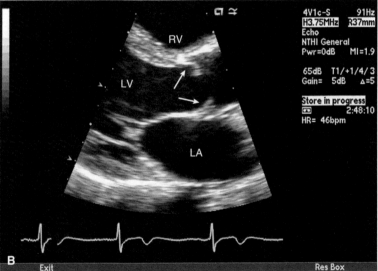

Figure 10-2. Movement of the aortic valve (AoV) and the importance of assessing number of cusps in systole. Images taken from a patient with bicuspid AoV. **A:** Parasternal long-axis (PLAX) view in diastole, AoV leaflets prolapse behind annular plane (*arrows*). **B:** PLAX in systole, doming of AoV leaflets signifying restricted motion (*arrows*). (*continued*)

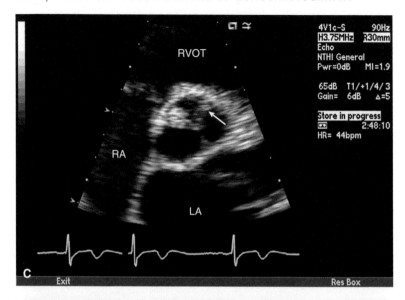

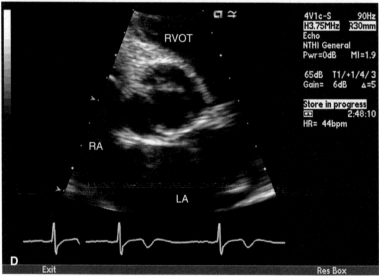

Figure 10-2. (*Continued*) **C:** Parasternal short-axis (PSAX) view in diastole, AoV appears to have three leaflets because of the presence of a raphe (*arrow*). **D:** PSAX in systole, "football"-shaped opening with fusion of right and left cusps.

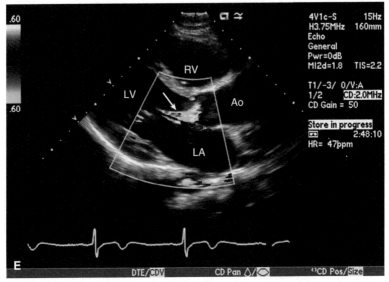

Figure 10-2. (*Continued*) **E:** PLAX in diastole with color Doppler showing eccentric posteriorly directed aortic regurgitation (*arrow*). Ao, aorta; LA, left atrium, LV, left ventricle; RA, right atrium; RV, right ventricle; RVOT, right ventricular outflow tract.

- In contrast, a dynamic obstruction is usually caused by systolic anterior motion of the anterior leaflet of the mitral valve being dragged into the LVOT during systole, causing a late peaking gradient. Dynamic means that provocative maneuvers that alter preload or afterload will alter the gradient.
  - *Supravalvular obstruction*
    - This is an uncommon congenital condition that is best visualized in the high PLAX view.
- ○ **Aortic root dimension**
  - Measure the dimension of the *sinuses of Valsalva, sinotubular junction,* and *ascending aorta during end diastole. The aortic annulus is measured at peak systole (i.e., when the AoV is open)* (Fig. 10-3).
  - Particularly **important in Marfan syndrome** (these patients develop a **"pear-shaped"** dilation of the aorta involving more of the sinuses and sinotubular junction than of the ascending aorta) **and BAV** (these patients can develop dilation of the aorta in the sinuses, sinotubular junction, or ascending aorta). Aortic dilation predisposes to dissection and rupture.
- ○ **LVOT dimension**
  - This measurement may be a significant source of error in the measurement of AVA in patients with AS (error is squared in the continuity equation).
    - Measure in the zoomed PLAX view during mid-systole (i.e., when aortic leaflets are open).
    - Measure just proximal to the AoV and parallel to the AoV plane.
  - The LVOT dimension is often ~2.0 cm (usual range: 1.6–2.4 cm), but precise measurement is critical and **should be reported** to increase accuracy of serial

Parasternal long-axis view

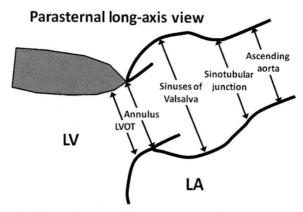

Figure 10-3. Left ventricular outflow tract (LVOT) and aortic root structures as a guide to location of measurements in a standard or high parasternal long-axis view. Note that the aortic annulus is measured in peak systole and the rest of the aortic root structures are measured in end-diastole. LA, left atrium; LV, left ventricle.

comparison of calculated valve areas (i.e., the LVOT dimension should remain constant during serial evaluations).
- ○ **Aortic annulus dimension**
  - – Measure from leaflet insertion to leaflet insertion in peak systole.
  - – This dimension is critical when considering transcatheter AoV replacement as it helps in the estimation of the size of the valve needed for implantation.
- ○ **LV dimensions**
  - – Patients with AS can develop significant ventricular hypertrophy and eventually dilation. This can have important management implications.
- ○ **LV function**
  - – LVEF is an important parameter to follow in patients with AS; even in asymptomatic patients, an LVEF ≤50% is a Class 1 indication for surgery.

- **Key Points:**
  1. *In the PLAX view, the right coronary cusp (closest to right ventricle [RV]) and typically the noncoronary cusp are seen. In the PSAX view, the noncoronary cusp lies near the interatrial septum, the right coronary cusp near the RVOT, and the left coronary cusp near the left atrium (LA).*
  2. *If the gradient across the AoV is higher than expected based on the 2D images of the valve, it is important to consider the possibility of a fixed or dynamic subvalvular obstruction.*
  3. *Aortic annulus is measured in peak systole.*
  4. *LVOT diameter is the greatest source of error when calculating AVA.*

- **Doppler assessment**
  - ○ **PW Doppler in the LVOT**
    - – In the A3C or A5C view, place the sample volume in the LVOT just proximal to the AoV such that only the closing click is seen and there is no spectral broadening or "feathering" of the Doppler profile (Fig. 10-4).

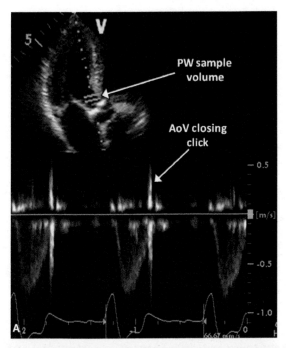

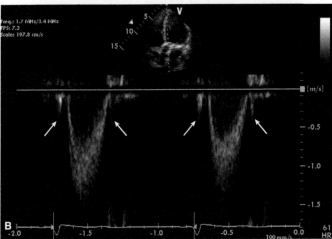

Figure 10-4. A: Correct positioning of the sample volume during pulsed-wave (PW) Doppler acquisition in the left ventricular outflow tract so that only the closing click of the aortic valve (AoV) is seen and there is little spectral broadening. **B:** Incorrect positioning of the sample volume too close to the AoV. Spectral Doppler shows both the opening and closing clicks of the AoV (*arrows*) and broadening of the Doppler jet, leading to overestimation of the velocity time integral.

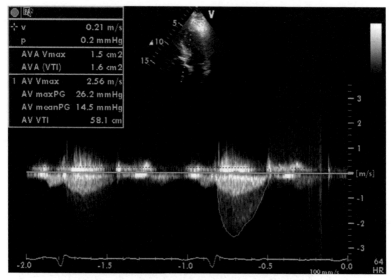

Figure 10-5. Continuous-wave Doppler across the left ventricular outflow tract (LVOT) showing two envelopes: Lighter envelope that is traced represents flow velocities across the aortic valve; brighter inner envelope represents flow velocities across the LVOT.

- Incorrect pulsed-wave (PW) Doppler location can lead to velocity time integral (VTI) and velocity measurement errors reducing the accuracy of the reported AVA using the continuity equation. Occasionally, as a "reality check," a very bright inner envelope is seen on continuous wave (CW) Doppler through the AoV that is representative of what the LVOT velocity and VTI should be (Fig. 10-5).
  ○ **CW Doppler through the AoV**
    - It is important to acquire the CW Doppler tracing from several locations (apex, suprasternal notch, and right parasternal) to ensure that the beam is parallel to the flow and the maximum jet velocity is obtained. The nonimaging probe (pedoff) should be used in each of these locations (Fig. 10-6).
    - **Mean gradient and peak velocity** is obtained when the CW Doppler signal is traced.
    - Mean gradient reflects the average gradient between the LV and aorta during systole; it is calculated by averaging the instantaneous gradients over the ejection period and requires tracing of the aortic Doppler envelope for machine calculation (see Fig. 10-6).
    - **Severe AS: Mean gradient >40 mm Hg**
  ○ **AVA**
    - AVA is calculated based on the continuity equation, which holds that the volume of blood ejected through the LVOT equals the volume of blood that crosses the AoV (Fig. 10-7):

$$AVA \times VTI_{AoV} = CSA_{LVOT} \times VTI_{LVOT}$$

  where CSA = cross-sectional area

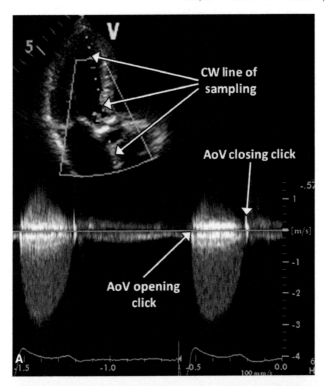

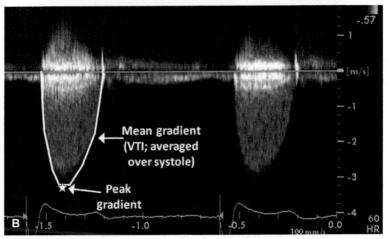

Figure 10-6. A: Continuous-wave (CW) Doppler across the aortic valve (AoV) allowing the highest velocity to be recorded. **B:** Measurement of mean and peak gradients from tracing the Doppler envelope. VTI, velocity time integral.

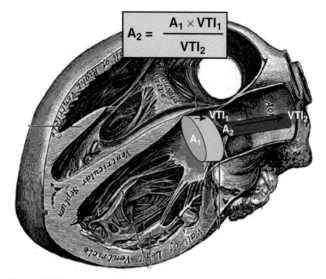

$$A_2 = \frac{A_1 \times VTI_1}{VTI_2}$$

Figure 10-7. Measurements used in the continuity equation to calculate aortic valve area. VTI, velocity time integral.

- Solving for AVA:

$$AVA = CSA_{LVOT} \times VTI_{LVOT}/VTI_{AoV}$$

- AVA should be indexed to body surface area (BSA) if patient is at extremes of body habitus.
- **Severe AS: AVA <1 cm², AVA/BSA <0.6 cm²/m²**
○ **Dimensionless index**
  - Since inaccurate measurement of the LVOT diameter leads to wide variability of calculated AVA, an index has been developed that does not rely on the diameter measurement.
  - This index takes the ratio of LVOT and AoV peak velocities. or VTIs.
  - **Severe AS: LVOT/AoV VTI ratio <0.25**
○ **Atrial fibrillation (and other irregular rhythms)**
  - Measure the VTI of the LVOT and AoV from at least six to eight successive beats and average the results for the determination of gradients and AVA.

• **Key Points:**
  1. *It is important to acquire the CW Doppler tracing from several locations (apex, suprasternal notch, and right parasternal) to ensure that the beam is parallel to the flow and the maximum jet velocity is obtained.*
  2. *Be sure to trace the modal (bright and clearly defined) Doppler envelope when measuring gradients. Spectral broadening or "feathering" of the envelope line can be exacerbated by contrast or inappropriate Doppler settings leading to overestimation of gradients.*

- **Advanced echocardiographic assessment of AS**
  - **Exercise testing**
    - ○ If the presence of symptoms is unclear when deciding on the optimal timing of surgical intervention, patients with severe AS may undergo an exercise stress test to assess functional capacity, symptoms, blood pressure response to exercise, and electrocardiographic changes.
  - **Low-dose dobutamine echocardiography for low flow, low gradient *reduced* LVEF AS**
    - ○ *Clinical problem:* In patients with significant LV dysfunction and reduced blood flow, the gradient generated across the AoV is often less than what is usually observed in severe AS (>40 mm Hg).
    - ○ **Low flow, low gradient, *reduced* LVEF severe AS is usually defined by: AVA <1 cm^2; LVEF <40%; and mean gradient <30–40 mm Hg.**
    - ○ Pseudosevere AS is when the reduced opening of the AoV is not primarily related to stiffened leaflets (as in "true" severe AS) but the inability of the LV to generate high enough transvalvular blood flow to fully open the leaflets.
    - ○ Differentiating "true" severe AS from pseudosevere AS is crucial to determining patient suitability for AoV replacement.
    - ○ *Why perform a dobutamine echocardiogram?* Dobutamine can enhance contractility and heart rate, both of which can increase transvalvular flow rate. This helps determine: (1) whether contractile reserve is present, and (2) whether there is true severe AS versus pseudosevere AS.
    - ○ *Contractile reserve:* defined as an increase in stroke volume ($CSA_{LVOT} \times VTI_{LVOT}$) by ≥20% with dobutamine; other measures include an improvement in wall motion, LVEF, or transvalvular flow rate. The absence of contractile reserve increases operative mortality.
    - ○ *Severe versus pseudosevere AS:* True severe AS is defined by the following: final AVA ≤1 cm^2 with dobutamine with an increase in stroke volume and gradient across the AoV.
  - **Low flow, low gradient *preserved* LVEF AS**
    - ○ *Clinical problem:* Seen in patients with normal to increased LVEF with significant LV concentric remodeling and **small cavity size** such that the total ventricular blood volume is markedly reduced.
      - ‐ This reduced volume results in reduced transvalvular blood flow and transvalvular gradients despite the presence of significant AS and normal LVEF.
      - ‐ If the calculated AVA is in the severe category, these patients have a similarly poor prognosis as patients with severe AS and markedly elevated gradients.
    - ○ It is important to first confirm that there have been no measurement errors (e.g., LVOT measured inaccurately small) in these cases before concluding that there is severe AS. A stress echocardiogram or computed tomography (CT) scan to evaluate AoV calcification may be helpful to clarify whether there is severe AS.
  - **Correlation with invasive measurements**
    - ○ A well-performed echocardiogram almost always provides adequate information for clinical management. When noninvasive testing is inconclusive or when there is a discrepancy between noninvasive test results and clinical findings regarding AS severity, invasive hemodynamics in the catheterization lab may be useful.

○ When comparing echocardiography-derived and invasive measurements, it is important to remember:
  - Reliable invasive hemodynamics requires the use of a dual-lumen pressure catheter to measure simultaneous pressures in the LV and aorta and not just an LV-to-aorta "pull back."
  - Invasive hemodynamics utilizes the Gorlin formula for a calculation of AVA, which is flow dependent and itself prone to various sources of error.
  - The popular peak-to-peak gradient measured invasively is a nonphysiologic value and is not the same as the peak instantaneous gradient measured by echocardiography (which will always be higher). Peak *instantaneous* gradients are comparable between both modalities.
  - Lower gradients measured invasively may result from **pressure recovery,** a phenomenon in which kinetic energy of the blood stream distal to the stenosis is recovered as pressure. As Doppler estimates the maximum pressure difference immediately distal to the valve, the pressure difference will be higher than when measured slightly downstream invasively when the pressure has been fully recovered. This is important in patients with small aortic roots (<3 cm).
  - **The mean transvalvular gradient is the best comparative measure between invasive and noninvasive techniques.**

• **Key Points:**
1. *When questions arise as to whether a patient with severe AS is symptomatic, an exercise echocardiogram can help clarify whether symptoms or other concerning features (e.g., drop in blood pressure with exercise) are present, indicating that surgery should be performed.*
2. *For patients with low flow, low gradient, reduced LVEF AS (classic low flow), a low dose dobutamine echocardiogram is helpful to clarify whether there is truly severe AS (vs. pseudosevere) and evaluate for contractile reserve.*
3. *When the AVA is in the severe range, but gradients are lower than expected, it is appropriate to first confirm that there have been no measurement errors.*

AORTIC REGURGITATION

• **Standard echocardiographic assessment of AR**
  • **Severity of AR**
    See Table 10-2.
  • **2D assessment**
    ○ **Leaflets**
      - Motion of the valve: Is there prolapse of one of the leaflets?
      - Leaflet number: Is this a factor (e.g., eccentric AR with BAV)?
      - Is there anything "extra" attached to the leaflets, (e.g., vegetation)?
      - Is there calcification present?
      - Aortic root dimensions and morphology: Is the support structure of the valve intact? Is there a suggestion of dissection? Is the root dilated?
    ○ **LV dimensions**
      - In chronic AR, the ventricle will dilate; the left ventricular end-systolic diameter (LVESD) and left ventricular end-diastolic diameter (LVEDD) are important to follow in these patients. Once the **LVESD reaches 5.0 cm**

TABLE 10-2	Severity of Aortic Regurgitation		
	Mild	**Moderate**	**Severe**
Structural parameters			
LA size	Normal[a]	Normal or dilated	Usually dilated[b]
Aortic leaflets	Normal or abnormal	Normal or abnormal	Abnormal/flail, or wide coaptation defect
Doppler parameters			
Jet width in LVOT—color flow[c]	Small in central jets	Intermediate	Large in central jets; variable in eccentric jets
Jet density—CW	Incomplete or faint	Dense	Dense
Jet deceleration rate—CW (PHT, msec)[d]	Slow >500	Medium 500–200	Steep <200
Diastolic flow reversal in descending aorta—PW	Brief, early diastolic reversal	Intermediate	Prominent holodiastolic reversal
Quantitative parameters[e]			
VC width, cm[c]	<0.3	0.3–0.6		>0.6
Jet width/LVOT width,%[c]	<25	25–45	46–64	≥65
Jet CSA/LVOT CSA,%[c]	<5	5–20	21–59	≥60
R Vol, mL/beat	<30	30–44	45–59	≥60
RF,%	<30	30–39	40–49	≥50
EROA, cm^2	<0.10	0.10–0.19	0.20–0.29	≥0.30

CSA, cross-sectional area; CW, continuous wave; EROA, effective regurgitant orifice area; LA, left atrium; LVOT, left ventricular outflow tract; PHT, pressure half-time; PW, pulsed wave; RF, regurgitant fraction; R Vol, regurgitant volume; VC, vena contracta.

[a]Unless there are other reasons for LV dilation. Normal 2D measurements: LV minor axis ≤2.8 cm/m^2, LV end-diastolic volumes ≤82 mL/m^2.

[b]Exception: Would be acute aortic regurgitation (AR), in which chambers have not had time to dilate.

[c]At a Nyquist limit of 50–60 cm/sec.

[d]PHT is shortened with increasing LV diastolic pressure and vasodilator therapy, and may be lengthened in chronic adaptation to severe AR.

[e]Quantitative parameters can subclassify the moderate regurgitation group into mild-to-moderate and moderate-to-severe regurgitation as shown.

Adapted from Baumgartner H, Hung J, Bermejo J, et al. Echocardiographic assessment of valve stenosis: EAE/ASE recommendations for clinical practice. *J Am Soc Echocardiogr.* 2009;22:1–23, with permission from Elsevier.

or the LVEDD reaches 7.0 cm, surgery should be considered, even in asymptomatic patients.

- In chronic AR, the ventricle develops **eccentric hypertrophy** (LV mass is increased, wall thickness increases, and the chamber dilates).
- In acute AR, the ventricle may be normal in size and shape and much less able to accommodate the large, sudden volume load, leading to a marked rise in LVEDP.

○ **LV function**
  - In chronic AR, the LVEF can remain relatively normal for a long period of time; however, surgery should be performed when the **LVEF is ≤50%,** even in asymptomatic patients.
  - **If the ventricle is hyperdynamic and the AR appears severe, the onset of the regurgitation is likely acute or subacute.**

○ **Doppler assessment:** A number of variables can affect the Doppler assessment of AR, including: volume status, filling pressures, eccentricity of the jet, coexisting regurgitant or stenotic valve lesions, and blood pressure. It is critical to *integrate all the information* obtained from the echocardiogram to determine the severity of regurgitation.

  - *Qualitative*
    ■ **Color Doppler jet width**
      □ **Width of the color jet versus width of the LVOT**
      □ Less accurate with highly eccentric jets (tends to underestimate severity)
      □ Measure in the PLAX or PSAX view (zoomed) or in the 120-degree long-axis view in TEE. (*Note:* Due to reduced lateral beam resolution, the jet will always seem broader in the apical views and therefore may be overestimated.)
      □ **<25% = mild AR; ≥65% = severe AR**
      □ **The length of the AR jet should not be used to assess AR severity** as it depends more on the driving pressure across the regurgitant orifice rather than the size of the orifice.

    ■ **Doppler vena contracta width**
      □ **Narrowest diameter of the regurgitant flow stream** reflects the diameter of the regurgitant orifice; relatively load and flow rate independent.
      □ For accurate measurement, **identification of all three components of the regurgitant jet** (i.e., proximal flow convergence, vena contracta, broadening in the LVOT) is key. This avoids erroneously measuring the jet as it rapidly expands in the LVOT as the vena contracta.
      □ Avoid overestimation of vena contracta by measuring **only the high velocity color width** and not lower velocity blood that is drawn to the regurgitant jet stream.
      □ Measure in the PLAX or PSAX view (zoomed) or in the 120-degree long-axis view in TEE.
      □ **Vena contracta <0.3 cm = mild AR; vena contracta >0.6 cm = severe AR** (Fig. 10-8).

    ■ **PHT**
      □ **Defined as the time it takes for the pressure difference between the aorta and LV to decrease by one-half during diastole.**
      □ Easy to measure using CW Doppler in the three- or five-chamber views.
      □ The intensity/density of the signal of the regurgitant Doppler profile is also a qualitative sign of the amount of AR.

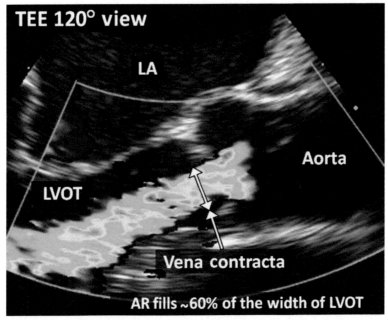

Figure 10-8. Transesophageal echocardiogram (TEE) long-axis midesophageal view of the left ventricular outflow tract (LVOT) showing image aortic regurgitation (AR) jet and measurement of the vena contracta. LA, left atrium.

- □ Can be influenced by numerous factors including LV compliance, LV filling pressure, presence of significant MR, and the chronicity of AR.
- □ **PHT <200 ms = severe AR, PHT >500 ms = mild AR** (Fig. 10-9).
- ▪ **Diastolic flow reversal in aorta**
  - □ Aortic flow reversal can be assessed with PW Doppler in the proximal descending thoracic aorta (suprasternal view) or in the abdominal aorta (in the subcostal view).
  - □ **Holodiastolic flow reversal suggests at least moderate AR,** with the greatest specificity being the presence of holodiastolic flow reversal in the abdominal aorta (Fig. 10-10).
  - □ Severe AR is suggested when the VTI of flow reversal approaches the VTI of forward flow in the aorta.

> • Key Point: *Early, brief diastolic flow reversal may be seen, especially in young patients with compliant aortas; this flow is NORMAL. It is important to distinguish this flow from HOLOdiastolic flow reversal, which is always ABNORMAL.*

- *Quantitative*
  - ▪ Unlike with MR, methods to quantify AR volume, while feasible, are not as frequently done. The severity of AR can often be determined by a combination of qualitative methods and the 2D assessment as previously described.

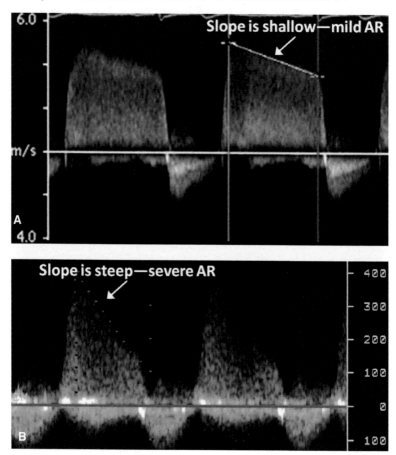

Figure 10-9. Measurement of pressure half-time of aortic regurgitation (AR) jet suggesting (**A**) mild or (**B**) severe regurgitation.

- **Proximal isovelocity surface area (PISA)**
  - □ Regurgitant flow accelerates in layers, or "surfaces," as it approaches the regurgitant orifice. Using color Doppler with a lowered aliasing velocity, the red–blue interface can be identified. The distance between the red–blue interface and the regurgitant orifice is the PISA radius. The PISA is the surface area of blood moving back from the aorta toward the closed AoV at the given aliasing velocity.
  - □ PISA = $2\pi \times$ (PISA radius)^2
  - □ Although difficult to measure, this should be performed on a "zoomed" A5C or ALAX view.
- **Regurgitant volume (R Vol)**
  - □ The volume of blood that regurgitates across the valve per beat

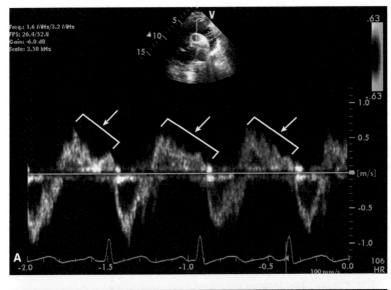

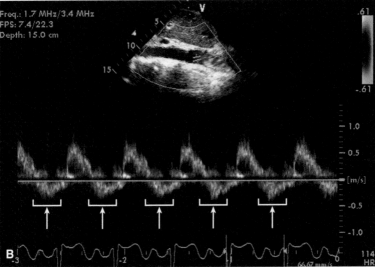

Figure 10-10. Pulsed-wave Doppler in the (**A**) proximal descending thoracic aorta and (**B**) abdominal aorta showing holodiastolic flow reversal (*arrows*) with similar velocity time integral to forward flow, suggestive of severe aortic regurgitation.

- **Calculated by three methods:**
  - □ Difference between transaortic and transmitral volume flow measured by PW Doppler
    - Transaortic volume is SV_{total} (forward volume and R Vol) and transmitral volume is $SV_{forward}$ (forward volume only), where SV = stroke volume.
    - $SV_{total} = CSA_{LVOT} \times VTI_{LVOT}$
    - $SV_{forward} = CSA_{mitral\ annulus} \times VTI_{mitral\ annulus}$
      (*Note: Use PW Doppler at the level of the mitral annulus.*)
    - $R\ Vol = SV_{total} - SV_{forward}$
    - Not valid when significant MR present
  - □ Another method for calculating SV_{total} uses 2D measurement of LV volumes.
    - $SV_{total} = LVEDV - LVESV$ (by Simpson method)
    - $R\ Vol = SV_{total} - SV_{forward}$
    - $R\ Vol = 2D\ LV\ SV - volume_{transmitral}$
  - □ PISA

$$R\ Vol = EROA \times VTI_{AR\ jet}$$

where EROA = effective regurgitant orifice area
  - **R Vol <30 mL/beat = mild AR, R Vol ≥60 mL/beat = severe AR**
- **Regurgitant fraction (RF)**
  - □ The ratio of the regurgitant flow to antegrade flow across the valve
  - □ $RF = R\ Vol/SV_{total}$ (where $SV_{total} = CSA_{LVOT} \times VTI_{LVOT}$)
  - □ **RF <30% = mild AR, RF ≥50% = severe AR**
- **Effective regurgitant orifice area**
  - □ EROA = PISA × aliasing velocity/peak AR velocity
    OR
  - □ $EROA = R\ Vol/VTI_{AR\ jet}$
  - □ **EROA <0.1 cm² = mild AR, EROA ≥0.3 cm² = severe AR**
  - ○ **TEE**
    - Can complement transthoracic echocardiography (TTE) in the assessment of AR
    - Provides better visualization of the valve morphology and aortic root dimension (e.g., endocarditis, aortic dissection)

- **Key Points:**
  1. *For complete aortic root measurement, moving the probe one intercostal space higher or tilting medially will often offer better visualization and acoustic definition.*
  2. *Significant AR may result from valvular pathology, aortic root dilation, or both.*
  3. *Assessment of the severity of AR requires an integrative approach, incorporating multiple qualitative and quantitative indices.*
  4. *When AR appears severe, but the LV chamber is normal in size and shape, suspect the possibility of acute AR and look for signs of aortic dissection or endocarditis.*

Mitral Valve Disease

Brian R. Lindman and Nishath Quader

MITRAL VALVE APPARATUS

The mitral valve (MV) apparatus consists of the mitral annulus, the leaflets, the chordae tendineae and the submitral apparatus, papillary muscles, and the LV wall into which the papillary muscles insert.

- **Leaflets**
  - Anterior and posterior leaflets each have three scallops (Fig. 11-1).
- **Annulus**
  - Annulus is the junction between atrium and ventricle and the place where the mitral leaflets insert.
  - There is an anterior and posterior portion of the annulus corresponding to the respective leaflets. The anterior portion is attached to the right and left fibrous trigones and is structurally more supported than the posterior portion.
  - The annulus may dilate (leading to functional regurgitation) or calcify (leading to stenosis).
  - Severe LA enlargement can also lead to annular dilation and thus MR.

Parasternal short-axis view
(mitral valve level)

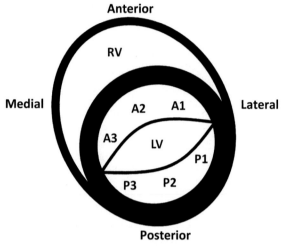

Figure 11-1. Diagram of parasternal short axis at the mitral valve level showing the different scallops numbered in ascending order from lateral to medial. RV, right ventricle.

- *Unlike the tricuspid and pulmonic valves, which are separated by the right ventricular (RV) infundibulum, the MV and aortic valve (AoV) are in direct continuity, separated only by a fibrous connection. This has ramifications for pathology, such as endocarditis, which can spread between the MV and AoV valves and cause annular and aortic root abscess.*
- **Subvalvular apparatus**
  - Papillary muscles: These are anterolateral and posteromedial; the anterolateral papillary muscle usually receives dual blood supply (left anterior descending and left circumflex artery), whereas the posteromedial papillary muscle usually has a single blood supply (either left circumflex or right coronary artery).
  - Chordae tendineae: Primary, secondary, and tertiary chords connect the papillary muscles to **both** valve leaflets; these can elongate, shorten, rupture, calcify, or fuse.
- **Ventricle**
  - The ventricular size and shape impact the function of the MV. As the ventricle dilates and becomes more spherical, the papillary muscles become apically and laterally displace. This is turn restricts the closure of the mitral leaflets, especially the posterior mitral leaflet, leading to posteriorly directed MR.

- **Key Points:**
  1. *The MV apparatus is a complex structure made up of the annulus, the leaflets, the submitral apparatus, and the insertion of the papillary muscles into the LV wall.*
  2. *MR can result when there is pathology of any of the components of the mitral apparatus.*
  3. *The anterolateral papillary muscle has a dual blood supply whereas the posteromedial papillary muscle has a single blood supply.*

MITRAL REGURGITATION

- *Causes of MR*

Degenerative/ MV prolapse syndrome	• Usually occurs as a primary condition (Barlow disease or fibro-elastic deficiency), but has also been associated with heritable connective tissue disorders (e.g., Marfan syndrome, Ehlers–Danlos syndrome, osteogenesis imperfecta) • Occurs in 1–2.5% of the population • Two-thirds are female • Posterior leaflet (P2 scallop) most commonly prolapses (Fig. 11-2) • Most common reason for MV surgery • Myxomatous proliferation and cartilage formation can occur in the leaflets, chordae tendineae, and/or annulus
Dilated cardiomyopathy	• Due to both annular dilation from LV enlargement and papillary muscle displacement from LV enlargement and spherical remodeling to prevent adequate leaflet coaptation • May occur in nonischemic- or ischemic-dilated cardiomyopathy (there are often multiple mechanistic reasons for MR in the setting of prior infarction)

Ischemic	• Primarily attributable to LV dysfunction—not papillary muscle dysfunction
	• Mechanism of MR usually involves one or both of the following:
	  – Annular dilation from LV enlargement
	  – Local LV remodeling with papillary muscle displacement (both the dilation of the LV and the akinesis/dyskinesis of the wall to which the papillary muscle is attached can apically displace leaflet coaptation, causing "tenting" of the leaflets) (Fig. 11-3)
	• Rarely, MR may develop acutely from papillary muscle rupture (usually the posteromedial papillary muscle because of its single blood supply)

Rheumatic	• May be pure MR or combined MR/MS • Caused by thickening and/or calcification of the leaflets and chordae
Infective endocarditis	• Usually caused by destruction of the leaflet tissue (i.e., perforation)
Other causes	• Congenital (e.g., cleft, parachute, or fenestrated MV) • Infiltrative diseases (e.g., amyloid) • Systemic lupus erythematosus (SLE; i.e., Libman—Sacks lesion) • Hypertrophic cardiomyopathy with LV outflow obstruction • Mitral annular calcification • Perivalvular MV prosthetic valve leak • Drug toxicity (e.g., phen-fen)
Acute causes	• Ruptured papillary muscle • Ruptured chordae tendineae • Infective endocarditis

- **Key Point:** *Be able to differentiate between primary and secondary causes of MR.*

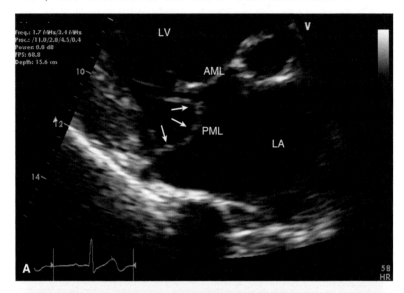

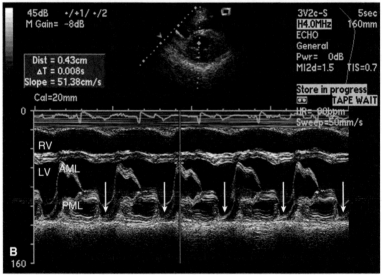

Figure 11-2. Posterior mitral valve leaflet (PML) prolapse (*arrows*) seen on (**A**) a zoomed two-dimensional image in the parasternal long-axis view and (**B**) M-mode echocardiography. AML, anterior mitral valve leaflet; LA, left atrium; LV, left ventricle; RV, right ventricle.

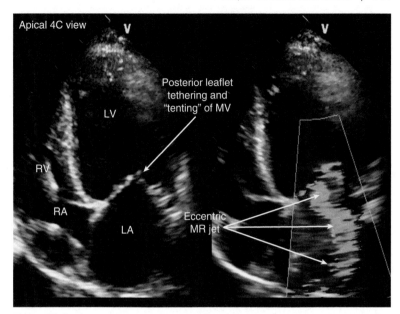

Figure 11-3. Tenting of the posterior mitral valve (MV) leaflet with apical and lateral displacement of leaflet coaptation resulting in eccentric posteriorly directed mitral regurgitation (MR). LA, left atrium; LV, left ventricle; RA, right atrium; RV, right ventricle.

- **Two-dimensional (2D) transthoracic echocardiography (TTE) assessment**
  - **Etiology**
    - Determining whether it is a primary mitral leaflet problem or a secondary mitral leaflet problem: Primary MR is due to a mitral leaflet problem (prolapse, perforation, flail) whereas secondary MR is a problem of the LV (leaflet tenting resulting from LV dilation). This has important management implications.
  - **Leaflets**
    - Motion of the valve: In prolapse, leaflet body bows >1 mm behind annular plane. If tenting is seen, leaflet coaptation occurs further into LV. With flail, leaflet tip points back to LA (Fig. 11-4).
    - Is there anything "extra" attached to the leaflets (e.g., vegetation) or a perforation?
    - Assess degree of calcification.
  - **Subvalvular apparatus**
    - Papillary muscle displacement
    - Torn or elongated chordae tendineae
  - **Mitral annulus**
    - Assess degree of dilation and/or calcification.
  - **LA dimension**
    - Chronic severe MR will lead to enlargement of the left atrium; the LA dimensions and volume can elucidate the chronicity and degree of volume overload.
  - **LV dimensions and function**
    - Measurement of the LV dimension at end-systole and end-diastole is important for assessing the ventricle's response to volume overload.

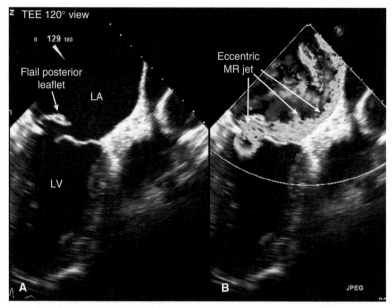

Figure 11-4. (**A**) Flail mitral valve with posterior leaflet pointing backward into left atrium (LA). By definition this anatomic finding results in severe mitral regurgitation (MR) as is seen in this case with color Doppler (**B**). Because the posterior leaflet is flail, the MR jet is anteriorly directed versus if there was prolapse/flail of the anterior leaflet, in which case the MR jet would be posteriorly directed. LV, left ventricle.

- ○ Chronic severe MR eventually leads to dilation of the ventricle. An enlarged end-systolic dimension (≥4.0 cm) is an indication for surgery even in the absence of symptoms per the American College of Cardiology/American Heart Association (ACC/AHA) guidelines.
- **Doppler**
  - **Color Doppler jet area**
    - ○ Color jet area depends on instrument settings, hemodynamics, jet eccentricity, orifice geometry, pulmonary venous counterflow, and LA size and compliance, and must be interpreted with caution.
    - ○ Measure in the apical four-chamber and PLAX views; usually this is assessed qualitatively. Both qualitative and quantitative criteria for assessing MR are noted in Table 11-1.
  - **Doppler vena contracta width**
    - ○ This is the narrowest diameter of the regurgitant flow stream and reflects the diameter of the regurgitant orifice. It is measured in the PLAX view in zoom mode and is the narrowest segment between the proximal flow convergence and the expansion of the regurgitant jet downstream (Fig. 11-5).
  - **Proximal isovelocity surface area**
    - ○ Regurgitant blood accelerates as "hemispheric layers" as it moves from the wider LV to the narrow MV orifice.

TABLE 11-1	Criteria for Determining Severity of Mitral Valve Regurgitation		
	Mild	**Moderate**	**Severe**
Specific signs of severity	• Small central jet <4 cm^2 or <20% of LA area^a • Vena contracta width <0.3 cm • No flow or minimal flow convergence^b	Signs of MR > mild present, but no criteria for severe MR	• Vena contracta width ≥0.7 cm *with* large central MR jet (area >40% of LA) or *with* a wall-impinging jet of any size, swirling in LA^a • Large flow convergence^b • Systolic reversal in pulmonary veins • Prominent flail MV leaflet or ruptured papillary muscle
Supportive signs	• Systolic dominant flow in pulmonary veins • A-wave dominant mitral inflow^c • Soft density, parabolic CW Doppler MR signal • Normal LV size^d	Intermediate signs/findings	• Dense, triangular CW Doppler MR jet • E-wave dominant mitral inflow (E >1.2 m/sec)^c • Enlarged LV and LA size^e (particularly when normal LV function is present).

Quantitative parameters^f

R Vol (mL/beat)	<30	30–44	45–59	≥60
RF (%)	<30	30–39	40–49	≥50
EROA (cm^2)	<0.20	0.20–0.29	0.30–0.39	≥0.40

CW, continuous wave; EROA, effective regurgitant orifice area; LA, left atrium; LV, left ventricle; MR, mitral regurgitation; MV, mitral valve; RF, regurgitant fraction; R Vol, regurgitant volume.

[a]At a Nyquist limit of 50–60 cm/sec.

[b]Minimal and large flow convergence defined as a flow convergence radius <0.4 cm and ≥0.9 cm for central jets, respectively, with a baseline shift at a Nyquist of 40 cm/sec; cut-offs for eccentric jets are higher, and should be angle corrected (see text).

[c]Usually above 50 years of age or in conditions of impaired relaxation, in the absence of mitral stenosis or other causes of elevated left atrial pressure.

[d]Left ventricular (LV) size applies only to chronic lesions. Normal two-dimensional measurements: LV minor axis ≤2.8 cm/m^2, LV end-diastolic volume ≤82 mL/m^2, maximal left atrial (LA) anteroposterior diameter ≤2.8 cm/m^2, maximal LA volume ≤36 mL/m^2 (2;33;35).

[e]In the absence of other etiologies of left ventricular and left atrial dilation and acute mitral regurgitation.

[f]Quantitative parameters can help subclassify the moderate regurgitation group into mild-to-moderate and moderate-to-severe as shown.

Adapted from Zoghbi WA, Enriquez-Sarano M, Foster E, et al. Recommendations for evaluation of the severity of native valvular regurgitation with two-dimensional and Doppler echocardiography. *J Am Soc Echocardiogr.* 2003;16:777–802, with permission from Elsevier.

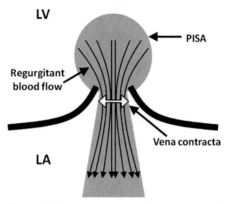

Figure 11-5. Diagram showing flow convergence of mitral regurgitant blood and the narrowest portion of the jet as the blood enters the left atrium (LA), called the vena contracta. LV, left ventricle; PISA, proximal isovelocity surface area.

- When the velocity exceeds the Nyquist limit, it aliases; that is, it changes from blue to red or red to blue depending on the direction of blood flow in relation to the probe.
- Using the continuity principle, the product of the surface area of the hemisphere as the blood aliases and the aliasing velocity must equal the product of the effective regurgitant orifice area (EROA) and the velocity of blood moving through the orifice (peak MR velocity).
- Surface area of a hemisphere $= 2\pi r^2$
- EROA $= 2\pi r^2 \times$ aliasing velocity/peak MR velocity.
  To increase the PISA radius for accurate measurement, the Nyquist limit baseline is moved in the direction of regurgitant blood flow so that the regurgitant blood aliases early. This direction therefore differs for TTE and TEE because of the different probe locations (Fig. 11-6).
- **Regurgitant volume**
  - Defined as the volume of blood that regurgitates across the valve per beat or second
  - Calculated by three methods:
    (1) Difference between transaortic and transmitral volume flow

    $$\text{Volume}_{\text{transaortic}} = \text{CSA}_{\text{LVOT}} \times \text{VTI}_{\text{LVOT}}$$
    $$\text{Volume}_{\text{transmitral}} = \text{CSA}_{\text{mitral annulus}} \times \text{VTI}_{\text{mitral annulus}}$$

    (Use PW Doppler at the level of the mitral annulus)

    $$\text{Regurgitant volume (R Vol)} = \text{Volume}_{\text{transmitral}} - \text{Volume}_{\text{transaortic}}$$

    (Not valid in the setting of significant aortic regurgitation [AR])
    (2) Difference between 2D LV stroke volume (SV) and forward SV

    $$\text{2D LV SV} = \text{LVEDV} - \text{LVESV (modified Simpson's)}$$
    $$\text{SV}_{\text{forward}} = \text{CSA}_{\text{LVOT}} \times \text{VTI}_{\text{LVOT}}$$
    $$\text{R Vol} = \text{2D LV SV} - \text{SV}_{\text{forward}}$$

    (3) PISA

    $$\text{EROA} = 2\pi r^2 \times \text{aliasing velocity/Peak MR velocity}$$
    $$\text{R Vol (mL)} = \text{EROA} \times \text{VTI}_{\text{MRjet}}$$

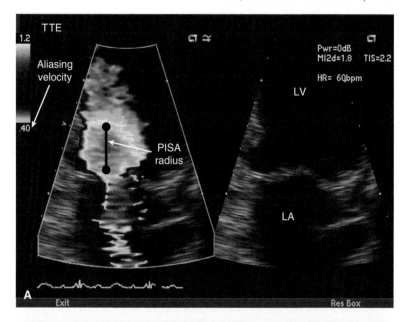

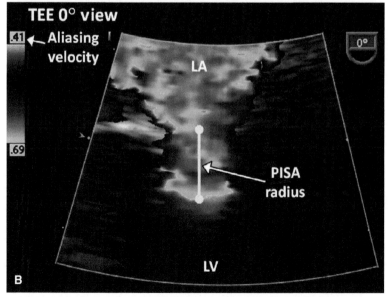

Figure 11-6. Measurement of proximal isovelocity surface area (PISA) radius with (**A**) a zoomed transthoracic echocardiogram (TTE) and (**B**) transesophageal echocardiogram (TEE) view. Note that the Nyquist baseline is shifted based on the direction of the mitral valve regurgitation in relation to the different probe locations. LA, left atrium; LV, left ventricle.

- **Regurgitant fraction (RF)**
  - ○ Defined as the ratio of the regurgitant flow to antegrade flow across the valve

$$RF = R\ Vol/SV_{total}\ (where\ SV_{total} = CSA_{mitral\ annulus} \times VTI_{mitral\ annulus})$$

- **EROA**

$$EROA = R\ Vol/VTI_{MR\ jet}$$

- **Indirect measures**
  - ○ In severe MR, the LA pressure is high; thus the E-wave in MV inflow should be high (>1.2 cm/sec). E/A reversal pattern (impaired myocardial relaxation) on MV inflow virtually excludes severe MR.
  - ○ The density (similar to inflow Doppler density) and shape (early peaking) of the MR jet on CW Doppler can be helpful.
    - ‒ The density/brightness of the CW Doppler envelope is proportional to the volume of blood. In severe MR, the MR jet has a similar density to the MV inflow.
    - ‒ The MR jet velocity is determined by the pressure gradient between LV and LA. In severe (usually acute) MR, the LA pressure is very high, thus the pressure difference between LV and LA will equilibrate quickly. This produces an MR jet with a sharp downslope in early systole (i.e., V-shaped) (Fig. 11-7A).
  - ○ Systolic flow reversal may be seen in the pulmonary veins and suggests severe MR (see Fig. 11-7B).
  - ○ Pulmonary pressures are invariably elevated in chronic severe MR. When following a patient with MR longitudinally, an increase in pulmonary artery pressures can be a marker that the MR has worsened.

- **Key Points:**
  1. *Qualitative methods to assess MR severity include: LV/LA dimensions, color Doppler, peak E wave velocity, density of the MR jet on CW Doppler, and pulmonary vein systolic flow reversals.*
  2. *Quantitative methods to assess MR severity include EROA, vena contracta, R Vol, and RF.*

- **Transesophageal echocardiography assessment**
  - TEE can provide important complementary information (to TTE) in the assessment of patients with acute or chronic MR.
  - Valve leaflets are better visualized to clarify which scallops are prolapsed or flail.
  - Higher-resolution images allow for more accurate assessment of PISA and vena contracta.
  - All the pulmonary veins can be interrogated for the evidence of systolic flow reversal, a marker of severe MR.
  - TEE is particularly helpful when assessing endocarditis, enabling an evaluation of the vegetation (size and mobility), leaflet damage (perforation), and extent of the infection (involvement of the fibrous continuum between the MV and AoV with abscess or fistula formation).
- **Three-dimensional (3D) echocardiography: advantages and pitfalls versus 2D echocardiography**
  - **Advantages**
    - ○ 3D echo allows for better communication between the surgeon and the echocardiographer by providing "the surgeon's view" of the MV.
    - ○ 3D echo provides excellent spatial and temporal resolution so that a very accurate assessment of the MV and dynamic changes can be recorded.

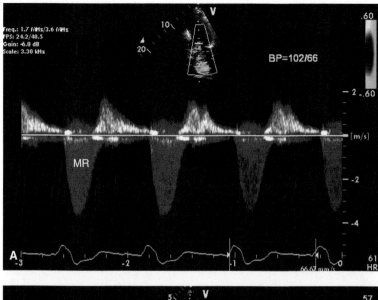

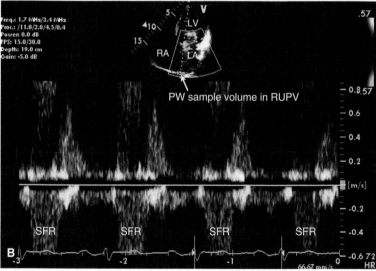

Figure 11-7. (**A**). Dense early peaking mitral regurgitation (MR) jet and (**B**) systolic flow reversal seen on pulsed-wave (PW) Doppler sampling of the right upper pulmonary vein (RUPV) suggest severe MR. LV, left ventricle; RA, right atrium.

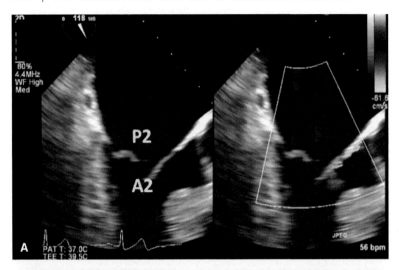

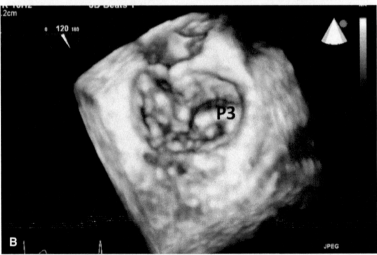

Figure 11-8. A: Two-dimensional transesophageal echocardiogram (TEE) shows flail posterior leaflet. At 120 degrees, one would assume that the P2 scallop of the posterior leaflet is flail. **B:** When three-dimensional TEE is utilized, one can clearly see that it is the P3 scallop of the mitral valve that is flail rather than the P2.

- ◦ Better characterization of lesions: As a result of the saddle shape of the mitral annulus, any distortions in the mitral anatomy can lead to misinterpretation of scallops if only 2D TEE is utilized (Fig. 11-8).
- ◦ 3D echo allows for better characterization of lesions such as mitral clefts (Fig. 11-9).

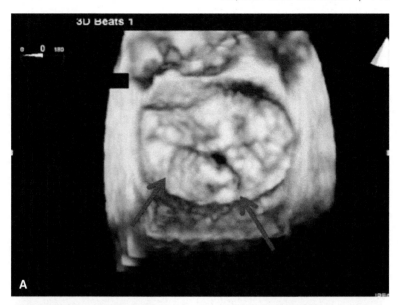

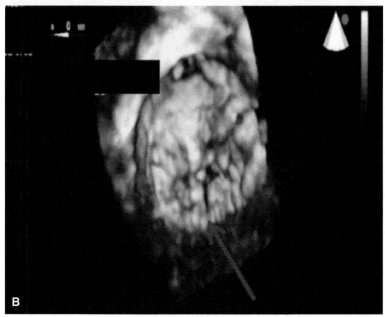

Figure 11-9. A: The mitral valve as viewed from the left atrial aspect. The *red arrows* point to indentations between the mitral scallops that extend to the annulus, which raises the suspicion for clefts. **B:** When the mitral valve is viewed from the ventricular aspect, one can clearly see the mitral clefts (*red arrows*). Two-dimensional transesophageal echocardiography cannot diagnose mitral clefts.

- **Disadvantages**
  - ○ The echocardiographer has to be familiar with image acquisition and manipulation.
  - ○ 3D echocardiography sometimes involves combining several volumes of image sectors; therefore any patient movement or irregular heart rhythm can produce what is termed "stitch artifact" (Fig. 11-10).
  - ○ 3D echocardiographic image dropout can lead to misinterpretation of lesions.

- **Key Points:**
  1. *TEE should be used to provide a more precise idea of the mitral scallops involved.*
  2. *Be aware of the advantages and disadvantages of 3D TEE when assessing the MV.*

MITRAL STENOSIS

- **Causes of MS (Table 11-2)**

Rheumatic	• Two-thirds are female • May be associated with MR • Stenotic orifice often shaped like a "fish mouth" (PSAX) (Fig. 11-11A), with doming of anterior leaflet (PLAX and apical views) (Fig. 11-12) and marked reduction in posterior leaflet motion • Can cause fibrosis, thickening, and calcification leading to fusion of the commissures, cusps, and/or chordae • Starts in the subvalvular apparatus and extends to the leaflets with increasingly severe disease, as opposed to calcific MS
Other causes	• Mitral annular calcification (i.e., calcific MS)—starts from annulus and extends to leaflets; significant calcification required to impact larger area of mitral annulus versus rheumatic MS (affects the leaflet tips) • Congenital MS • Chest radiation • MV prosthesis dysfunction • Mucopolysaccharidoses • Malignant carcinoid • SLE • Rheumatoid arthritis • Iatrogenic as a result of surgery for MR: oversewn mitral annuloplasty ring, MV clip/Alfieri stitch • "Functional MS" caused by restriction of LA outflow (MV leaflets are normal): 　– Tumor (typically atrial myxoma) 　– LA thrombus 　– Endocarditis with large vegetation 　– Cor triatriatum (congenital LA membrane)

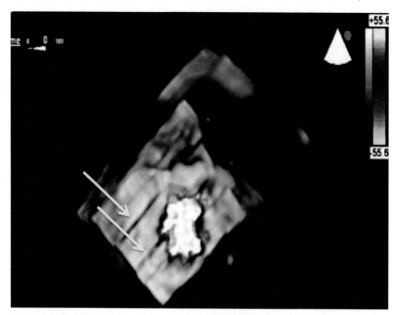

Figure 11-10. Three-dimensional color Doppler of the mitral valve showing stitch artifact (*yellow arrows*).

- Key Points:
  1. *Rheumatic MS is characterized by thickening and calcification that begins at the leaflet tips and extends into the subvalvular apparatus.*
  2. *Calcific MS primarily involves the annulus, with some relative sparing of the leaflet tips.*
  3. *Chest radiation–induced MS involves the anterior mitral leaflet to a greater extent than the posterior mitral leaflet as a result of the proximity of the anterior structures to the chest wall/radiation source.*

- **2D TTE assessment**
  - **Leaflets**
    - ○ Motion/mobility of the valve
    - ○ Thickening
    - ○ Calcification
  - **Subvalvular apparatus**
    - ○ Chordal fusion, shortening, fibrosis, and calcification
  - **MVA planimetry**
    - ○ The MV orifice is traced in the PSAX view, usually during mid-diastole.
    - ○ This can be a way to assess the severity of MS that is independent of flow, chamber compliance, and other valve lesions; however, it is also prone to error. While in the PSAX view, scanning should be done from apex to base to ensure that planimetry is being done at the leaflet tips. Sometimes, reviewing

TABLE 11-2	Stages of Mitral Stenosis			
	Stage A (at risk of MS)	Stage B (progressive MS)	Stage C (asymptomatic severe MS)	Stage D (symptomatic severe MS)
Valve anatomy	Mild MV doming during diastole	Rheumatic changes with commissural fusion; diastolic doming of the MV leaflets; MVA >1.5 cm^2	Rheumatic changes with commissural fusion; diastolic doming of the MV leaflets; MVA ≤1.5 cm^2 (MVA ≤1.0 cm^2 with very severe MS)	Rheumatic changes with commissural fusion; diastolic doming of the MV leaflets; MVA ≤1.5 cm^2
Valve hemodynamics	Normal transmitral flow velocity	Increased transmitral flow velocities; PHT <150 msec	PHT ≥150 msec; PHT ≥220 msec with very severe MS	PHT ≥150 msec; PHT ≥220 msec with very severe MS
Hemodynamic consequence	None	Mild-to-moderate LAE; normal PASP at rest	Severe LAE; PASP >30 mm Hg	Severe LAE; PASP >30 mm Hg
Symptoms	None	None	None	Decreased exercise tolerance; exertional dyspnea

LAE, left atrial enlargement; MS, mitral stenosis; MV, mitral valve; MVA, mitral valve area; PASP, pulmonary artery systolic pressure; PHT: pressure half-time.
Adapted from Nishimura RA, Otto CM, Bonow RO, et al. 2014 AHA/ACC guidelines for the management of patients with valvular heart disease. *Circulation.* 2014;129:2440–92.

the anatomy from the PLAX view can help identify the right plane in the short-axis view. 3D imaging is particularly helpful in enhancing accuracy (see Fig. 11-11B).

- **LA dimension**
  - Significant MS can lead to substantial dilation of the LA, predisposing the patient to atrial arrhythmias and thrombus formation.
- **Doppler**
- **MVA**
  - **Pressure half-time (PHT) method:** Defined as the time it takes for the pressure across the MV to decrease by one-half its original maximal value; it is measured by tracing the deceleration slope of the E wave on the CW Doppler profile through the MV:

$$MVA = 220/PHT$$

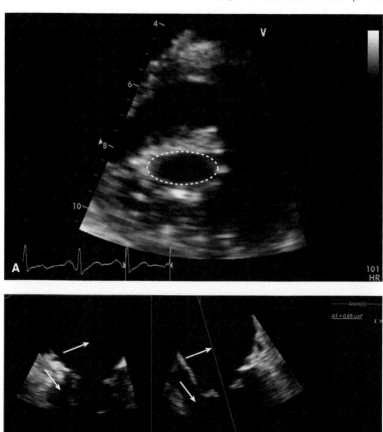

Figure 11-11. A: Two-dimensional parasternal short-axis (PSAX) view at the mitral valve (MV) leaflet tips with planimetry of the orifice in mid-diastole. **B:** Three-dimensional (3D) PSAX view for planimetry of a MV that is severely stenotic. Note the ability to easily determine the correct position of the orifice in the 3D example by manipulation of the planes in the biplanar transesophageal echocardiogram images (*arrows*).

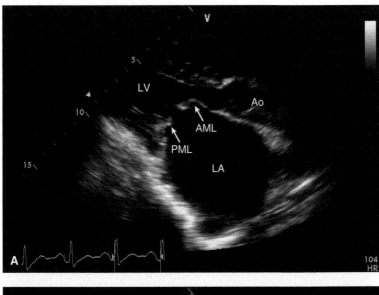

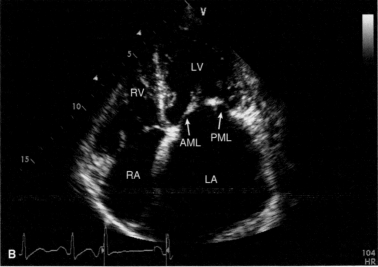

Figure 11-12. Parasternal long-axis (**A**) and apical four-chamber (**B**) views showing doming of the anterior mitral leaflet (AML) and a thickened and fixed posterior mitral leaflet (PML) consistent with rheumatic mitral valve disease (*arrows*). (**C**) M-mode shows the classic features of thickened mitral valve leaflets, "tracking" of the posterior leaflet, and reduced E-F slope. Ao, aorta; LA, left atrium; LV, left ventricle; RA, right atrium; RV, right ventricle.

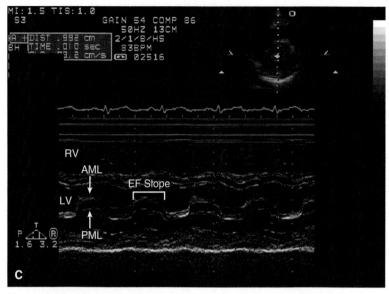

Figure 11-12. (*Continued*)

- PHT should not be used to estimate MVA in the following circumstances: Immediately postvalvuloplasty (first ~72 hours), if MV is prosthetic, in the presence of an atrial septal defect, if severe AR is present, or when LV filling pressures are very high (Fig. 11-13).
- *If the Doppler profile contains a brief steep slope and then longer less steep slope, measure the latter. The so called "ski slope" beginning is not indicative of the true gradient between LA and LV during filling.*

○ **Continuity equation method:** Analogous to measuring aortic valve area (AVA) utilizing measurements of the left ventricular outflow tract (LVOT) and AoV, this is calculated as follows:

$$MVA = \pi \times (D_{LVOT}/2)^2 \times (VTI_{LVOT}/VTI_{mitral})$$

where D_{LVOT} is the LVOT diameter (in cm), VTI_{LVOT} is measured from the PW Doppler in the LVOT, and VTI_{mitral} is measured from the CW Doppler through the MV.

- This method is not accurate in the setting of atrial fibrillation or ≥ moderate MR or AR.

○ **PISA method:** Uses a zoom view of MV with baseline of the Nyquist limit moved in the direction of mitral inflow to allow earlier aliasing of color and a larger flow convergence radius (r) to be measured.

$$MVA = (\pi r^2 \times V_{aliasing}/V_{peak\ mitral\ E}) \times \alpha/180°$$

where α = opening angle of mitral leaflets.

- This method is of limited use because of errors in accurately measuring r and α.

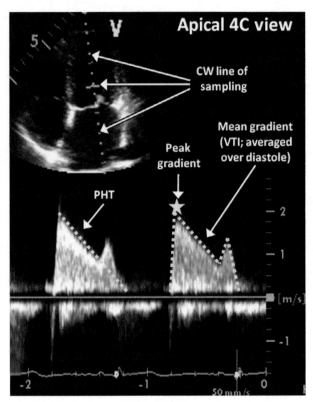

Figure 11-13. Continuous-wave (CW) Doppler of mitral inflow with pressure half-time (PHT) measured. VTI, velocity time integral.

- **Mean and peak MV gradients**
  - The CW Doppler signal is obtained through the MV in the apical window; this Doppler profile is traced for calculation of the gradient.
  - Peak gradient is calculated using peak velocity in the modified Bernoulli equation: $\Delta P = 4 \times v^2$
- Mean gradient reflects the average gradient between LA and LV during diastole; it is calculated by averaging the instantaneous gradients (tracing the CW Doppler MV envelope).
- **Mean gradient is more useful clinically;** however, it is important to realize that it is influenced by heart rate, diastolic filling time, cardiac output, and associated MR (Fig. 11-14).
  - *In reporting MV gradients, the heart rate should always be included to allow comparison between serial studies and to alert the referring physician to the influence that this may have on the diastolic filling period.*
- **Pulmonary artery pressure**
  - The estimated pulmonary artery systolic pressure and mean pulmonary artery pressure should be measured.

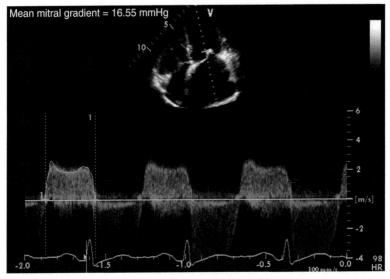

Figure 11-14. Continuous-wave Doppler of mitral inflow traced to measure the mean mitral gradient.

- **Atrial fibrillation (and other irregular rhythms)**
  - Average results over several beats (preferably 6–10) when measuring PHT and mitral gradients

---

- **Key Points:**
  1. *MVA = 220/PHT*
  2. *Always report mean gradients along with the heart rate at which the gradient is recorded.*
  3. *PHT and mean gradient can be affected by heart rate (tachycardia) or high output states.*
  4. *PSAX at the MV level can be used to determine MVA via planimetry.*

- **TEE assessment**
  - Provides a better look at the MV and subvalvular anatomy to assess candidacy for percutaneous balloon valvuloplasty
  - Assesses degree of MR before and after balloon valvuloplasty
  - Assesses for LA or left atrial appendage (LAA) thrombus
- **Percutaneous mitral balloon valvuloplasty (PMBV)**
  - PMBV is contraindicated if moderate-to-severe MR or LA thrombus is present.
  - The Wilkins score (Table 11-3) is used to assess candidacy for PMBV, and echocardiography is essential to determine if a patient has a favorable anatomy for PMBV (Wilkins score ≤8) or where PMBV should not be attempted (Wilkins score ≥12).
- **Exercise testing**
  - This can be very helpful to determine functional capacity and the hemodynamic impact of a stenotic MV in the setting of exertion.

TABLE 11-3	Wilkins Score Grading			
Grade	Mobility	Thickening	Calcification	Subvalvular thickening
1	Highly mobile valve with only leaflet tips restricted	Leaflets near normal in thickness (4–5 mm)	A single area of increased echo brightness	Minimal thickening just below the mitral leaflets
2	Leaflet mid and base portions have normal mobility	Midleaflets normal, considerable thickening of margins (5–8 mm)	Scattered areas of brightness confined to leaflet margins	Thickening of chordal structures extending to one-third of the chordal length
3	Valve continues to move forward in diastole mainly from base	Thickening extending through entire leaflet (5–8 mm)	Brightness extending into mid-portions of leaflets	Thickening extended to distal third of chords
4	No or minimal forward movement of leaflets in diastole	Considerable thickening of all leaflet tissue (>8–10 mm)	Extensive brightness throughout much of leaflet tissue	Extensive thickening and shortening of all chordal structures extending down to papillary muscles

Adapted from Baumgartner H, Hung J, Bermejo J, et al. Echocardiographic assessment of valve stenosis: EAE/ASE recommendations for clinical practice. *J Am Soc Echocardiogr.* 2009;22:1–23, with permission from Elsevier.

- Measurement of **mean MV gradient** and **pulmonary artery pressure** are the most important parts of the exercise echocardiogram for patients with MS.
  - Exercise time should be recorded.
  - When the mean mitral gradient is reported at peak exercise, the heart rate at which the mitral gradient was determined should also be reported.
- **Correlation with invasive catheterization measurements**
  - Can provide an invasive assessment of pulmonary artery pressures if they are unclear by echocardiography.
  - The mean mitral gradient is most accurately calculated with simultaneous pressure recordings in the LA (utilizing a trans-septal puncture) and the LV.
  - Pulmonary capillary wedge pressure should not be used to determine mitral gradient.

- Key Points:
  1. *Wilkins score is used to assess suitability for PMBV.*
  2. *TEE should be performed to better assess the MV prior to PMBV.*
  3. *Moderate or more MR or a LA/LAA thrombus is a contraindication to PMBV.*
  4. *In a symptomatic patient where the clinical picture and echocardiographic findings are discordant, exercise stress test can be useful.*

12 Pulmonic Valve

Tyson K. Turner, Kathryn J. Lindley, and Julio E. Pérez

HIGH-YIELD CONCEPTS

- Pulmonic stenosis (PS) is usually found in conjunction with other **congenital heart diseases**.
- PS may occur at the valvular, subvalvular, or supravalvular levels.
- Carcinoid disease is a common cause of **acquired** pulmonic valve disease and can cause both stenosis and regurgitation.
- Severe pulmonic regurgitation (PR) is most often seen in the setting of repaired congenital heart disease, such as tetralogy of Fallot.
- With severe PR, continuous-wave (CW) Doppler shows **rapid deceleration** of the PR jet. Presystolic forward flow can be seen with severe PR owing to premature opening of the pulmonic valve (PV) as a result of high right ventricular end-diastolic pressure (RVEDP).

KEY VIEWS

Transthoracic echocardiography (TTE)
- Parasternal long-axis (PLAX) and parasternal short-axis (PSAX) views tilted toward right ventricular outflow tract (RVOT)
- Subcostal view: anterior angulation

Transesophageal echocardiography (TEE)
- High esophageal view at 0–20 degrees
- Mid esophageal level at 50–90 degrees (RV inflow/outflow view)
- Deep transgastric view at 110–140 degrees

GENERAL PRINCIPLES

- The PV is a trileaflet valve similar to the aortic valve (AoV).
- The pulmonary artery (PA) and aorta (Ao) arise parallel to each other developmentally; however, the two arteries rotate so that the PA then wraps around the Ao.
- Echocardiography can usually help assess two cusps of the PV; sometimes the subcostal view can show the three PV cusps.
  - Due to the pulmonic leaflets being frequently thin and pliable, all three cusps are sometimes difficult to visualize by echocardiography.
- The PV should always be assessed in conjunction with the RVOT.
- Besides two-dimensional (2D) echocardiography, pulsed-wave (PW) and CW Doppler should also be used to assess the PV.

- Doppler interrogation of the PV is done at the PSAX view.
- Normal PV outflow tract velocity is approximately 1.0 m/sec.
- Acceleration time (AT) should be assessed. In normal individuals this is usually greater than 140 msec.

- **Key Points:**
  1. *PV should be assessed along with the RVOT.*
  2. *Normal PV outflow tract velocities are low (approximately 1.0 m/sec).*
  3. *PV AT is usually greater than or equal to 120 msec in normal individuals.*

PULMONIC VALVE STENOSIS

- PS is usually a congenital lesion that is typically quantified by echocardiography.
- Obstruction can be subvalvular, valvular, or supravalvular.
  - Valvular: dysplastic, bicuspid, or unicuspid valves; stenosis of pulmonary homograft
  - Subvalvular: narrowing of infundibulum/RVOT, which can be seen in tetralogy of Fallot or double-chambered right ventricle, congenital ventricular septal defects, severe RV hypertrophy, external compression by mass or tumor
  - Supravalvular: obstruction at the level of the main PA or its more distal branches (e.g., Noonan syndrome and Williams syndrome) (Fig. 12-1).

Etiology

Congenital heart disease (most common)	• Tetralogy of Fallot • Transposition of great arteries • Isolated valvular PS • Noonan syndrome (60% with PS) • Williams syndrome (40% with PA stenosis)
Other causes (rare)	• Carcinoid syndrome • Rheumatic heart disease • External compression by sinus of Valsalva aneurysms, aortic graft aneurysms, or large mediastinal tumors • Cardiac tumors compressing RVOT

2D Echocardiography

- Thickening and doming of the PV usually seen
- RV hypertrophy (normal RV free wall thickness is <5 mm at end-diastole) with markedly increased trabeculations of the RV walls (Fig. 12-2A)
- With severe PS, see septal flattening and RV enlargement (see Fig. 12-2B,C)
- Poststenotic dilation of PA

M-mode

- Exaggerated "a" wave amplitude (>6 mm) of PV during diastole
  - With atrial contraction, elevated RVOT pressure is transmitted to the PV.

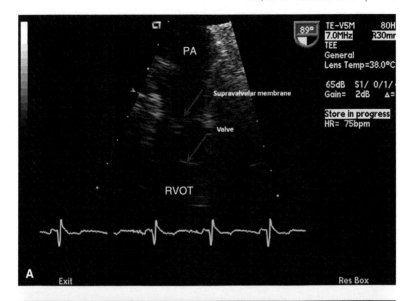

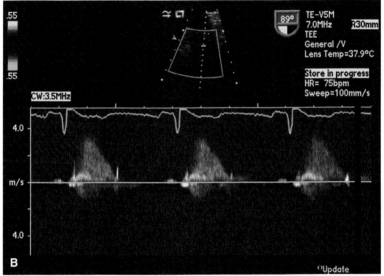

Figure 12-1. A: Patient with supravalvular stenosis with zoomed transesophageal echocardiogram image demonstrating location of supravalvular membrane compared to the valve leaflets. **B:** Continuous-wave Doppler showing elevated gradient. PA, pulmonary artery; RVOT, right ventricular outflow tract.

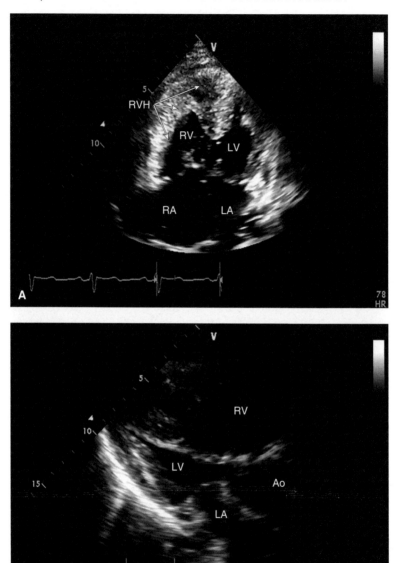

Figure 12-2. A: Apical four-chamber view from patient with atrioventricular canal defect showing massive right ventricular hypertrophy (RVH) (*arrows*). **B, C:** Parasternal long-axis and short-axis (PSAX) views, respectively, from patient with severe primary pulmonary hypertension showing marked RV dilation and remodeling. Note in PSAX how ventricles have "swapped" shapes (i.e., small crescent-like, "D-shaped" left ventricle (LV), and thickened, spherical RV. These changes reflect marked elevation in right heart pressures. Ao, aorta; LA, left atrium; RA, right atrium.

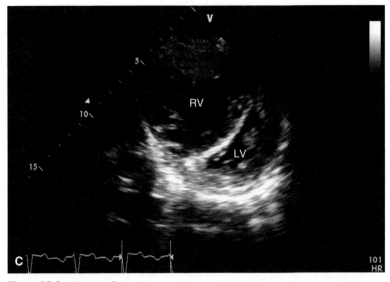

Figure 12-2. (*Continued*)

- This results in accentuated presystolic opening of the PV.
- M-mode of the PV only indicates presence of PS, but does not provide quantitative information.

Color Doppler
- Useful in determining direction and location of stenotic jet for alignment of PW and CW Doppler
- Turbulent flow may be noted

PW and CW Doppler
- Normally the systolic gradient across the PV is low.
    - *Dynamic infundibular stenosis can often be distinguished from valvular stenosis as in the former scenario, the jet tends to be "dagger shaped" and late peaking in systole, indicating dynamic obstruction, whereas in valvular stenosis the jet peaks earlier in systole and does not change with hemodynamic maneuvers.*
- Calculate peak transvalvular gradient via the modified Bernoulli equation: $\Delta P = 4v^2$ using CW Doppler. The best images are usually obtained in PSAX view with the Doppler sampling parallel to flow (Fig. 12-3).
- In cases of PS, PW Doppler should be used to determine the anatomic level of the obstruction.
- PA systolic pressure = (RV systolic pressure – peak systolic pressure gradient across PV) + right atrial pressure (RAP).
- See Table 12-1 for classification of PS.

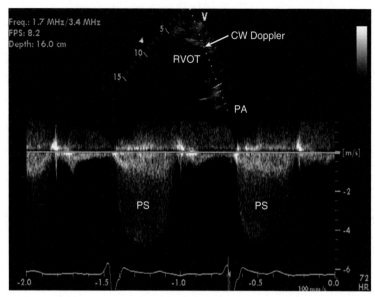

Figure 12-3. Continuous-wave (CW) Doppler showing severe pulmonic stenosis (PS) with peak gradient >4 m/sec. PA, pulmonary artery; RVOT, right ventricular outflow tract.

• Key Points:

1. *2D echocardiography usually demonstrates thickening and doming of the PV if PS is present.*

2. *M-mode may demonstrate presystolic "a" wave accentuation.*

3. *Peak pressure is determined by CW Doppler using the modified Bernoulli equation.*

PULMONIC REGURGITATION

PR is usually an incidental finding. Trace-to-mild PR, usually detected by color Doppler, is found in nearly all individuals and is usually not a pathologic finding. The next section lists some of the pathologic causes of PR. Table 12-2 lists the echocardiographic evaluation of PR.

TABLE 12-1	Parameters for Determining Severity of Pulmonic Stenosis	
	Peak gradient	**Peak velocity**
Mild PS	<36 mm Hg	<3 m/sec
Moderate PS	36–64 mm Hg	3–4 m/sec
Severe PS	>64 mm Hg	>4 m/sec

PS, pulmonic stenosis.
From Baumgartner H, Hung J, Bermejo J, et al. Echocardiographic assessment of valve stenosis: EAE/ASE recommendations for clinical practice. *J Am Soc Echocardiogr.* 2009;22:19–20, with permission from Elsevier.

TABLE 12-2	Echocardiographic Assessment of Pulmonary Regurgitation		
Parameter	**Mild**	**Moderate**	**Severe**
Pulmonic valve	Normal	May be abnormal	Abnormal
RV size	Normal	Can be dilated	Dilated
Jet size by color Doppler	Narrow origin	Intermediate	Usually large with a wide origin
Jet density and deceleration time by CW	Soft and slow deceleration	Dense, variable deceleration	Dense, steep deceleration, early termination of diastolic flow
Pulmonic systolic flow compared to systemic flow by PW	Slightly increased	Intermediate	Greatly increased

CW, continuous wave; PW, pulsed wave; RV, right ventricle.
From Zoghbi WA, Enriquez-Sarano M, Foster E, et al. Recommendations for evaluation of the severity of native valvular regurgitation with two dimensional and Doppler echocardiography. *J Am Soc Echocardiogr.* 2003;16:777–802.

Etiology

Adult congenital heart disease	• Tetralogy of Fallot (especially with a history of transannular patch repair) • Congenital absence or redundancy of PV • Pulmonary autograft following Ross procedure • Truncus arteriosus (conduit valve regurgitation)
Other causes	• PA dilation from pulmonary hypertension • Infective endocarditis (rare) • Carcinoid heart disease (usually occurs when liver metastases present and with tricuspid valve involvement) • Medications (methysergide, pergolide, fenfluramine) • Rheumatic disease • Trauma (e.g., from Swan–Ganz catheter or balloon valvuloplasty)

2D Echocardiography

- RV enlargement suggestive of RV volume overload
- Enlarged RVOT, main PA
- PV leaflet malcoaptation
- PV vegetations in endocarditis
- Diastolic flattening of the interventricular septum
- RV systolic dysfunction (late finding).

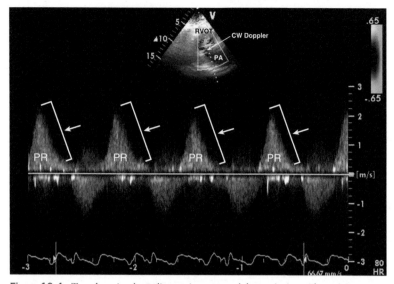

Figure 12-4. Transthoracic echocardiogram in parasternal short-axis view with continuous-wave (CW) Doppler of pulmonic valve showing dense diastolic jet with short deceleration time (*arrows*), suggestive of severe pulmonic regurgitation (PR). PA, pulmonary artery; RVOT, right ventricular outflow tract.

M-mode

- RV enlargement (most often seen with chronic PR)
- Diastolic septal flattening suggesting RV volume overload (not specific sign for PR)

CW and PW Doppler

- Determine PA end-diastolic pressure using end-diastolic flow velocity of the pulmonic regurgitant jet: $\Delta P = 4v^2 + RA$ pressure
- Mean PA pressure can then be calculated if PA systolic pressure is known using the formula:

$$PA_{mean} = (PA_{systolic} + 2PA_{diastolic})/3$$

- There are no specific quantifiable guidelines used in the assessment of PR.
- **Dense** jet with **steep deceleration** and **early termination of diastolic flow** suggests severe PR (Fig. 12-4).
  - The deceleration time can be shortened if the RVEDP is elevated in the absence of severe PR.
  - Rapid equalization of RV and PA pressures can result in a "to and from" signal (sine wave pattern).
- Presystolic forward flow across the PV suggests elevated RVEDP (Fig. 12-5).

Color Doppler

- Color Doppler can be misleading and can underestimate severity when there is wide open PR present.

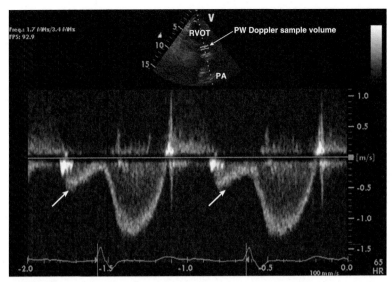

Figure 12-5. Transthoracic echocardiogram in parasternal short-axis view with pulsed-wave (PW) Doppler of right ventricular outflow tract (RVOT) showing presystolic forward flow (*arrows*) resulting from premature equalization of RV and pulmonary artery (PA) pressures in diastole. This can be seen in severe pulmonic regurgitation with premature opening of the pulmonic valve.

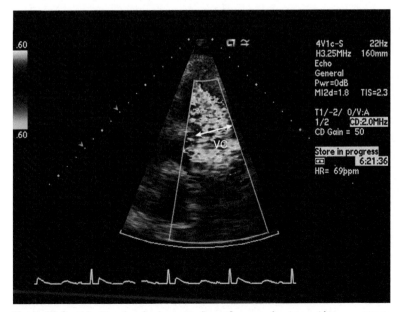

Figure 12-6. Color Doppler of right ventricular outflow tract showing a wide vena contracta (VC) associated with severe pulmonic regurgitation.

- Because the pulmonary system is a relatively low pressure system, occasionally color Doppler will not demonstrate a distinct zone of flow convergence.
  - CW can be used to identify the distinct to and fro flow.
- Diastolic regurgitant jet is directed toward the RV, beginning at the line of leaflet coaptation.
- The width of the jet is narrow in mild PR and arises at the valve commissure with a narrow vena contracta.
- As the PR gets worse, the **width of the jet increases** and can fill the RVOT (Fig. 12-6).

- **Key Points:**
  1. *Look for RV enlargement and eventual dysfunction as a sequalae of severe PR.*
  2. *The PR jet can be used to assess PA end-diastolic pressure.*
  3. *A dense PR signal with a steep deceleration may be suggestive of significant PR.*
  4. *Severe PR may result in a "to and from" signal on CW Doppler as a result of rapid equalization of RV and PA pressures.*

13

Tricuspid Valve Disorders

Nishtha Sodhi and Julio E. Pérez

HIGH-YIELD CONCEPTS

Severe tricuspid regurgitation (TR)
- Vena contracta width > 0.7 cm
- Right atrial (RA) area occupied by TR jet >10 cm^2
- Gross leaflet malcoaptation
- Tricuspid valve (TV) annulus dilation ≥4 cm
- Dense, early peaking TR continuous-wave (CW) Doppler envelope
- Hepatic vein systolic flow reversal
- RA/right ventricular (RV) enlargement
- Evidence of RV volume overload

Severe tricuspid stenosis (TS)
- Leaflets thickened, calcified, fused, immobile
- Diastolic leaflet doming
- RA enlargement
- Dilated inferior vena cava (IVC)
- Mean TV gradient ≥5 mm Hg
- Pressure half-time (PHT) ≥190 msec

KEY VIEWS

- Parasternal RV inflow tract
- Parasternal short-axis (PSAX) RV inflow/outflow
- Apical four-chamber (A4C)
- Subcostal four-chamber

GENERAL PRINCIPLES

- The TV consists of three anatomically distinct and asymmetric leaflets (anterior, inferior/posterior, and septal) that vary in shape between triangular and semicircular.
- These leaflets are thinner and the TV annulus is larger than the mitral valve (MV) annulus.
- The TV is more anterior and rightward than the MV. It is also more apically displaced in location compared to the MV and is not in direct continuity with the pulmonic valve (PV) owing to the presence of the infundibulum.
  - *The atrioventricular (AV) valves are always associated with their respective ventricle.*
  - *In patients with congenital heart disease where the ventricular position may be altered, the more apically displaced TV helps in recognition of the RV.*

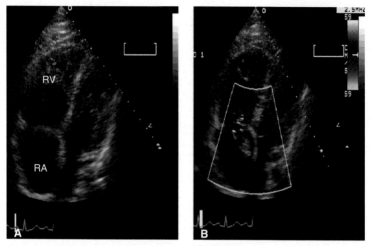

Figure 13-1. A: Right atrium (RA) and right ventricle (RV) enlargement along with tricuspid annular dilation. **B:** Tricuspid regurgitation associated with a dilated tricuspid annulus.

- *The AV valves being on the same plane suggests an AV canal defect.*
- *Ebstein anomaly is recognized by the septal tricuspid leaflet being markedly apically displaced.*
- In contrast to the right-sided AV valves, the left-sided AV valves are separated only by a fibrous continuum, allowing for pathology such as endocarditis to easily spread to either valve, potentially causing annular or root abscesses.
- **Primary valvular causes** of TV disease include Ebstein anomaly, carcinoid tumors, endocarditis, myxomatous degeneration, and rheumatic disease.
- **Secondary causes** include any process that leads to tricuspid annulus dilation as a result of RV and/or RA enlargement (Fig. 13-1) (e.g., **pulmonary hypertension,** left ventricular (LV) dysfunction, left-to-right shunts, RV infarction).
- TS is rare and almost always associated with rheumatic heart disease. It is extremely rare to find in isolation (i.e., in the absence of MV or aortic valve disease).
  - Less common causes: congenital abnormalities, endocarditis, carcinoid disease, and large RA masses that may mimic TS.

- **Key Points:**
  1. *TV consists of three leaflets.*
  2. *TV is more apically displaced compared to the MV unless the patient has an AV canal defect.*
  3. *Be familiar with the primary and secondary causes of TV disease.*

TWO-DIMENSIONAL ASSESSMENT

TV Leaflets and Chordae

- Tricuspid leaflet **location, thickness, mobility, and coaptation** should be assessed in all available views.
  - The RV inflow is the one view where the **posterior leaflet** is seen along with the anterior leaflet (Fig. 13-2A); the anterior and septal leaflets are seen in the A4C view.

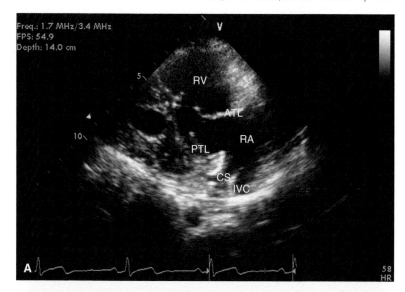

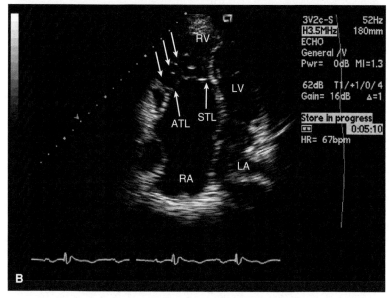

Figure 13-2. A: Right ventricular (RV) inflow view showing posterior tricuspid leaflet (PTL) and anterior tricuspid leaflet (ATL) in patient without tricuspid valve disease. **B:** Apical four-chamber view showing apically displaced septal tricuspid leaflet (STL) and long, "sail"-like ATL tethered to the RV free wall (*arrows*), in patient with Ebstein anomaly. CS, coronary sinus; IVC, inferior vena cava; LA, left atrium; LV, left ventricle.

- With Ebstein anomaly, there is (a) apical displacement (>0.8 cm/m^2) of the septal leaflet, (b) a large, "sail-like" anterior leaflet with a variable number of tethering attachments to the anterior RV free wall, and (c) atrialization of the RV secondary to apically displaced TV coaptation (see Fig. 13-2B).
- Rheumatic disease of the TV produces thickened chordae progressing to leaflet tip thickening/fusion and restricted movement. **It is rarely seen in the absence of MV involvement.**
  - Leaflet thickening, fusion of the commissures, and retraction and thickening of the subvalvular apparatus are features of rheumatic heart disease.
  - Diastolic "doming" of the leaflets is characteristic of rheumatic TS (Fig. 13-3).
- Carcinoid tumors cause a serotonin-induced fibrosis that results in short, thickened, and restricted tricuspid leaflets that are **"club"**-like in appearance and fixed in an open position (Fig. 13-4).
  - *The serotonin-like substance is deactivated in the pulmonary circulation; therefore, right-sided valves are only typically affected.*
  - *However, left-sided valves may also be involved in the presence of an interatrial shunt with right-to-left flow.*
- Flail leaflets can be seen in the setting of endocarditis, repeated endomyocardial biopsies (e.g., heart transplant patients; Fig. 13-5), myxomatous degeneration, and blunt chest trauma.

Chamber Dimensions and Ventricular Function

- RA and RV enlargement are common in severe TR.
- TV annulus dilation ≥4 cm is often seen in severe TR unless it is acute.

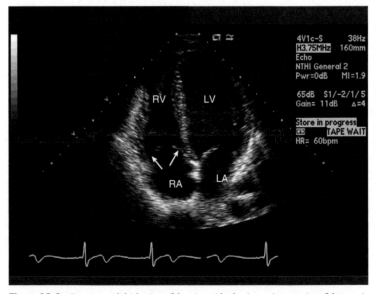

Figure 13-3. Doming and thickening of the tricuspid valve (*arrows*) suggestive of rheumatic tricuspid stenosis. LA, left atrium; LV, left ventricle; RA, right atrium; RV, right ventricle.

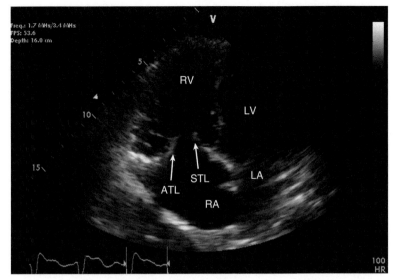

Figure 13-4. Apical four-chamber, "right ventricle (RV)-focused" view showing thickened, "club-like" septal tricuspid leaflet (STL) and anterior tricuspid leaflet (ATL) fixed in an open position (*arrows*). This appearance is suggestive of carcinoid disease. LA, left atrium; LV, left ventricle; RA, right atrium.

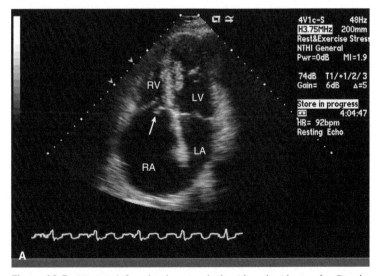

Figure 13-5. (**A**) Apical four-chamber view both with and without color Doppler acquired from cardiac transplant patient (biatrial elongation because of atrial anastomoses). A flail septal leaflet of the tricuspid valve (*arrow*) is seen with consequential severe eccentric tricuspid regurgitation (TR) (*continued*)

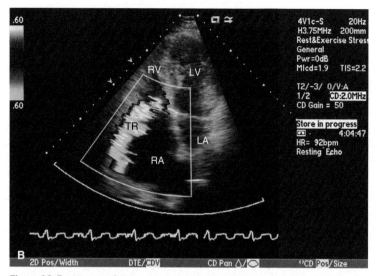

Figure 13-5. (*Continued*) (**B**) as a complication of cardiac biopsy. Typical of a flail leaflet, the jet is directed to the opposite side from the affected leaflet. LA, left atrium; LV, left ventricle; RA, right atrium; RV, right ventricle.

- RV systolic function can be compromised in the setting of pulmonary hypertension, LV failure, and RV infarction.

Interventricular Septum

- **Diastolic flattening** of the interventricular septum is seen in RV *volume* overload.
- RV *pressure* and volume overload may eventually develop, causing a "D-shaped" LV resulting from flattening of the septum in both systole and diastole.

IVC

- Dilation (>2.1 cm) with no respiratory collapse may be seen in severe TR and TS.

Intracardiac Catheters or Pacemaker/Defibrillator Leads

- Look for vegetations or thrombus.
- The leads can also interfere with TV coaptation leading to TR.

- **Key Points:**
  1. *Tricuspid leaflet location, thickness, mobility, and coaptation should be assessed in all available views.*
  2. *RA and RV enlargement are common in severe TR.*
  3. *RV pressure and volume overload may eventually develop, causing a "D-shaped" LV resulting from flattening of the septum in both systole and diastole.*
  4. *Dilation (>2.1 cm) with no respiratory collapse may be seen in severe TR.*

TRICUSPID VALVE REGURGITATION

See Tables 13-1 and 13-2.

TABLE 13-1	Tricuspid Valve Regurgitation Evaluation		
Stages of TR	Valve anatomy	Valve hemodynamics	Hemodynamic consequences
A	**Primary:** Mild rheumatic change, mild prolapse, vegetation, early carcinoid deposition, early radiation changes, RV pacemaker or ICD lead or status post endomyocardial biopsy **Functional:** Normal anatomy or early annular dilation	No or trace TR	None
B	**Primary:** Progressive leaflet destruction, moderate-to-severe prolapse, limited chordal rupture **Functional:** Early annular dilation, moderate leaflet tethering	**Mild TR** • Central jet area <5.0 cm^2 • Vena contracta width not defined • CW jet density and contour: soft and parabolic • Hepatic vein flow: systolic dominance **Moderate TR** • Central jet area 5–10 cm^2 • Vena contracta width not defined but <0.70 cm • CW jet density and contour: dense, variable contour • Hepatic vein flow: systolic blunting	**Mild TR** • RV/RA/IVC size normal **Moderate TR** • No RV enlargement • No or mild RA enlargement • No or mild IVC enlargement with normal respirophasic variation • Normal RA pressure
C	**Primary:** Flail or grossly distorted leaflet **Functional:** Severe annular dilation (>40 mm or 21 mm/m^2), marked leaflet tethering	• Central jet area >10.0 cm^2 • Vena contracta width > 0.7 cm • CW jet density and contour: dense, triangular with early peak • Hepatic vein flow: systolic reversal	• RV/RA/IVC dilated with decreased IVC respirophasic variation • Elevated RA pressure with "c-v" wave • Diastolic interventricular septal flattening may be present

(continued)

TABLE 13-1	Tricuspid Valve Regurgitation Evaluation (*Continued*)		
Stages of TR	Valve anatomy	Valve hemodynamics	Hemodynamic consequences
D	**Primary:** Flail or grossly distorted leaflets **Functional:** Severe annular dilation (>40 mm or >21 mm/m^2), marked leaflet tethering	• Central jet area >10.0 cm • Vena contracta width >0.70 cm • CW jet density and contour: dense, triangular with early peak • Hepatic vein flow: systolic reversal	• RV/RA/IVC dilated with decreased IVC respirophasic variation • Elevated RA pressure with "c-v" wave • Diastolic interventricular septal flattening • Reduced RV systolic function in late phase

CW, continuous wave; ICD, implantable cardiac defibrillator; IVC, inferior vena cava; RA, right atrium; RV, right ventricle; TR, tricuspid regurgitation.
From Nishimura RA, Otto CM, Bonow RO, et al. 2014 AHA/ACC guideline for the management of patients with valvular heart disease. *J Am Coll Cardiol.* 2014;63:e57–e185.

Color Doppler

• Severe TR: Regurgitant jet area >10 cm^2 and vena contracta width >0.7 cm (Fig. 13-6A)
• **Proximal isovelocity surface area (PISA) method** (not commonly used)
  • Severe TR: PISA radius >0.9 cm for a Nyquist limit of 28 cm/sec.

TABLE 13-2	Classification of Tricuspid Stenosis		
Stages of TS	Valve anatomy	Valve hemodynamics	Hemodynamics consequences
C, D	Thickened, distorted calcified valves with fusion of the commissures and retraction and thickening of the subvalvular apparatus	Reduced E-F slope Elevated TV inflow velocity >1 m/sec Mean TV gradient: moderate 2 to 5 mm Hg Severe ≥5 mm Hg Pressure half-time ≥190 msec Valve area ≤1 cm^2	RA enlargement and IVC dilation

IVC, inferior vena cava; RA, right atrium; TS, tricuspid stenosis; TV, tricuspid valve.
From Nishimura RA, Otto CM, Bonow RO, et al. 2014 AHA/ACC guideline for the management of patients with valvular heart disease. *J Am Coll Cardiol.* 2014;63:e57–e185.

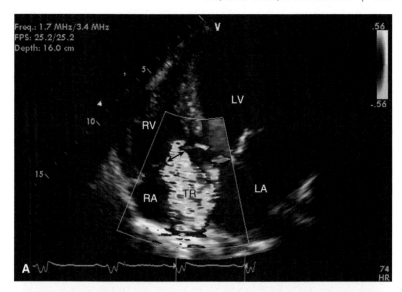

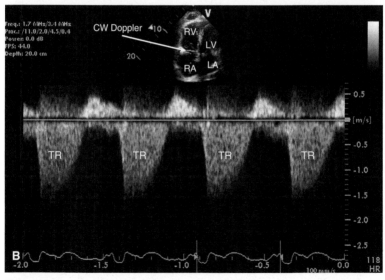

Figure 13-6. A: Apical four-chamber view with severe tricuspid regurgitation (TR) seen on color Doppler with wide vena contracta (*arrow*) and jet filling a large portion of the right atrium (RA). **B:** Spectral Doppler of TR showing early peaking, low velocity, dense Doppler envelope. LA, left atrium; LV, left ventricle; RV, right ventricle.

Pulse and CW Doppler

- Density of the CW TR envelope correlates with TR severity.
  - Severe TR is when the TR envelope is as **dense** as TV inflow and is **early peaking** because of rapid equilibration of pressures between RA and RV (see Fig. 13-6B).
  - The antegrade and retrograde CW signals across the valve may almost be mirror images of each other.
- Pulsed-wave (PW) Doppler of early diastolic tricuspid E velocity >1.0 m/sec.
- PW of the hepatic veins (subcostal view)
  - Normal or mild TR: systolic predominance
  - Moderate TR: systolic blunting
  - Severe TR: **systolic flow reversal**
  - **However, other conditions can cause systolic blunting (i.e., atrial fibrillation, elevated right atrial pressure [RAP]).**
- **Estimated pulmonary artery systolic pressure (PASP)**
  - CW Doppler of TR (modified Bernoulli equation):

$$4v^2 + \text{mean RAP}$$

- **Key Points:**
  1. *Severe TR: Regurgitant jet area >10 cm² and vena contracta width >0.7 cm.*
  2. *Severe TR envelope on CW appears as a dense, early peaking signal.*
  3. *Severe TR is associated with systolic flow reversals in hepatic veins.*
  4. *Other causes of systolic blunting in hepatic veins include atrial fibrillation and elevated RA pressure.*

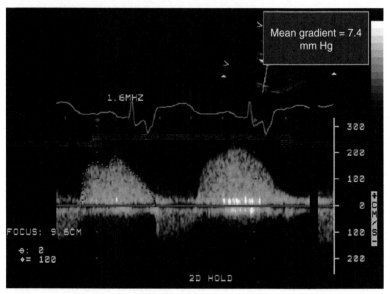

Figure 13-7. Tricuspid stenosis with dense, flat inflow profile on spectral Doppler. Mean gradient is markedly elevated (~7.4 mm Hg).

TRICUSPID STENOSIS

M-mode

- **Reduced E-F slope** reflects the restricted leaflet motion in TS.

Doppler

- Tricuspid inflow velocity should be recorded from a PSAX, RV inflow, or A4C view.
- Since tricuspid flow varies by inspiration, a few cardiac cycles should be recorded and averaged for measurement, or measurements should be done at end expiration.
- In atrial fibrillation, five cardiac cycles should be averaged.
- Elevated TV inflow velocity >1 m/sec, occasionally approaching 2 m/sec with inspiration (Fig. 13-7)
- Inflow time-velocity integral >60 cm
- **Mean TV gradient:** severe TS ≥5 mm Hg
- **PHT ≥190 msec** consistent with severe TS
- A valve area ≤1 cm^2 is indicative of severe TS.
  - However, the valve area can be underestimated when significant TR is present.

14 Evaluation of Prosthetic Valves

Jose A. Madrazo

HIGH-YIELD CONCEPTS

- Whenever possible, know the type, size, and age of the prosthesis being evaluated.
- Serial echocardiographic evaluation of prosthetic valves should be referenced to a **baseline study** performed early after implantation.
- High gradients across a valve may be due to:
  - Valve dysfunction/obstruction
  - Increased flow:
    - Regurgitation
    - High output states
  - Patient–prosthesis mismatch (PPM)
- The ultrasound beam cannot penetrate the dense material of prosthetic valves. **Multiple views** are required to allow the beam to interrogate chambers without interference from prosthesis-related artifact. **In patients with multiple prosthetic valves, transesphogeal echocardiography (TEE) is often necessary** if clinical suspicion of prosthetic valve dysfunction is high.

KEY POINTS

- The following should raise concern for **severe** prosthesis malfunction:
  - Prosthetic **aortic** valve (AoV):
    - Stenosis
      - Peak velocity >3.0 m/sec
      - Left ventricular outflow tract (LVOT)/ AoV velocity or velocity time integral (VTI) ratio <0.25
      - Aortic acceleration time (AT) >100 msec (rounded velocity contour)
    - Regurgitation
      - Dense regurgitant jet with pressure half-time (PHT) <200 msec
      - Jet width ≥65% of the LVOT
      - Regurgitant volume (R Vol) >60 mL/beat; regurgitant fraction (RF) >50%
      - Prominent holodiastolic flow reversal in the descending aorta
      - Leak involving >20% of the sewing ring or evidence of dehisence
  - Prosthetic **mitral** valve (MV):
    - Stenosis
      - Peak velocity ≥2.5 m/sec
      - Mean gradient >10 mm Hg
      - MV inflow PHT >200 msec

- o Regurgitation
  - Dense early, peaking continuous-wave (CW) Doppler jet (triangular)
  - Preserved left ventricular ejection fraction (LVEF) with reduced LVOT stroke volume (SV)
  - Effective regurgitant orifice area (EROA) ≥0.5 cm^2
  - Regurgitant jet of ≥8 cm^2 area
  - Perivalvular leak vena contracta (VC) ≥0.6 cm
  - R Vol ≥60 mL/beat; RF >50%
  - Pulmonary vein systolic flow reversal in one or more veins
  - MV/LVOT VTI ratio >2.5
- Prosthetic pulmonary valve (PV)
  - o Stenosis
    - Cusp or leaflet thickening/immobility
    - Peak prosthetic velocity >3 m/sec
    - Peak velocity through homograft >2 m/sec
    - Increase in peak velocity on serial studies
    - Impaired RV function or elevetad right ventricular systolic pressure (RVSP)
  - o Regurgitation
    - Evidence of RV volume overload
    - Jet >50% of annulus
    - Dense and steep deceleration on CW
    - To and fro CW pattern
    - RF >50%
    - Diastolic flow reversal in the pulmonary artery (PA)
- Prosthetic tricuspid valve (TV)
  - o Stenosis
    - Peak velocity >1.7 m/sec
    - Mean gradient ≥6 mm Hg
    - PHT ≥230 msec
  - o Regurgitation
    - Valve dehiscence
    - Jet area >10 cm^2
    - VC >0.7 cm
    - Dense early peaking CW jet contour
    - Holosystolic reversals in hepatic vein
    - Dilated inferior vena cava (IVC)

GENERAL PRINCIPLES

- The echocardiographic evaluation of prosthetic valves is a challenging task as there are many different types of prostheses and they frequently impart imaging artifacts and shadowing (Fig. 14-1).
- Understanding the types of valves available helps determine the expected appearance, gradients, and physiologic regurgitation.
- Valves are generally divided into bioprosthetic and mechanical.
  - Bioprosthetic valves may be stented, stentless, homografts, or xenografts.
  - Mechanical valves may be ball-cage or tilting disk (single or double).

Diastole   Systole

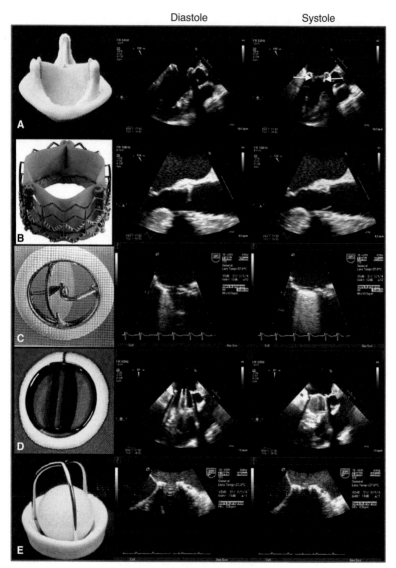

Figure 14-1. Transesophageal echocardiography (TEE) images of prosthetic valve types and TEE images during diastole and systole. **A:** Bioprosthesis in the mitral position. Note the prominent struts (*arrows*). **B:** Edwards SAPIEN transcathether aortic valve. (From Baim DS. *Grossman's Cardiac Catheterization, Angiography, and Intervention.* 7th ed. Philadelphia, PA: Lippincott Williams & Wilkins; 2006.) **C:** Single tilting disk valve. (From Weyman AE. *Principles and Practice of Echocardiography.* 2nd ed. Philadelphia, PA: Lea & Febiger; 1994.) **D:** Bileaflet tilting disk valve. **E:** Ball and cage valve.

ECHOCARDIOGRAPHIC EVALUATION

General Evaluation

- Start evaluation by identifying the valve and confirming the expected appearance.
- Look for **stability** of the valve and ring.
  - Excessive movement of the entire prosthesis ("**rocking**") suggests dehiscence.
- Evaluate leaflet/disk motion when they are visible.
  - Pay attention to the presence of calcifications, thrombi, or vegetations.
- Prosthetic valves will cause shadowing distal to the ultrasound beam and make those areas difficult to inspect visually. Standard and off-axis views should be selected to **interrogate areas of interest first and then the prosthesis to minimize shadowing** (e.g., for evaluating mitral regurgitation [MR] for a mitral prosthesis, the pasternal long-axis [PLAX] and subcostal images can visualize the left atrium [LA] without significant artifact compared to the apical four-chamber [A4C] view).
  - TEE is often necessary when clinical suspicion of prosthetic valve dysfunction is high, especially when multiple prostheses are present (Fig. 14-2).
- In addition to TEE, traditional fluoroscopy or gated computed tomography (CT) scanning can be used to assess leaflet opening and closure angles with mechanical disk valves.
  - Pannus (exuberant scar formation) or thrombus may impair valve disk motion and lead to pathologic obstruction and regurgitation.

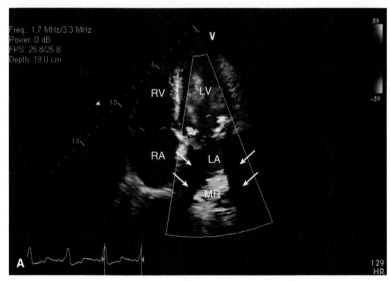

Figure 14-2. Severe perivalvular mitral regurgitation (MR) can be missed. Ultrasound beam attenuation artifact (*arrows*) allows only distal segments of the MR jet to be visualized in these apical four-chamber (**A**) and apical long-axis (**B**) images. The MR jet reaches to the back of the left atrium (LA) with pulmonary vein systolic flow reversal (SFR) (**C**), elevated mean mitral gradient (**D**), and an mitral valve (MV) velocity time integral (VTI) that is close to 2.5 times the measured left ventricular outflow tract (LVOT) VTI (**E**), which is consistent with severe MR. Ao, aorta; CW, continuous wave; LVOT, left ventricular outflow tract; PUL, pulmonary; PW, pulsed wave; RA, right atrium; RUPV, right upper pulmonary vein; RV, right ventricle. (*continued*)

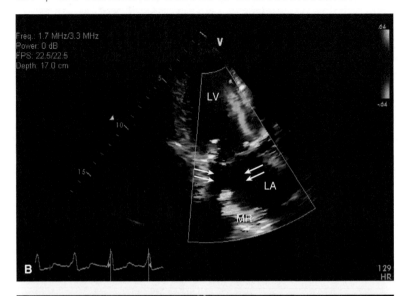

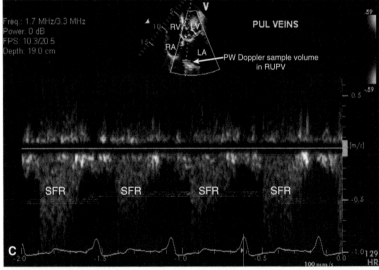

Figure 14-2. (*Continued*)

Regurgitation

- Most mechanical valves will have some built in **"physiologic" regurgitation** (Fig. 14-3). Knowing the type of valve will help determine the expected pattern of regurgitation. Some common examples:
  - Bileaflet tilting disk valves will have two small lateral (and one small central for St. Jude's) jets of regurgitation that are angled inward.

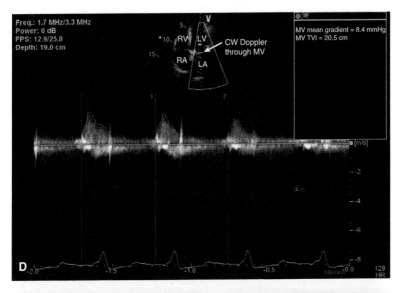

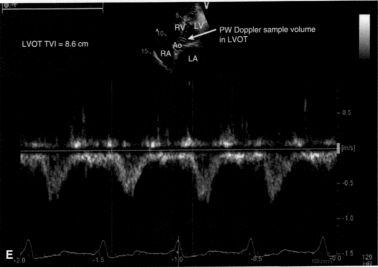

Figure 14-2. (*Continued*)

- Single tilting disk valves will have a central area of regurgitation around the hinge-point (that is larger than what is seen in bileaflet valves).
- Perivalvular leak (typically unilateral, eccentric, turbulent jet) is in contrast **pathologic** (Fig. 14-4) and occurs most often when extensive calcium debridement is required prior to valve implantation (newer percutaneously inserted valves will not uncommonly have a small perivalvular regurgitant jet).
  - *In general, "physiologic" regurgitation **are low velocity jets and not turbulent.***

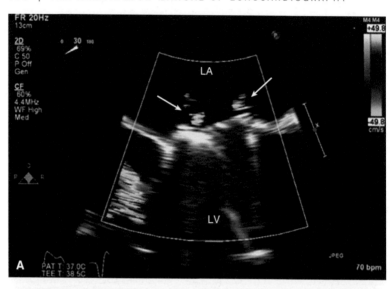

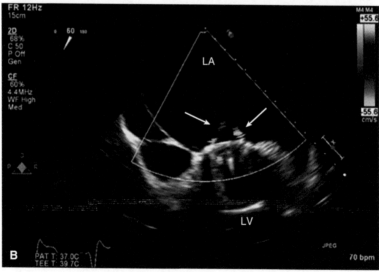

Figure 14-3. Transesophageal echocardiography images of normal "physiologic" regurgitation. **A,B:** Small peripheral regurgitant jets in bileaflet tilting disk valve (*arrows*).

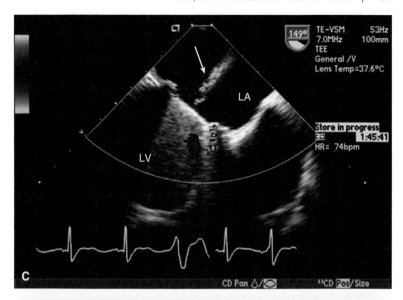

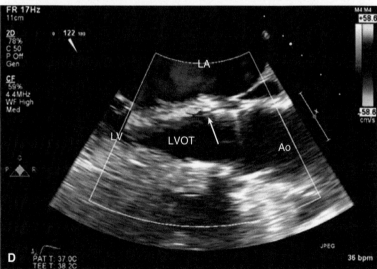

Figure 14-3. (*Continued*) **C:** Larger central jet in single tilting disk valve (*arrow*). **D:** Perivalvular regurgitation in Edwards SAPIEN percutaneously implanted valve (*arrow*). Ao, aorta; LA, left atrium; LV, left ventricle; LVOT, left ventricular outflow tract.

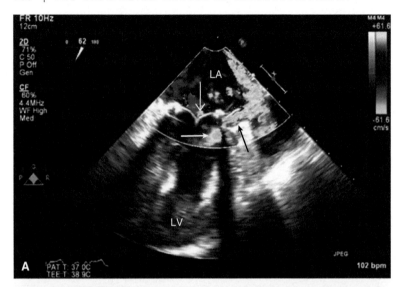

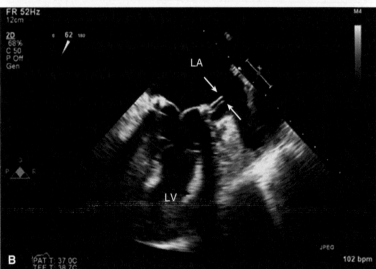

Figure 14-4. Pathologic perivalvular regurgitation. **A:** Transesophageal echocardiography images at 60 degrees of a bioprosthetic valve in the mitral position demonstrating severe peri-alvular regurgitation (*black arrow*) and mild "physiologic" central regurgitation (*open white arrow*). Note the area of flow convergence (proximal isovelocity surface area) on the ventricular side (*solid white arrow*). **B:** Suture dehiscence clearly seen (*white arrows*). LA, left atrium; LV, left ventricle.

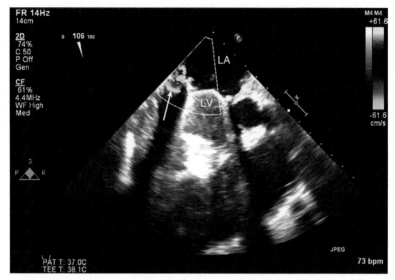

Figure 14-5. Severe perivalvular mitral regurgitation. Transesophageal echocardiography view showing an area of flow convergence with aliasing on the ventricular surface (*arrow*) of a bileaflet tilting disk valve in the mitral position in a patient with severe regurgitation. LA, left atrium; LV, left ventricle.

Color Doppler

- Look for flow pattern and velocity during the open phase of the valve.
  - Flow convergence with aliasing may be the first clue that the valve is stenosed or there is increased flow through it.
- Assess for regurgitation during the closed phase of the valve. Pay attention to the origin and direction of regurgitant leaks if present.
  - An area of flow convergence on the opposite surface of the valve (e.g., LV surface of MV prosthesis) is always abnormal and may be the only clear sign of perivalvular leak (Fig. 14-5).

High Gradients

- It is important to know the type of valve a patient has as well as its size.
  - This will dictate the expected effective orifice area (EOA) and gradients for that valve.
  - There are tables that can be referenced to know these expected values. The EOA should preferably be indexed to body surface area (EOAi).
- The age of the valve since implantation can help predict clinical complications (bioprosthetic valves tend to degenerate earlier than mechanical valves and pannus formation can occur in older valves of either type).
- Always compare findings to the baseline Doppler derived gradients and valve area performed soon after valve implantation.
- Table 14-1 provides some normal expected values for aortic and mitral prosthesis.
- An increasing gradient across a valve over time may be the only clue that a problem exists.

TABLE 14-1	Expected Values for Normally Functioning Aortic and Mitral Prosthetic Valves		
Valve type	Peak velocity (m/sec)	Peak gradient (mm Hg)	Mean gradient (mm Hg)
Aortic position			
St. Jude	2.3 ± 0.6	22 ± 12	12 ± 7
Bjork–Shiley	2.6 ± 0.5	27 ± 9	14 ± 6
Starr–Edwards	3.2 ± 0.2	40 ± 3	24 ± 4
Tissue	2.1 ± 0.5	19 ± 9	11 ± 5
Mitral position			
St. Jude	1.6 ± 0.3	11 ± 4.0	5 ± 2.0
Bjork–Shiley	1.6 ± 0.3	10 ± 3	5 ± 2
Starr–Edwards	1.8 ± 0.4	13 ± 5	5 ± 2
Beall	1.8 ± 0.2	13 ± 4	6 ± 2
Tissue	1.5 ± 0.3	9.9 ± 3.4	4.8 ± 1.7

Adapted from Nanda NC, Cooper JW, Mahan EF, et al. Echocardiographic assessment of prosthetic valves. *Circulation.* 1991;84(Suppl 1):228–39, with permission.

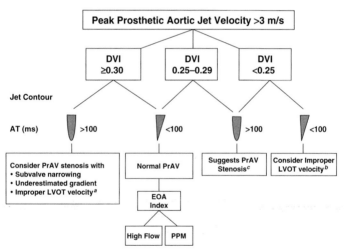

Figure 14-6. Algorithm for the evaluation of elevated peak prosthetic aortic jet velocity incorporating dimensionless valve index (DVI), jet contour, and acceleration time (AT). AVR, aortic valve replacement, EOA, effective orifice area; LVOT, left ventricular outflow tract; PPM, patient prosthesis mismatch; PrAV, prosthetic aortic valve. [a]Pulsed-wave (PW) Doppler sample too close to the valve (particularly when jet velocity by continuous-wave Doppler is ≥4 m/sec). [b]PW Doppler sample too far (apical) from the valve (particularly when jet velocity is 3.0–3.9 m/sec). [c]Stenosis further substantiated by EOA derivation compared with reference values if valve type and size are known. Fluoroscopy and transesophageal echocardiography TEE are helpful for further assessment, particularly in bileaflet valves. Adapted from Zoghbi, Chambers JB, Dumesnil JG, et al. Recommendations for evaluation of prosthetic valves with echocardiography and Doppler ultrasound. *J Am Soc Echocardiogr.* 2009;22:975–1014).

- A high gradient may be observed as a result of stenosis or increased flow across the valve (such as in significant regurgitation or a hyperdynamic state).
- All valves are **inherently stenotic** compared to native valves. At its extreme, a valve may be too small compared to the patient's body surface area and hemodynamic requirements, known as PPM.
  - **PPM is severe when EOAi <0.65 cm²/m² for the AoV or <1.2 cm²/m² for the MV.**
- Using the principles discussed, a systematic approach for assessing high gradients for prosthetic valves in the aortic (Fig. 14-6) as well as mitral (Table 14-2) position has been provided by the American Society of Echocardiography guidelines.

- **Key Points:**
  1. *Be able to differentiate normal "physiologic" regurgitation from pathologic regurgitation.*
  2. *Look for excessive flow convergence by color Doppler that could indicate prosthetic valve stenosis or regurgitation.*
  3. *Elevated gradients with normal AT or PHT are suggestive of regurgitation, high flow states, PPM, or technical aspects like pressure recovery rather than valvular obstruction (Fig. 14-7).*

Pressure Recovery

- In general, the maximal instantaneous gradient recorded on cardiac catheterization corresponds to the peak instantaneous gradient measured by CW Doppler on echocardiography (Fig. 14-8).

TABLE 14-2	Expected Parameters for a Normal Mitral Valve Prosthesis and Parameters Suggesting Possible or Significant Stenosis		
	Normal[a]	Possible stenosis[c]	Suggests significant stenosis[a,c]
Peak velocity (m/sec)[b,d]	<1.9	1.9–2.5	≥2.5
Mean gradient (mm Hg) [b,d]	≤5	6–10	>10
VTI_{prMV}/VTI_{Lvo}[b,d]	<2.2	2.2–2.5	>2.5
EOA (cm²)	≥2.0	1–2	<1
PHT (msec)	<130	130–200	>200

EOA, effective orifice area; PHT, pressure half-time; PrMV, prosthetic mitral valve; VTI, velocity time integral.
[a]Best specificity for normality or abnormality is seen if the majority of the parameters listed are normal or abnormal, respectively.
[b]Slightly higher cutoff values than shown may be seen in some bioprosthetic valves.
[c]Values of the parameters should prompt a closer evaluation of valve function and/or other considerations such as increased flow, increased heart rate, or patient prosthesis mismatch.
[d]These parameters are also abnormal in the presence of significant prosthetic mitral regurgitation.
From Zoghbi WA, Chambers JB, Dumesnil JG, et al. Recommendations for evaluation of prosthetic valves with echocardiography and Doppler ultrasound. *J Am Soc Echocardiogr.* 2009;22:975–1014, with permission from Elsevier.

Increased gradient due to:	High flow/normal valve	Valve stenosis
Mitral Doppler	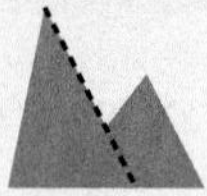	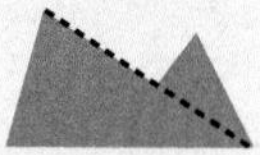
Pressure half-time (PHT)	Normal (<130 ms)	Increased (>200 ms)
Aortic Doppler	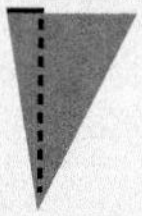	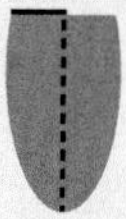
Acceleration time (AT):	Normal (<100 ms) Triangular	Increased (>100 ms) Rounded contour

Figure 14-7. Doppler profiles of prosthetic valves with elevated gradients resulting from high flow versus stenosis; ms, milliseconds.

- Occasionally, in some prosthetic valves and when the ascending aorta is small, pressure recovery phenomenon is known to occur.
- According to Bernoulli principle, as the flow of a fluid accelerates toward a narrowing, there is a loss of pressure (the fluid gains kinetic energy but loses pressure energy). As the fluid moves distal to the narrowing, it slows down and regains some of that lost pressure energy. This is called *pressure recovery.*

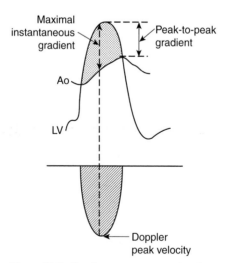

Figure 14-8. Simultaneous pressure tracings from the left ventricle (LV) and aorta (Ao) invasively measured compared with Doppler-derived pressure gradients.

- Thus, the Doppler measured peak instantaneous gradient may be significantly higher than one measured by cardiac catheterization (where the sampling is performed in the aorta after pressure has recovered).
- Pressure recovery is most pronounced with higher velocities through small bileaflet mechanical valves (e.g., 19 mm valves), in patients with caged-ball valves, and in patients with small aortas (diameter ≤3 cm) where laminar flow is preserved.
- This discrepancy is exacerbated as CW Doppler may measure **localized high velocities** within the mechanical bileaflet valve (side orifices are smaller than the central orifice); the resultant instantaneous gradient is not a true reflection of the overall gradient between the aorta and LV.

- **Key Points:**
  1. *Maximal instantaneous gradient recorded on cardiac catheterization corresponds to the peak instantaneous gradient measured by CW Doppler on echocardiography.*
  2. *Pressure recovery phenomenon in a bileaflet mechanical valve or a caged-ball valve can lead to a discrepancy between catheter and echo-derived peak gradients.*

15 Infective Endocarditis

Mirnela Byku, Majesh Makan, and Nishath Quader

HIGH-YIELD CONCEPTS

- The clinical presentation should always be considered when interpreting the description of valvular and annular masses on echocardiography.
- When the clinical suspicion for endocarditis is high, a transesophageal echocardiogram (TEE) is the test of choice.
- Concurrent mitral valve (MV) and aortic valve (AoV) infection is common as they are in direct continuity, separated only by a fibrous band of tissue. Therefore, examine the aortic root carefully for an abscess.
- Vegetations often have an echodensity similar to tissue, demonstrate independent movement, and have a predilection for the lower pressure side of native valve leaflets.
- Endocarditis involving native valves often arises from the leaflets, whereas endocarditis of prosthetic valves often arises where the sewing ring and annulus meet.

INTRODUCTION

Infective endocarditis (IE) describes a microbial infection of the endothelial surface of the heart. Valvular involvement is common and characterized by the presence of **vegetations**. Infection is also common on any implanted or prosthetic material such as valves, conduits, grafts, or pacing wires. Complications include, but are not limited to, valvular insufficiency, root abscess, fistula formation, pericardial effusion, arrhythmia, embolic phenomenon, and congestive heart failure. Factors that predispose a patient to IE include structural abnormality of a heart valve (e.g., bicuspid AoV), ventricular septal defect, prosthetic valve, intravenous drug use, hemodialysis, diabetes, and poor dental hygiene.

Persistently positive blood cultures, presence of intravascular devices, physical examination, and history should be taken into account when assessing patients who may have IE. The Duke criteria state evidence of endocardial involvement on echocardiography as a major criterion for IE. TEE is recommended as a first-line test in patients with suspected prosthetic valve endocarditis or suspected complications such as an aortic root abscess. The following are defined as positive findings on TEE by the Duke criteria:

1. *Presence of vegetation (tissue-like echodensity with independent motion implanted on the valve, prosthetic material, or endocardium in the trajectory of a regurgitant jet in the absence of alternative anatomic explanation)*
2. *Presence of an abscess*
3. *New dehiscence of a valve prosthesis*

• **Key Points:**

1. *Complications of IE: valvular insufficiency, root abscess, fistula formation, pericardial effusion, arrhythmia, embolic phenomenon, and congestive heart failure*
2. *Factors that predispose a patient to IE: structural abnormality of a heart valve, ventricular septal defect, prosthetic valve, intravenous drug use, hemodialysis, diabetes, and poor dental hygiene*

TRANSTHORACIC VERSUS TRANSESOPHAGEAL ECHOCARDIOGRAPHY

• Transthoracic echocardiography (TTE) is the initial diagnostic test for the evaluation of intermediate-risk patients for IE (Fig. 15-1). However, keep in mind the following:
  • TTE has lower resolution than TEE and can miss vegetations <0.5 cm in size.
  • Sensitivity of TTE for IE ranges from 40% to 63%, with a specificity of 90% to 98%.
  • If IE is diagnosed with TTE, it should be followed by TEE to evaluate other valves and complications of IE such as abscess, fistula formation, mycotic aneurysm, pseudoaneursym, and leaflet perforation.
• TEE is the preferred initial study in high-risk patients by Duke criteria, or in patients who have suboptimal TTE images.
  • High-risk patients are defined as those with prosthetic heart valves, congenital heart disease, previous endocarditis, new murmur with a clinical suspicion for IE, heart failure, or stigmata of IE.
  • Proximity of a high frequency TEE probe to the heart allows excellent visualization of valvular structures and the aortic root.
  • Sensitivity of TEE for IE is 90–99%, with a specificity of 91–99%.
  • Since IE is a dynamic disease, a repeat TEE in 7–10 days in patients with a strong suspicion of IE and TEE with no obvious vegetations may be considered to reassess for vegetations.

VEGETATIONS

• Vegetations from IE are often a mixture of microorganisms, inflammatory cells, platelets, and fibrin (Table 15-1).
• They are often found on the leading edge of the affected native valve on the lower pressure side or grow from the annulus if a prosthetic valve is present.
  • Rarely, infections will extend to adjacent structures such as the chamber wall.

TABLE 15-1	Echo Criteria for Defining Vegetation	
Positive feature	**Negative feature**
Low reflectance	High echogenicity
Attached to valve, upstream side	Nonvalvular location
Irregular shape	Smooth surface
Mobile, oscillating	Fibrillar structure
Associated tissue changes	Nonmobile
Associated valvular regurgitation	Absence of regurgitation

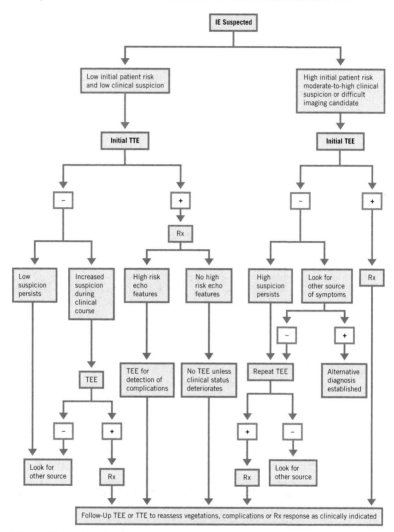

Figure 15-1. Algorithm for the use of transthoracic echocardiogram (TTE) in evaluation of a patient suspected of infective endocarditis (IE). TEE, transesophageal echocardiogram. (From AHA Scientific Statement: Infective endocarditis: diagnosis, antimicrobial therapy, and management of complications: a statement for healthcare professionals from the Committee on Rheumatic Fever, Endocarditis, and Kawasaki Disease, Council on Cardiovascular Disease in the Young, and the Councils on Clinical Cardiology, Stroke, and Cardiovascular Surgery and Anesthesia, American Heart Association: Endorsed by the Infectious Diseases Society of America. *Circulation.* 2005;111:e394–e434.)

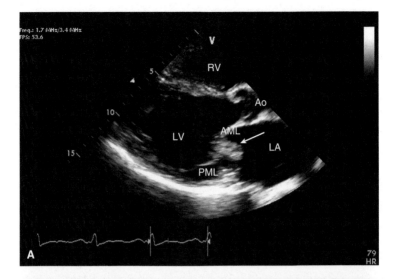

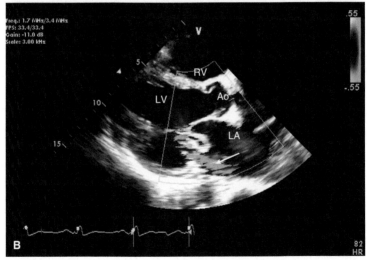

Figure 15-2. A: Parasternal long-axis view with mass seen on atrial surface of the anterior mitral leaflet (AML) consistent with vegetation (*arrow*). **B:** This causes mitral valve malcoaptation and moderate-severe posteriorly directed mitral regurgitation (*arrow*). Ao, aorta; LA, left atrium; LV, left ventricle; PML, posterior mitral leaflet; RV, right ventricle.

- **Because of leaflet malcoaptation or destruction, valvular regurgitation is almost always an accompanying feature** (Fig. 15-2).
  - *Consider alternative diagnoses for masses that appear close to a heart valve but are not associated with valvular regurgitation (e.g., a partially visualized myxoma growing from the interatrial septum to the valve)* (Fig. 15-3).

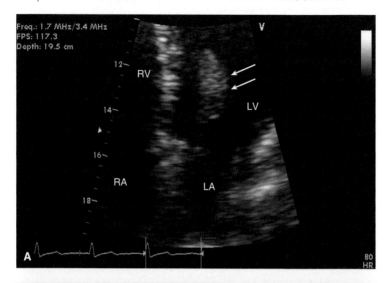

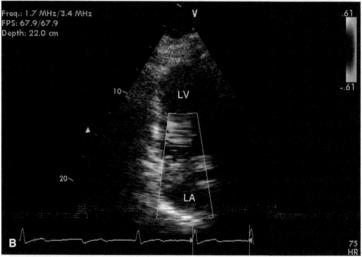

Figure 15-3. A: Apical four-chamber view with zoom of mitral valve shows mass (*arrows*) that appears to be attached to the anterior mitral leaflet, suggestive of vegetation. **B:** Apical two-chamber color Doppler shows no associated mitral regurgitation.

- Vegetations may also be seen where regurgitant flow or flow from a fistula strikes the endocardial wall (i.e., so-called "jet vegetations").
  - *If the regurgitant jet of an infected valve strikes the endocardial wall, that area should be closely inspected for further vegetations.*
- Occasionally, vegetations can cause obstruction and mimic valvular stenosis.

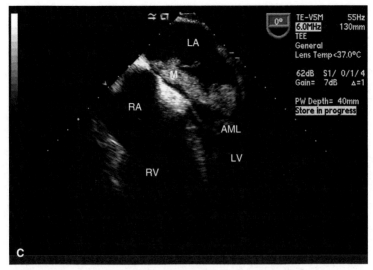

Figure 15-3. (*Continued*) **C:** Transesophageal echocardiogram performed in same patient shows that the mass is, in fact, larger than appreciated on transthoracic echocardiogram and is attached to the interatrial septum projecting into the mitral orifice. The diagnosis of left atrial (LA) myxoma was confirmed on pathology. LV, left ventricle; RA, right atrium; RV, right ventricle.

- Echocardiographic images should be captured with attention to the following:
  - Presence, size, shape, and location of vegetations
  - Valvular hemodynamics:
    - Carefully assess the entire valve apparatus to find abnormalities such as regurgitation, chordal rupture, and perforation.
    - Perforation may manifest as multiple jets with turbulence seen on the high-pressure surface of the valve leaflet (Fig. 15-4).
    - Assess for degree of regurgitation or stenosis.
    - Table 15-2 lists some of the complications of IE.
- Pacing wires and catheters should also be carefully inspected for vegetations (Fig. 15-5). TEE is the preferred imaging modality to visualize lead infections and also to determine whether the tricuspid valve is affected.

- **Key Points:**
  1. *Vegetations usually occur on the lower pressure side of a valve (atrial aspect for MV vegetations, ventricular aspect for AoV vegetations).*
  2. *Vegetations can cause valvular regurgitation as well as stenosis.*
  3. *Perforation is a common complication of vegetations and should be assessed carefully.*
  4. *Pacing wires and dialysis catheters in the right side chambers of the heart should be assessed carefully for vegetations.*

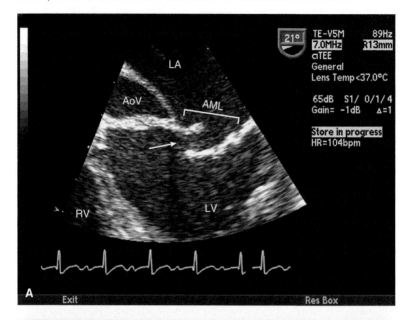

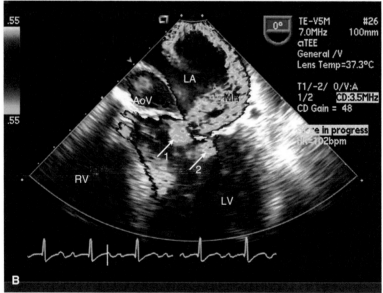

Figure 15-4. A: Transesophageal echocardiogram (midesophageal view) zoomed on anterior mitral leaflet (AML). There is an area of discontinuity suggestive of perforation (*arrow*). **B:** This is confirmed on color Doppler where a separate flow acceleration and mitral regurgitation (MR) jet is seen (*arrow-1*) in addition to the jet that occurs at leaflet coaptation (*arrow-2*). AoV, aortic valve; LA, left atrium; LV, left ventricle; RV, right ventricle.

TABLE 15-2	Complications of Endocarditis	
Structural	**Hemodynamic**
Leaflet rupture	Acute valvular vegetation
Flail leaflet	Valve obstruction
Leaflet perforation	Heart failure
Abscess	Intracardiac shunt
Aneurysm	Perivalvular regurgitation
Fistula	Tamponade
Prosthetic valve dehiscence	
Embolization	
Pericardial effusion	

Adapted from Armstrong WF, Ryan T, Feigenbaum H. *Feigenbaum's Echocardiography*. 7th ed. Philadelphia, PA: Wolters Kluwer Health/Lippincott Williams and Wilkins; 2010.

ABSCESSES

- Abscesses are more commonly seen in left rather than right-sided endocarditis, with a disposition for the **aortomitral continuity** (between the aortic and mitral annulus).
- **TEE is the test of choice to identify an abscess.** Sensitivity of TTE for abscess is <25%.
- Look for increased thickening of the aortic root; occasionally an abscess may be associated with a fistula, which can be diagnosed using 2D echocardiography and color Doppler (Fig. 15-6).

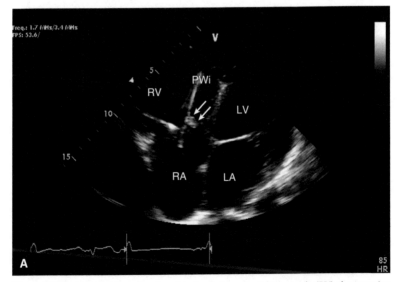

Figure 15-5. A: Apical four-chamber view focused on the right ventricle (RV) shows pacing wire (PWi) with small vegetation near the tricuspid valve (TV) (*arrows*). (*continued*)

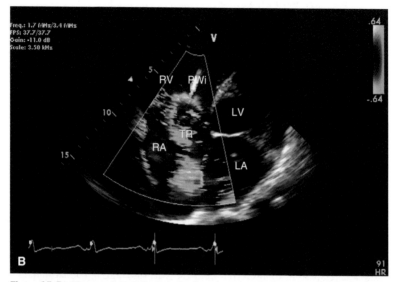

Figure 15-5. (*Continued*) **B:** Color Doppler shows severe tricuspid regurgitation (TR) suggestive of TV involvement and leaflet destruction. LA, left atrium; LV, left ventricle; RA, right atrium.

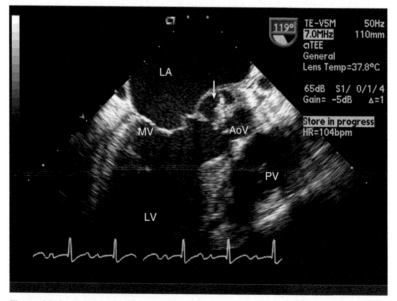

Figure 15-6. Transesophageal echocardiogram 120-degree, left ventricle (LV) long-axis view showing an abnormal septated cavity (*arrow*) between the mitral valve (MV) and aortic valve (AoV) (fibrous continuum) extending to the aortic root consistent with aortic root abscess. LA, left atrium; PV, pulmonic valve.

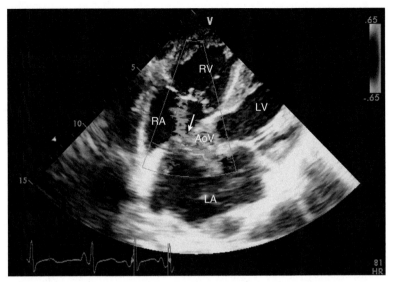

Figure 15-7. Apical five-chamber view with color Doppler shows high velocity jet originating from the right coronary sinus (*arrow*) and directed to the right atrium (RA). AoV, aortic valve; LA, left atrium; LV, left ventricle; RV, right ventricle.

- *An aortic abscess has to be differentiated from thickening of the aortic root seen in patients with recent AoV replacement. When evaluating a prosthetic valve for endocarditis, make sure to review the postoperative TEE to compare any changes that could suggest an aortic root abscess.*

FISTULAS

- Fistulas should be considered particularly when a continuous murmur is heard in a patient with IE.
- Abscess at the right coronary sinus tends to fistulize to the right ventricle (RV) and/or right atrium (RA) (Fig. 15-7).
- Abscess near the noncoronary cusp tends to fistulize to the left atrium (LA) through the aortomitral continuity.
- Fistulas may connect the aortic root with the LA.
  - *Check continuous wave (CW) Doppler through the fistulous tract. Peak flow velocity should be consistent with the pressure difference between the aorta and the connecting chamber.*

- **Key Points:**
  1. *Look for aortic root abscesses by carefully evaluating the aortomitral continuity and aortic root.*
  2. *Review postoperative TEEs in patients with prosthetic AoVs.*
  3. *Abscesses can sometimes be associated with fistulas. Color and CW Doppler should be utilized to determine if a fistula is present.*

PROSTHETIC VALVES

- Because of artifacts related to the prosthesis leading to incomplete evaluation of prosthetic valves by TTE, patients suspected of having IE with prosthetic valves should undergo TEE for further evaluation.
- Sensitivity of TEE for prosthetic valve IE is 86–94%, with a specificity of 88–99%.
- **Compared to native valves, in prosthetic valves the annulus instead of the leaflets is the more common initial site of infection.**
- Multiple components of the prosthesis need to be examined carefully.
  - Sewing ring: Check for a regular contour without an abnormal disruption. Both pannus and thrombus can disrupt the outline of the sewing ring in a similar fashion. Pannus tends to be echogenic/brighter compared to vegetations or thrombus.
  - Bioprosthetic leaflets: Examine the leaflets carefully for vegetations. Be aware that such leaflets can degenerate without any infectious cause over the natural life of the valve. Such degeneration can look similar to that of damage secondary to infection.
  - Mechanical leaflets: Examination can be difficult secondary to acoustic shadowing from the valve. Check the leaflets for symmetrical opening and closing angles. Examine whether a nonphysiologic gradient exists across the valve suggestive of obstruction. Also assess for perivalvular regurgitation (PVL).
  - Valve apparatus: Check for dehiscence of the valve apparatus from the myocardium that may cause a "rocking" motion of the valve if the dehiscence is large. The resulting PVL is seen as an asymmetric turbulent jet on color Doppler (Fig. 15-8). Note that dehiscence can occur from infection and also disrupted sutures, friable myocardium, and excessive calcification. Finally, examine the perivalvular area for echolucent areas suggestive of abscess. Be aware that echo artifact from the valve may cause similar echolucency, but will not be accompanied by a regurgitant jet.

> - **Key Point:** *TEE is preferable for the evaluation of prosthetic valve or mechanical lead infection.*

INFECTED INTRACARDIAC DEVICES

- As with prosthetic valves, infection can occur on intracardiac devices such as pacemakers/defibrillator leads.
  - TEE is the preferred diagnostic test in most cases.
- Presence of a mobile mass attached to an indwelling catheter or chamber wall suggests possible endocarditis; however, it is impossible to distinguish vegetation from thrombus on echocardiographic grounds alone. Clinical correlation is therefore paramount.

EMBOLIZATION

- Embolization of vegetations remains a source of considerable morbidity and mortality.

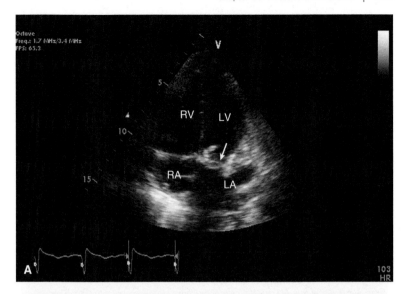

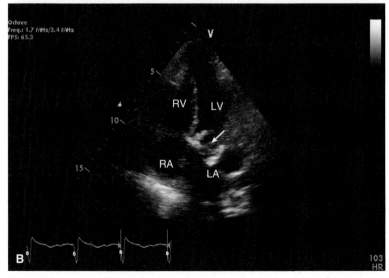

Figure 15-8. A: Apical four-chamber view with mitral valve bioprosthesis (*arrow*) tilted toward the anterolateral wall in diastole. **B:** In systole, the bioprosthesis tilts further. This movement backward and forward throughout the cardiac cycle is called "rocking" and is suggestive of significant valve dehiscence. (*continued*)

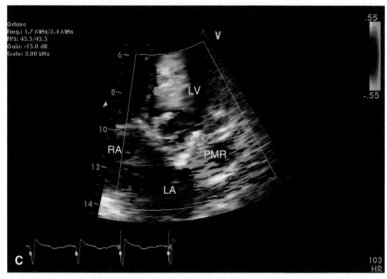

Figure 15-8. (*Continued*) **C:** Significant perivalvular mitral regurgitation (PMR) is seen on color Doppler. LA, left atrium; LV, left ventricle; RA, right atrium; RV, right ventricle.

- **Criteria associated with increased risk of embolization include right-sided endocarditis, vegetation length >10 mm, MV involvement (particularly anterior mitral leaflet [AML]), significantly mobile vegetations, and perivalvular extension.**

INDICATIONS FOR SURGICAL CONSULTATION

- Congestive heart failure secondary to valvular insufficiency that is refractory to medical therapy
- Fungal IE (except *Histoplasma capsulatum*)
- Persistent sepsis (>72 hours) despite appropriate antibiotic therapy
- Valve dehiscence, rupture, abscess, or fistula
- AML infection in the setting of AoV IE
- Heart block caused by abscess
- Prosthetic valve endocarditis
- Highly mobile, large (>10 mm) vegetations

MONITORING OF INFECTIVE ENDOCARDITIS

- Diagnosis of IE made by TTE should be followed by TEE to assess for other valve involvement and complications that may not be visible by TTE.
- If the patient's clinical course deteriorates, TEE should be repeated.
- Following completion of therapy, TTE is preferred so as to establish a new baseline for comparison to future studies.

FALSE POSITIVES FOR INFECTIVE ENDOCARDITIS

- Not all valvular vegetations are secondary to IE. Clinical correlation is necessary to assist in differentiating the following from IE:
  - Libman–Sacks endocarditis
  - Lambl excrescences
  - Myxoma
  - Papillary fibroelastoma
  - Acute rheumatic carditis
  - Prosthetic valve suture, pannus, or thrombus
  - Nodules of Arantius

16 Pericardial Disease and Cardiac Tamponade

Marc Sintek and Michael Yeung

HIGH-YIELD CONCEPTS

In tamponade assess for these findings:
- Amount of pericardial fluid (large >2 cm)
- Right atrial (RA) systolic collapse (>1/3 systolic period)
- Right ventricular (RV) diastolic collapse
- Respiratory variation in tricuspid (>40%) and mitral (>25%) inflow
- Fixed and dilated inferior vena cava (IVC) (>2.1 cm)

KEY VIEWS

- *Parasternal long axis (PLAX)*—initial screening of effusion/differentiation between pleural effusion (PLeff) and pericardial effusion
- *Parasternal short axis (PSAX)*—assessment of RV diastolic collapse
- *Apical four chamber (A4C)*—use respirometer for the evaluation of TV/MV respiratory variation
- *Subcostal*—good view for sizing full extent of pericardial effusion as well as assessment of RA systolic collapse and RV diastolic collapse

DEFINITIONS

- Cardiac tamponade is a syndrome of **low cardiac output** resulting from impaired ventricular filling secondary to increase intrapericardial pressure from a pericardial effusion.
- Constrictive pericarditis is a **chronic** heart failure syndrome of impaired ventricular filling and elevated systemic venous pressures secondary to a noncompliant, scared pericardium.

ANATOMY AND PHYSIOLOGY OF THE PERICARDIUM

- The pericardium consists of two layers: the **visceral pericardium**, which is adjacent to the epicardial surface of the heart, and the **parietal pericardium**, which is a thicker, fibrous layer that encases most of the heart.
- The **pericardial space**, located between these two layers, contains approximately 10–50 mL of pericardial fluid and allows the transmission of changes in intrathoracic pressure to the cardiac chambers. Therefore, during inspiration, for example, the intrathoracic pressure, pulmonary capillary wedge pressure (PCWP), and left ventricular (LV) diastolic pressure fall in concert with minimal change in LV filling.

- The **pericardium** serves as a mechanical barrier between the heart and its adjacent mediastinal structures, a lubricant between the pericardial layers, and a mechanical restraint on cardiac volume. This restraint is the rationale for **ventricular interdependence**; the pressure and volume changes of one ventricle affect the other.

- In the **normal respiratory cycle**, inspiration leads to a decrease in intrathoracic pressure, allowing for an increase in blood flow through the right side of the heart. Under normal conditions, the cardiac chambers and pericardium are compliant enough to accommodate this increase in blood flow.

- In **tamponade/constriction, ventricular interdependence is exaggerated** as transmission of changes in intrathoracic pressure to the ventricles and ventricular compliance is diminished by an increase in intrapericardial pressure or pericardial scarring. During inspiration, intrathoracic pressure decreases with a decrease in PCWP. LV diastolic pressure, however, does not decrease to the same degree because of increased intrapericardial pressure. This results in a reduced gradient (PCWP-LV diastolic pressure) and reduction in LV filling pressure, which is reflected in a reduced mitral E wave peak velocity. Increased venous return and reduced LV filling promotes increased RV filling, which is reflected in an increased tricuspid E wave peak velocity. Reciprocal changes occur during expiration, where LV filling is promoted to the detriment of RV filling.

- In constriction, there is prominent, rapid early diastolic filling as a result of markedly elevated atrial pressures with abrupt cessation of filling as the pericardium constrains ventricular volumes. This rapid filling and abrupt cessation is manifested as prominent Y descent on atrial wave forms and diastolic flattening (or "square root sign") on ventricular waveforms.

- Kussmaul sign is a lack of decrease in central venous pressure with inspiration and can be seen in constriction. With cardiac tamponade, jugular veins are distended and show a prominent x descent and an absent y descent. Conversely, patients with constrictive pericarditis have a prominent x and y descent.

- **Pulsus paradoxus** is a clinical manifestation of increased ventricular interdependence in tamponade (and occasionally in constriction). A **decrease in systolic blood pressure >12 mm Hg during inspiration** is highly suggestive of tamponade and a decrease of >25 mm Hg is virtually diagnostic of severe tamponade.

- The electrocardiographic sign of **electrical alternans** corresponds to the pendulum-like swinging of the heart within a large pericardial effusion.

- Once intrapericardial pressures exceed intracardiac pressures, chamber collapse is seen, beginning with the lowest-pressure chambers.

- The **rate of accumulation** is just as important as the size of the pericardial effusion. A small but rapidly accumulating effusion may lead to tamponade with as little as 200 cc, whereas a chronic effusion can accommodate much more pericardial fluid before presenting with hemodynamic compromise.

- **Key Points:**
  1. *In tamponade/constriction, there is exaggerated ventricular interdependence.*
  2. *RA wave forms in constriction demonstrate a prominent x and y descent and ventricular waveforms in this disease demonstrate diastolic flattening ("square root sign").*
  3. *Kussmaul sign is a lack of decrease in central venous pressure with inspiration and is specific for constriction.*
  4. *Pulsus paradoxus is a clinical manifestation of increased ventricular interdependence in tamponade.*
  5. *The rate of accumulation is just as important as the size of the pericardial effusion.*

ETIOLOGY OF PERICARDIAL DISEASE AND EFFUSIONS

- **Idiopathic**
- **Infectious**
  - **Viral:** echovirus, coxsackievirus, adenovirus, hepatitis B, human immunodeficiency virus
  - **Bacterial:** Pneumococcus, Staphylococcus, Streptococcus, Mycobacterium
  - **Fungal:** histoplasmosis, coccidiomycosis
- **Immune/inflammatory**
  - **Connective tissue disease:** systemic lupus erythematosus, rheumatoid arthritis, scleroderma
  - **Postmyocardial infarction:** Dressler syndrome
  - **Uremic**
  - **Postcardiac surgery**
  - **Drug-induced:** procainamide, hydralazine, isoniazid, cyclosporine
- **Neoplastic disease**
  - **Direct extension:** lung carcinoma, breast carcinoma
  - **Metastatic:** lymphoma, melanoma
  - **Primary cardiac tumor**
- **Mechanical**
  - **Blunt chest trauma**
  - **Procedure-related:** percutaneous coronary intervention, implantation of pacemakers/defibrillators
  - **Postmyocardial infarction free wall rupture**

DIFFERENTIAL DIAGNOSIS OF ECHOLUCENT SPACE SURROUNDING THE HEART

- **Epicardial fat:** Usually presents as an isolated echolucent area anterior to the RV free wall and spares the posterior pericardium. Epicardial fat can sometimes be identified as having a granular or speckled appearance when compared with blood or pericardial fluid. Epicardial fat is more prevalent in the elderly, females, diabetics, patients with dyslipidemia, and the obese.
- **PLeff:** In the PLAX view, effusions seen anterior to the proximal descending thoracic aorta are pericardial, whereas effusions that track posterior to the thoracic aorta are left-sided PLeffs (Fig. 16-1). Left PLeffs tend to localize primarily in the posterior–lateral aspect of the heart, whereas most pericardial effusions are present circumferentially unless loculated as a result of adhesions from surgery or an inflammatory process.
- **Simple pericardial effusion:** This tends to initially accumulate posteriorly in the oblique sinus. It is best seen in the PLAX view.
- **Loculated pericardial effusion:** This is often seen after cardiac surgery or mediastinal radiation, or resulting from a long-standing inflammatory condition that allows fibrin strands and adhesions to deposit along the pericardial space. This may lead to a localized increase in intrapericardial pressure with the absence of traditional echocardiographic signs of respiratory variation and diastolic collapse because of the absence of free-flowing fluid.
  - *Pericardial effusion and hematoma may be difficult to visualize immediately after cardiac surgery. Additional examination by transesophageal echocardiography (TEE) should be considered if clinical suspicion for tamponade is high.*

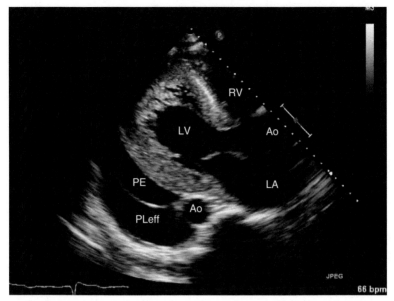

Figure 16-1. Parasternal long-axis (PLAX) view of a pericardial effusion (PE) anterior to the descending aorta and a pleural effusion (PLeff) posterior to the aorta. Ao, aorta; LA, left atrium; LV, left ventricle; RV, right ventricle.

- **Key Points:**
  1. *In PLAX views, pericardial effusion is found anterior to the descending thoracic aorta and PLeff is posterior to the descending thoracic aorta.*
  2. *Epicardial fat is commonly seen on echo and has to be differentiated from pericardial effusion based on the granular/speckled appearance.*
  3. *Pericardial effusion and hematoma can be difficult to assess immediately after surgery by transthoracic echocardiography (TTE). Additional imaging modalities such as TEE may be needed if clinical suspicion is high.*

ECHOCARDIOGRAPHIC ASSESSMENT OF CARDIAC TAMPONADE

- **Two-dimensional (2D) echocardiography**
  - **Pericardial effusion** is seen on 2D echocardiography as an echolucent space surrounding the heart (Fig. 16-2). A complex effusion is characterized by the presence of loculations, fibrinous strands, and thrombus (Fig. 16-3).
  - **The size** of the pericardial effusion can be estimated in the PLAX, A4C, and subcostal views. Measurements are taken in diastole and the effusion is generally classified as:
    - Small: if <1.0 cm from the LV wall
    - Moderate: if 1.0–2.0 cm from the LV wall
    - Large: if ≥2 cm from the LV wall
    - Very large: ≥20 mm and compressing the heart

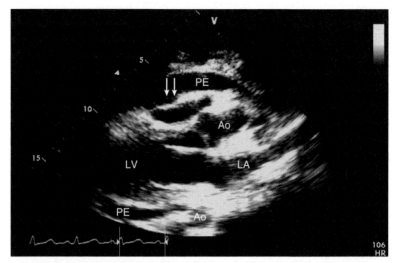

Figure 16-2. Simple concentric pericardial effusion (PE) in the parasternal long-axis (PLAX) view. Note diastolic compression of right ventricle (*arrows*), suggestive of tamponade. Ao, aorta; LA, left atrium; LV, left ventricle.

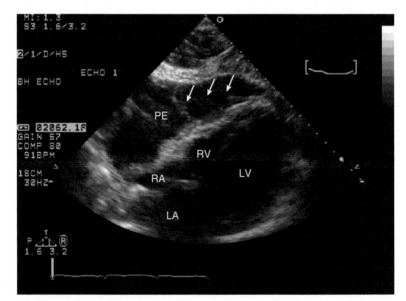

Figure 16-3. Complex pericardial effusion (PE) seen in the subcostal view with linear echodensities (*arrows*) attached along the compressed right atrial (RA) and right ventricular (RV) free wall. LA, left atrium; LV, left ventricle.

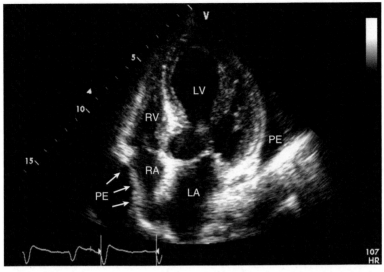

Figure 16-4. Marked right atrial (RA) collapse (*arrows*) in the apical four-chamber (A4C) view. LA, left atrium; LV, left ventricle; PE, pericardial effusion; RV, right ventricle.

- **RA inversion** is best visualized in the A4C and subcostal views. RA inversion begins to manifest when intrapericardial pressure is higher than in the right atrium. This presents **prior to the hemodynamic changes** that lead to RV diastolic collapse, given that RA pressure is lower than RV pressure. The right atrium normally contracts with atrial systole. When intrapericardial pressure is elevated, the RA wall remains collapsed throughout ventricular diastole (Fig. 16-4). This is a specific finding in cardiac tamponade.
- **RV diastolic collapse** should be evaluated from multiple acoustic windows. M-mode shows a characteristic "dipping" of the anterior RV free wall during diastole (Fig. 16-5). As in RA inversion, this occurs when intrapericardial pressure exceeds RV pressure. This finding is a sensitive and specific finding for cardiac tamponade.
  - *Patients with conditions that predispose them to elevated RV pressure or wall stiffness, as seen in pulmonary hypertension, infiltrative diseases, or atrial septal defects, will have a less pronounced or even absent RV diastolic collapse, despite an elevated intrapericardial pressure.*
- **"Septal bounce"** or exaggerated septal motion can be seen due to ventricular interdependence. During inspiration, LV filling decreases and RV filling increases. This leads to the septum moving to the left. However, during expiration, LV filling increases and RV filling decreases. This causes the septum to move to the right. In patients with diseases of the pericardium, the septal bounce is best appreciated in the A4C view. Other common causes of abnormal septal motion are left bundle branch block, previous cardiac surgery, RV pressure, or volume overload.
- In the subcostal view, visualization of a **dilated IVC** >2.1 cm with <50% collapse during inspiration as well as dilated hepatic veins with expiratory diastolic

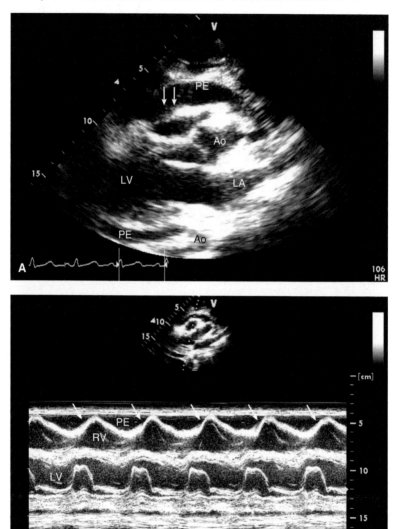

Figure 16-5. (**A**) Right ventricular (RV) diastolic collapse in the parasternal long-axis (PLAX) view with corresponding M-mode image (*arrows*) (**B**). Ao, aorta; LA, left atrium; LV, left ventricle; PE, pericardial effusion.

flow reversals suggests increased RA pressure, lending support to the diagnosis of elevated intracardiac pressures secondary to pericardial disease. IVC assessment is limited in patients who are undergoing mechanical ventilation.

- Key Points:
  1. *Size of the effusion is measured in diastole.*
  2. *RA collapse in systole is a specific sign for cardiac tamponade; however, RV collapse is a sensitive and specific sign for this disease.*
  3. *Patients with pulmonary hypertension and RV hypertrophy may not have RV diastolic collapse in tamponade.*
  4. *Exaggerated septal motion ("septal bounce") is seen due to ventricular interdependence.*
  5. *Dilated IVC with minimal collapse on inspiration is suggestive of tamponade in the appropriate clinical context.*

- **Doppler echocardiography**
  - **Mitral and tricuspid respiratory variation:** In the A4C view, assessment of the mitral and tricuspid valve inflow velocities using pulsed-wave (PW) Doppler at the leaflet tips is performed. At the respiratory physiology menu, **slow the sweep speed to 25 cm/sec** to allow for an increased number of cardiac and respiratory cycles to be displayed. In tamponade, the increased blood flow entering the RV during inspiration corresponds to an increase in tricuspid valve inflow velocity of approximately 40% or greater. Reciprocally, a decrease in mitral inflow velocity of approximately 25% or greater is seen.

- Key Point: *Typically these changes occur on the first beat after the beginning of inspiration or expiration, differentiating tamponade from variation that occurs with diseases that result in large changes in intrathoracic pressures. For example, with severe obstructive airways disease, changes in mitral and tricuspid inflow occur several beats after inspiration or expiration. Also, variation could be related to an irregular heart rhythm such as atrial fibrillation, which causes changes in the cardiac filling pattern unrelated to tamponade physiology (Fig. 16-6).*

GENERAL CONSIDERATIONS

These echocardiographic signs are dependent on the balance between intrapericardial and intracardiac pressures. Patients with RV hypertrophy or pulmonary hypertension, for example, may require higher intrapericardial pressures for 2D and Doppler signs of tamponade to manifest.

Variation in mitral and tricuspid inflow is **volume** dependent and may not be present in patients with hypovolemia.

Most important, cardiac tamponade is a **clinical diagnosis** and the echocardiographic signs described are only a "snapshot" and guide to the clinical status of the patient.

- Key Point: *Uncommonly, other pathology may mimic pericardial tamponade. For example, large PLeffs or pneumothorax can compress the mediastinum, thus increasing ventricular interdependence and producing physiology similar to pericardial tamponade.*

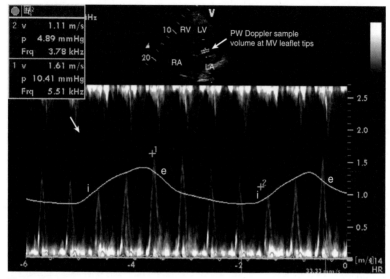

Figure 16-6. Pulsed-wave (PW) Doppler with sample volume at mitral leaflet tips recorded at a slow sweep speed. The green line indicates respirations, with the beginning of inspiration (i) and expiration (e) labeled. There is significant respiratory variation in the mitral valve Doppler inflow. Note timing of change in Doppler peak velocities compared with patient's respirations. LA, left atrium; LV, left ventricle; RA, right atrium; RV, right ventricle.

EVALUATION OF CONSTRICTIVE PERICARDITIS

- Constrictive pericarditis should be considered in the evaluation of patients who present with heart failure despite normal LV systolic function and evidence of systemic venous congestion.
- Most common causes of constriction are prior cardiac surgery, mediastinal radiation, mediastinal infections, and collagen vascular diseases.
- Pericardial thickening and calcification typically have to be severe to be recognized on 2D echocardiographic images.
- Although nonspecific, **bi-atrial enlargement** representing elevated filling pressures, along with a normal systolic function, may be indicative of constriction.
- Other features include rapid expansion and then sudden diastolic flattening of the LV inferolateral wall ("heart in a box"), late diastolic interventricular septal bounce (septal movement reflects ventricular interdependence as the ventricles share a fixed pericardial volume—if one expands the other must shrink), IVC dilation, increased hepatic Doppler flow reversal during **expiration**, and significant atrioventricular valve inflow respiratory variation in the **absence of a pericardial effusion** (Fig. 16-7). More subtle findings of increased intracardiac filling pressures such as premature opening of the pulmonic valve may also be present.
- Pulmonary pressures are often normal in patients with constrictive pericarditis as opposed to restrictive cardiomyopathy, where pulmonary pressures >60 mm Hg are commonly seen.

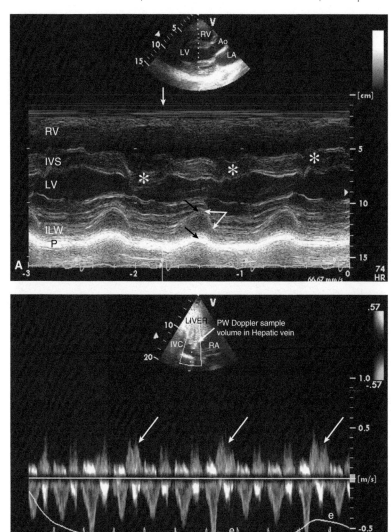

Figure 16-7. Patient with constrictive pericarditis. **A:** Parasternal long-axis (PLAX) M-mode at the base of the ventricles shows exaggerated inferolateral wall motion with rapid and abrupt cessation of motion during diastole without further expansion (*double headed arrow*). "Tracking" of the pericardium with the inferior–lateral wall (ILW) is seen, suggesting attachment (*short black arrows*). Interventricular late diastolic dip back toward the left ventricle (LV) is seen (*). **B:** Hepatic Doppler shows increased flow reversals (*long arrows*) during expiration (e). Ao, aorta; IVC, inferior vena cava; IVS, interventricular septum; LA, left atrium; RA, right atrium; RV, right ventricle.

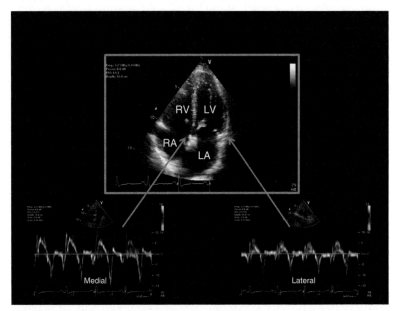

Figure 16-8. Patient with constrictive pericarditis with "annulus paradoxus." The mitral annular peak early velocity is greater than the lateral annulus (reverse of normal). This is due to adherent pericardium reducing lateral motion and compensatory exaggerated septal motion. LA, left atrium; LV, left ventricle; RA, right atrium; RV, right ventricle.

- **"Annulus paradoxus"** refers to the phenomenon in constrictive pericarditis whereby the mitral septal annular velocity is normal (≥8 cm/sec) and greater than the lateral mitral annular velocity despite evidence for increased filling pressures (e/e′ >15). In constriction, alterations in ventricular filling are related to an abnormal, less compliant pericardium with the **myocardium being normal.** This is in contrast to infiltrative disease or restriction whereby ventricular filling is impaired secondary to abnormal myocardial relaxation, reflected in reduced annular velocities.

- **Key Point:** *In contrast to normal hearts, in constrictive pericarditis the mitral septal annular velocity (e′) may be higher than the lateral annulus secondary to (1) tethering of the lateral wall from the adjacent thickened, adherent pericardium, and (2) exaggerated motion of the unencumbered septal wall ("annulus reversus") (Fig. 16-8).*

DIFFERENTIATION OF CONSTRICTIVE PERICARDITIS AND RESTRICTIVE CARDIOMYOPATHY

- Adjunct modalities such as cardiac catheterization, computed tomography, or magnetic resonance imaging may be needed to aid in the differentiation of constrictive pericarditis from restrictive cardiomyopathy.
- Left ventricular myocardial thickness is often increased in restrictive cardiomyopathy in contrast to constrictive disease where the pericardium is abnormally thickened or calcified.

- Both conditions exhibit elevated left and right atrial filling pressures.
- Pulmonary artery systolic pressures are elevated in restrictive cardiomyopathy (>60 mm Hg), whereas this is often normal in constrictive pericarditis.
- Because ventricular compliance is impaired, the diastolic filling pattern is similar in both constrictive pericarditis and advanced restrictive cardiomyopathy.
- Both conditions display diastolic flow reversal of the hepatic vein Doppler. The hepatic vein flow reversal is more prominent during **inspiration** for the restrictive cardiomyopathies ("sick RV" cannot accommodate increased venous return). In contrast, the diastolic flow reversal is increased more prominently during **expiration** for constrictive pericarditis (RV volume is limited by expansion of the LV— ventricular interdependence).
- Left ventricular strain analysis can be applied to differentiate both conditions. A reduced circumferential strain and early diastolic apical untwisting velocities are consistent with pericardial constriction (**outer fibers** involved in these movements). In contrast, restrictive cardiomyopathy displays a reduced longitudinal displacement and e′ (subendocardial fibers involved in these movements).

OTHER PERICARDIAL PATHOLOGY

Absent **congenital pericardium** occurs partially on the left side, whereas the complete absence of pericardium is extremely rare. Most patients are free of symptoms. Echocardiographically, this entity may manifest as exaggerated cardiac movement, abnormal ventricular septal motion, or partial displacement of cardiac structures to the left, giving the impression of right-sided enlargement and overload.

Pericardial cysts are typically benign and found incidentally. These cysts may be found predominantly by the left or right costophrenic angle. This is seen as a round, echo-free structure filled with fluid.

17 Diseases of the Great Vessels: Aorta and Pulmonary Artery

Praveen K. Rao and Nishath Quader

- Aortic root measurements are made in a modified parasternal long-axis (PLAX) view at end-diastole.
- It is important to index aortic size for body surface area (BSA).
- With aortic dissection, determine where flow in systole is occurring—this usually identifies the true lumen (TL).
- Intramural hematomas are treated similarly to aortic dissection.
- McConnell sign in combination with 60/60 sign is specific for pulmonary emboli.

KEY TRANSTHORACIC ECHOCARDIOGRAHY VIEWS: AORTA AND PULMONARY ARTERY

- Standard PLAX: Descending aorta in cross-section
- Modified PLAX (probe is placed in a superior rib space than standard PLAX): Aortic valve annulus, sinuses of Valsalva, sinotubular junction, ascending aorta
- Right ventricular outflow tract (RVOT): Main pulmonary artery (PA)
- Parasternal short axis (PSAX): Aortic valve leaflets, sinuses of Valsalva, RVOT, and main PA
- Off-axis apical four chamber (A4C) and apical two chamber (A2C) (posterior tilt): Descending aorta
- Subcostal view (long axis): Proximal abdominal aorta
- Suprasternal notch: Aortic arch, identification of branch vessels (innominate, carotid, and subclavian arteries), descending aorta, and right pulmonary artery (RPA)

Whereas transthoracic echocardiography (TTE) provides useful serial measurement of the great vessels, transesophageal echocardiography (TEE) is the ultrasound modality of choice in comprehensive imaging of these structures, especially in emergency situations or in patients with poor echocardiographic windows.

AORTA

Anatomy

- The aorta is divided into the thoracic and abdominal aorta.
- The thoracic aorta is further divided into the aortic root, arch, ascending, and descending aorta.

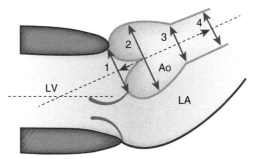

Figure 17-1. The four sites in the parasternal long-axis (PSAX) view where the aortic root should be measured: (1) the aortic annulus, (2) the sinus of Valsalva, (3) the sino-tubular junction, and (4) the proximal ascending aorta. Ao, aorta; LA, left atrium; LV, left ventricle. (From Lang RM, Badano LP, Mor-Avi V, et al. Recommendations for cardiac chamber quantification by echocardiography in adults: an update from the American Society of Echocadiography and the Europeans Association of Cardiovascular Imaging. *J Am Soc Echocardiogr.* 2015;28:1–39.)

- The aortic root consists of the aortic annulus, the sinuses of Valsalva, and the sino-tubular junction, which joins the proximal ascending portion of the thoracic aorta (Fig. 17-1). Note the four sites of measurements that should be made of the aortic root and proximal ascending aorta in the PLAX view.
- Figure 17-2 gives 95% confidence intervals for aortic root at the sinus of Valsalva based on BSA and age.

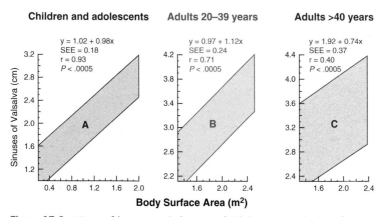

Figure 17-2. 95% confidence intervals for sinus of Valsalva based on body surface area (**A**) in children and adolescents, (**B**) in people ages 20–39 years old, and (**C**) in adults >40 years of age. (From Lang RM, Badano LP, Mor-Avi V, et al. Recommendations for cardiac chamber quantification by echocardiography in adults: an update from the American Society of Echocadiography and the Europeans Association of Cardiovascular Imaging. *J Am Soc Echocardiogr.* 2015;28:1–39.)

TABLE 17-1	Normal Aortic Root Measurements for Men and Women Indexed to Body Surface Area			
	Absolute values (cm)		Indexed values (cm/m²)	
Aortic root	Men	Women	Men	Women
Annulus	2.6 ± 0.3	2.3 ± 0.2	1.3 ± 0.1	1.3 ± 0.1
Sinuses of Valsalva	3.4 ± 0.3	3.0 ± 0.3	1.7 ± 0.2	1.8 ± 0.2
Sinotubular junction	2.9 + 0.3	2.6 ± 0.3	1.5 ± 0.2	1.5 ± 0.2
Proximal ascending aorta	3.0 ± 0.4	2.7 ± 0.4	1.5 ± 0.2	1.6 ± 0.3

From Lang RM, Badano LP, Mor-Avi V, et al. Recommendations for cardiac chamber quantification by echocardiography in adults: an update from the American Society of Echocadiography and the Europeans Association of Cardiovascular Imaging. *J Am Soc Echocardiogr.* 2015;28:1–39.

- Table 17-1 provides indexed values for the aortic root based on gender.
- The ascending portion continues until the origin of the innominate artery.
- The aortic arch gives rise to the innominate, left carotid, and left subclavian arteries.
- The descending aorta begins after the origin of the left subclavian artery and continues past the diaphragm, becoming the abdominal aorta (Fig. 17-3). The ligamentum arteriosum is just distal to the left subclavian artery. The area between the left subclavian artery and ligamentum arteriosum is a common location for abnormalities such as coarctation, patent ductus arteriosus, and dissections resulting from trauma or deceleration injury.

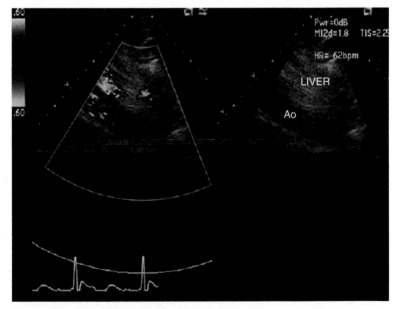

Figure 17-3. Subcostal view of the abdominal aorta.

- **Key Points:**
  1. *Indexed measurements (to BSA) of the aortic root are crucial and these are specific for gender.*
  2. *The aortic root consists of aortic annulus, the sinuses of Valsalva, and the sinotubular junction, which joins the proximal ascending portion of the thoracic aorta.*

Key TTE Views

- PLAX: The aortic root and proximal ascending aorta as well as the descending thoracic aorta can be visualized.
- PSAX: By tilting the probe away from the aortic valve (AoV) superiorly, one can visualize the proximal ascending aorta and the main PA.
- A4C and A2C: Tilting of the probe can help visualize the descending thoracic aorta.
- Subcostal view: The abdominal aorta can be visualized and pulsed-wave (PW) Doppler can be used to assess for severity of aortic regurgitation (AR) and coarctation.
- Suprasternal notch: The aortic arch is visualized along with assessment for narrowing of the descending aorta that could suggest coarctation. PW Doppler can again be utilized to assess holodiastolic flow reversals as a marker for severe AR. In addition, PW Doppler can be used to assess for coarctation.

Key TEE Views

TEE is an excellent modality to image the entire aorta apart from a small "blind-spot" where the air-filled trachea shields a segment of the distal ascending aorta as it becomes the proximal aortic arch.

- High esophageal views (20 cm) 0-degree: Ascending aorta along with the main PA and its bifurcation
- Upper esophageal (20–25 cm) 0-degree long axis: Aortic arch
- Upper esophageal (20–25 cm) 90-degree short axis: Aortic arch along with PA
- Midesophageal (30–40 cm) 30- to 40-degree short axis: Aortic valve
- Midesophageal (30–40 cm) 100- to 120-degree LV long-axis view: Aortic valve and root
- Deep transgastric view (45–50 cm) 0- to 20-degree flexion: Aortic valve and root
- Turning probe posteriorly: Transgastric to upper esophageal views; 0- and 90-degree views of thoracic aorta.

Pathology

Aortic Aneurysm

- Dilation of the aorta at any segment should alert the clinician to evaluate the entire aorta.
- An aortic aneurysm is defined as presence of dilation to >1.5 times the normal dimension for that segment.
- Primary aortic diseases include those that may be associated with connective tissue diseases and Marfan syndrome. There is involvement of the medial layers with subsequent dilation of the aorta.
- Marfan syndrome is characterized by disproportionate dilation of the sinuses (Fig. 17-4) and maybe be associated with AR resulting from loss of normal aortic cusp coaptation. Mitral valve prolapse is also frequently seen in this syndrome.
- Other disease states (secondary causes) that can cause aortic dilation include hypertension, AR from chronic volume overload, and aortic stenosis where poststenotic dilation can be seen.

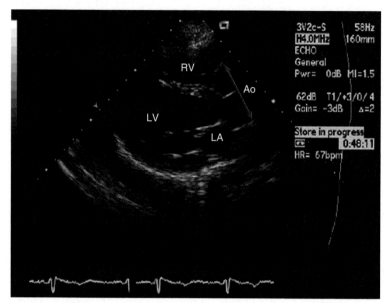

Figure 17-4. Parasternal long-axis (PLAX) view showing aortic root dilation at the sinus of Valsalva (*double-headed arrow*) in a patient with Marfan syndrome. Ao, aorta; LA, left atrium; LV, left ventricle; RV, right ventricle.

- Aneurysms of the descending aorta may be associated with dissections, thrombus, and significant protruding atheroma.

- **Key Points:**
  1. *Dilation of one part of the aorta should prompt evaluation of the rest of the aorta.*
  2. *An aortic aneurysm is dilation of the aorta to >1.5 times the normal value.*
  3. *Know the various causes of aortic dilation.*

Sinus of Valsalva Aneurysm
- These aneurysms commonly arise from the right coronary sinus (Fig. 17-5), can project into the right atrium, and appear as a "windsock" deformity.
- Sinus of Valsalva aneurysms can also arise from the noncoronary sinus, where they are noted projecting into the interventricular septum and rarely can also arise from the left coronary sinus.
- One of the major complications of a sinus of Valsalva aneurysm is rupture. Other complications include malcoaptation of the AoV cusps with resultant aortic insufficiency and thrombosis of the aneurysm.

- **Key Points:**
  1. *Common site for the formation of sinus of Valsalva aneurysms is the right coronary sinus.*
  2. *Right coronary sinus of Valsalva aneurysms project into the right atrium.*
  3. *Some complications of these aneurysms include rupture, thrombosis, and AR.*

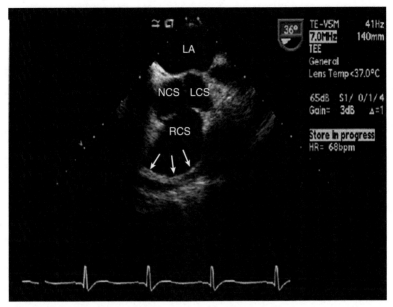

Figure 17-5. Transesophageal echocardiography (TEE) short-axis image of the aortic valve demonstrating a large right coronary sinus (RCS) of Valsalva aneurysm. LA, left atrium, LCS, left coronary sinus; NCS, noncoronary sinus.

Acute Aortic Syndromes

Aortic Dissection

- The typical aortic dissection consists of a tear of the intima extending into the media. As the column of blood propagates between the two layers, it propagates the dissection even further.
- Spontaneous aortic hematoma is considered a type of aortic dissection as it presents similarly to the classic dissection. Hemorrhage within the media does not communicate with the lumen, but there is a risk of it extending into the adventitia (Fig. 17-6).
- Factors that predispose patients to dissection include hypertension, bicuspid AoV, cystic medial necrosis, trauma, pregnancy, cocaine use, connective tissue disease, prolonged steroid use, inflammatory arteritis such as giant cell arteritis, and iatrogenic trauma.
- Two main classification systems have been used to describe aortic dissections: the Stanford and DeBakey systems.
- DeBakey I originates in the ascending aorta propagating to the arch. It may involve other sections of the aorta as well. DeBakey II is limited to the ascending aorta and DeBakey III involves the descending aorta only.
- With the Stanford system, Type A is any dissection involving the ascending aorta (including DeBakey I and II) and Type B only involves the descending aorta (DeBakey III) (Fig. 17-7).

- **Key Point:** *Aortic hematomas have a similar presentation to aortic dissection and in general are treated similar to aortic dissections.*

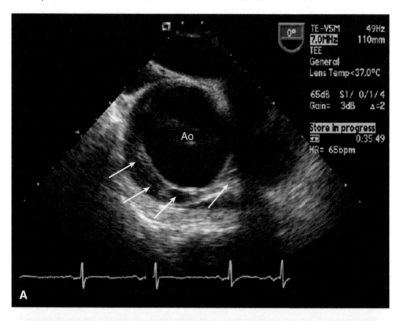

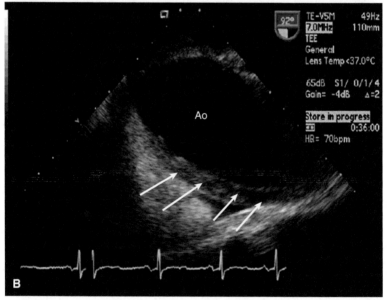

Figure 17-6. A: Transesophageal echocardiography (TEE) short-axis image of the descending thoracic aorta showing the classic crescent shape of an intramural hematoma (*arrows*). **B:** This is also seen on the corresponding 90-degree view. Ao, aorta.

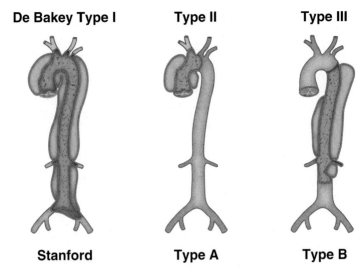

De Bakey Type I	Type II	Type III
Stanford	**Type A**	**Type B**

Figure 17-7. The DeBakey and Stanford classifications for aortic dissections. (From Tsai TT, Nienaber CA, Eagle KA. Contemporary reviews in cardiovascular medicine: acute aortic syndromes. *Circulation.* 2005;112:3802–3813.)

Two-dimensional (2D) and Doppler Findings

- TTE is usually inadequate in diagnosing an aortic dissection. It can be used to assess complications of aortic dissection such as AR, pericardial effusion, wall motion abnormalities due to the dissection extending into the coronary (usually the right coronary artery).
- Other abnormalities that can be detected by TTE:
  - Dilated aortic root.
  - Linear mobile echodensity representing an intimal flap
  - *In the suprasternal view, at times, the innominate vein can be mistaken for a dissection flap. Color Doppler of the area can be used to distinguish vein from a dissection flap. It is important to recognize this as a* normal *anatomic finding* (Fig. 17-8).
- Given that the esophagus lies in close proximity to the thoracic aorta, the higher spatial resolution of TEE has a very high sensitivity and specificity (99% and 98%) for the diagnosis of aortic dissection (Figs. 17-9 and 17-10).
  - The echocardiographer has to be able to differentiate artifacts arising from the aortic wall from a dissection flap.
  - TEE can image the most of the aorta except a "blind-spot" where the air-filled trachea shields a segment of the distal ascending aorta as it becomes the proximal aortic arch.
- Differential color Doppler in false lumen (FL) and TL: the TL usually fills with blood during systole, whereas the FL has variable flow (Fig. 17-11). Entry points between the two lumens may be seen as areas of turbulence on color Doppler. Occasionally swirling, low-velocity flow may be noted in the FL, with areas of partial or complete thrombosis.

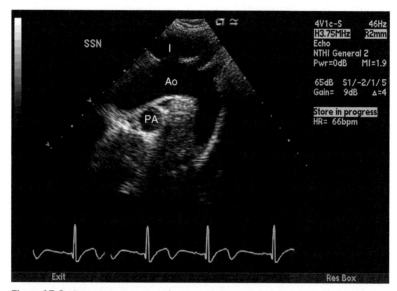

Figure 17-8. Innominate vein seen adjacent to the aortic arch in the suprasternal notch view. Ao, aorta; PA, pulmonary artery.

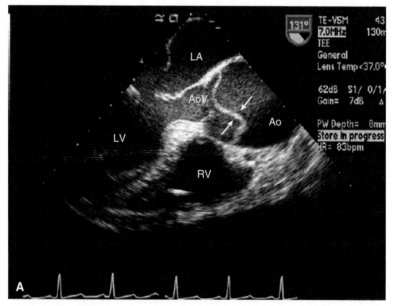

Figure 17-9. A: Transesophageal echocardiography (TEE) left ventricular (LV) long-axis image demonstrating a dissection flap (*arrows*) in the aortic root causing a flail noncoronary cusp of the aortic valve.

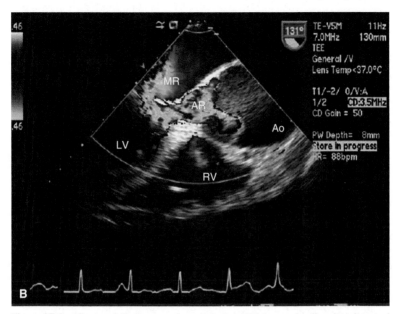

Figure 17-9. (*Continued*) **B:** Severe aortic regurgitation (AR) is seen as well as diastolic mitral regurgitation (MR) secondary to elevated LV end-diastolic pressure. Ao, aorta; RV, right ventricle.

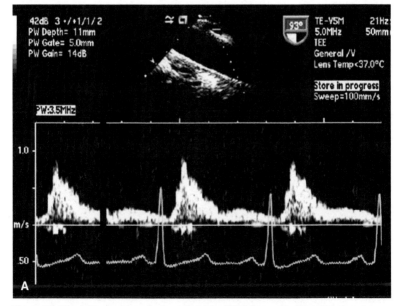

Figure 17-10. **A:** Transesophageal echocardiography (TEE) image of a descending thoracic aorta dissection at 90 degrees, with color Doppler demonstrating flow in the true lumen (TL). (*continued*)

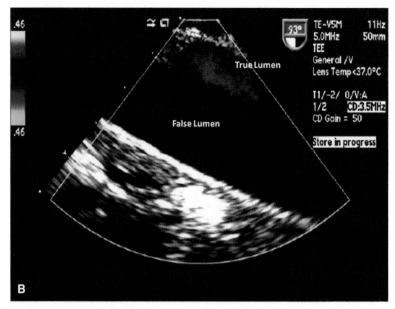

Figure 17-10. (*Continued*) **B:** Pulsed-wave Doppler confirms systolic flow in the TL.

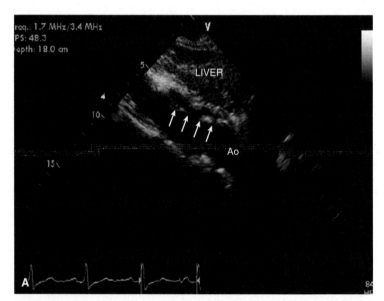

Figure 17-11. (**A**) Subcostal view demonstrating a dissection flap (*arrows*) in the abdominal aorta with (**B**) flow seen in the true lumen (TL) on color Doppler. FL, false lumen.

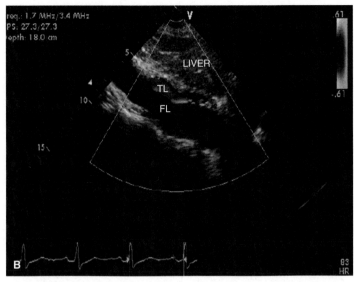

Figure 17-11. (*Continued*)

- Although it is sometimes difficult to distinguish the TL from the FL, the following are distinguishing features:
  - The FL is usually larger than the TL in diastole, with the TL expanding during systole.
  - The TL usually has a more regular shape (either circular or oval).
  - The TL, especially in the descending aorta, is usually the smaller of the two lumens.
  - There is usually spontaneous echo contrast or thrombus present in the FL.
  - The FL may contain small fibrinous strands.

- **Key Points:**
  1. *Know the complications of aortic dissection that can be detected by TTE.*
  2. *Be able to distinguish the innominate vein from a true dissection flap in the suprasternal view.*
  3. *Know the limitations of TEE in detecting aortic dissections.*
  4. *Be able to distinguish the TL from the FL.*

Coarctation of the aorta

This is a congenital condition involving narrowing of the descending aorta at the site of the ligamentum arteriosum, immediately distal to the left subclavian artery. Associated conditions include Turner syndrome, bicuspid aortic valve, patent ductus arteriosus, ventricular septal defect (VSD), and intracranial aneurysms. There are three types of coarctation:

- Preductal: Narrowing proximal to ductus arteriosus
- Ductal: Narrowing at insertion of ductus arteriosus
- Postductal: Narrowing distal to ductus arteriosus
- Coarctation of the aorta is best seen in the suprasternal view by TTE and in high esophageal views by TEE.

2D Findings

- Suprasternal view: Tapering or discrete area of narrowing of the proximal descending aorta (Fig. 17-12A).
- Poststenotic dilation possible
- LV hypertrophy

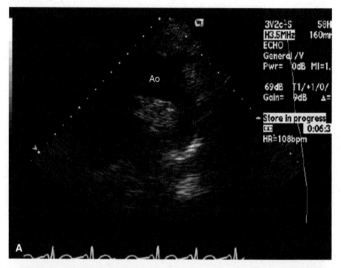

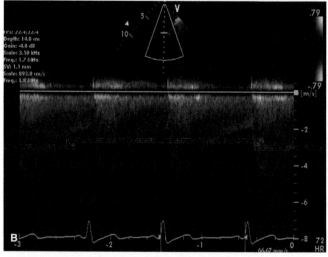

Figure 17-12. A: Suprasternal notch view of the aortic arch with a marked reduction in caliber of the lumen seen at the proximal descending aorta (Ao, *arrow*). **B:** Continuous-wave Doppler demonstrates the classic "shark-tooth" pattern associated with aortic coarctation. There is an early elevated peak velocity followed by a slow taper of the Doppler envelope related to diastolic "run-off" in the collateral circulation.

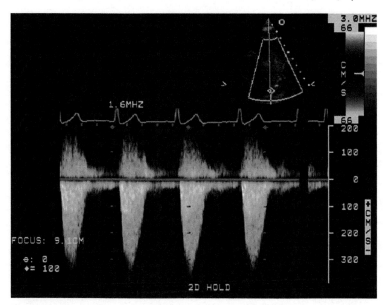

Figure 17-13. Continuous-wave Doppler in the suprasternal notch view of the aorta in a patient with a history of *coarctation repair*. Note the high peak velocities seen in the descending without diastolic "run-off" related to residual narrowing of the aorta.

CW and PW Doppler

- "Shark-tooth" pattern describes a systolic peak with slowly decremental diastolic flow related to distal diastolic run-off if significant collateral circulation is present (see Fig. 17-12B).
- There will be increased velocity across coarctation in descending aorta (Fig. 17-13).
- Estimate peak gradient across coarctation with modified Bernoulli equation:

$$\Delta P = 4 \times v^2$$

- *Be aware of different Doppler patterns in the suprasternal notch view (Fig. 17-14).*

- **Key Points:**
  1. *2D TEE or TTE can be used to visualize the coarctation.*
  2. *CW Doppler shows a classic pattern in coarctation, with flow seen in systole and diastole.*

Aortic Atherosclerosis

Aortic atherosclerosis is a known risk factor for ischemic stroke and peripheral embolic events, and is correlated with coronary artery disease. TEE is an excellent imaging modality to identify aortic atherosclerotic plaque as it allows for detailed visualization of the entire thoracic aorta (Fig. 17-15).

- **Key Point:** *Atheromas that measure >5 mm; are mobile, pedunculated, or protruding; and have an irregular, intimal surface have been demonstrated to more likely result in embolic events.*

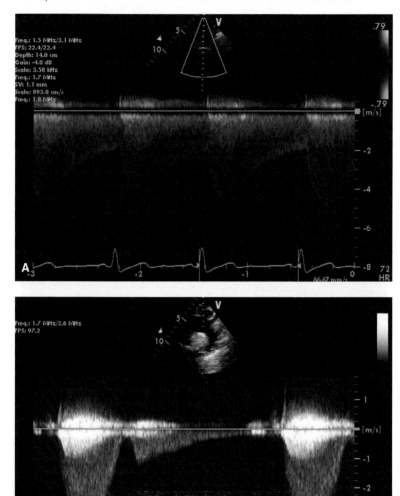

Figure 17-14. Comparison of abnormal Doppler patterns acquired from the suprasternal notch view. **A:** Continuous-wave (CW) Doppler of the descending aorta demonstrating the classic pattern of aortic coarctation. **B:** CW Doppler detecting an elevated systolic velocity secondary to right pulmonary artery (RPA) stenosis.

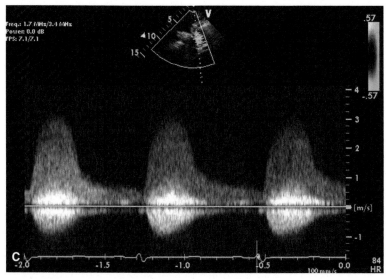

Figure 17-14. (*Continued*) **C:** CW Doppler detecting an elevated systolic velocity (note, toward the probe) secondary to significant stenosis of the left subclavian artery.

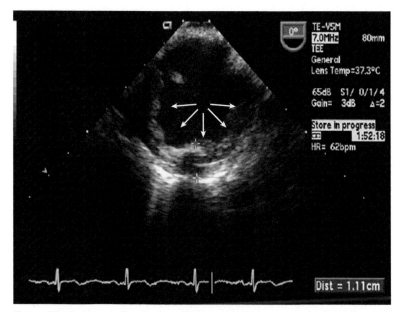

Figure 17-15. Transesophageal echocardiography (TEE) short-axis view of the descending thoracic aorta demonstrating severe aortic atherosclerosis (*arrows*).

PULMONARY ARTERY

Anatomy

The main PA begins at the base of the RV and gives rise to right and left main stem branches.

Key Views

- PLAX RVOT view: Main PA
- PSAX at the level of the AoV: RVOT, main PA, and bifurcation (Fig. 17-16)
- Suprasternal view: RPA visualized in cross section posterior to ascending aorta and beneath aortic arch

Pathology

Pulmonary Artery Dilation

Dilation of the PA can be found in conjunction with a number of conditions, including right-sided volume overload, pulmonary hypertension (Fig. 17-17), and congenital forms.

Pulmonary Embolism

Whereas TTE is not recommended as a routine test to confirm pulmonary embolism (PE), useful signs suggest this diagnosis and these findings are important for risk stratification and management. Acute PE can affect right-sided heart function resulting from a sudden increase in pulmonary arterial resistance. Echocardiographic findings

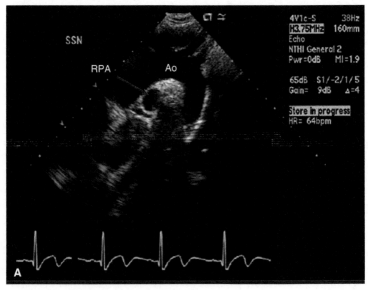

Figure 17-16. A: Suprasternal notch view with the right pulmonary artery (RPA) seen underneath the aortic arch.

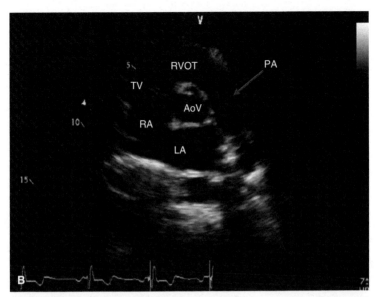

Figure 17-16. (*Continued*) **B:** Parasternal short-axis (PSAX) view at the aortic level showing the main pulmonary artery (PA) (*arrow*) prior to bifurcation. Ao, aorta; AoV, aortic valve; LA, left atrium; RA, right atrium; RVOT, right ventricular outflow tract; TV, tricuspid valve.

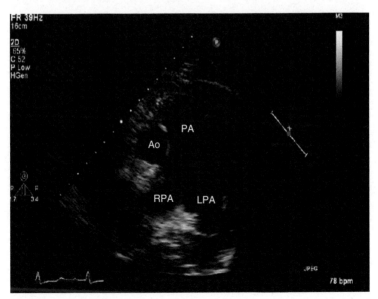

Figure 17-17. Parasternal short-axis (PSAX) at the base of the heart showing a dilated pulmonary artery (PA) in a patient with primary pulmonary hypertension. LPA, left pulmonary artery; RPA, right pulmonary artery. Ao, aorta.

of right heart strain have been well documented to carry a worse prognosis and may indicate a need for more aggressive measures such as thrombectomy or intravenous thrombolytic therapy.

2D and Doppler Findings of PE

- Free-floating thrombus in RV or "clot in transit"—very rare, but diagnostic of PE (main PA/saddle embolism) (Fig. 17-18)
- RV enlargement, free wall hypokinesis
  - Abrupt rise in PA pressure
  - McConnell sign: Normal to hyperdynamic motion of the RV apex, with akinesis of the RV mid free wall; high specificity for PE (Fig. 17-19)
  - Interventricular paradoxic septal movement: "D-shaped" septum in PSAX, suggestive of pulmonary hypertension; often, LV cavity is small (Fig. 17-20).
  - "60/60 sign": RV systolic pressure <60 mm Hg + RVOT acceleration time <60 msec (Fig. 17-21). With an acute rise in PA pressures, the RV does not have a chance to generate pressures >60 mm Hg. In addition, the time from onset to peak flow velocity (acceleration time) across the RVOT is shortened as a result of the elevated afterload the RV encounters.

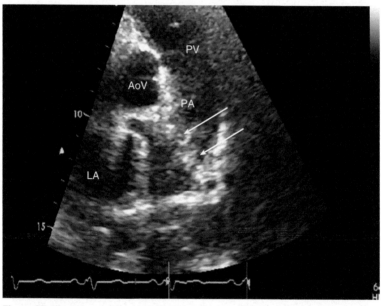

Figure 17-18. Parasternal short-axis (PSAX) at the base of the heart with a saddle embolism (*arrows*) seen in the pulmonary artery (PA). AoV, aortic valve; LA, left atrium; PV, pulmonic valve.

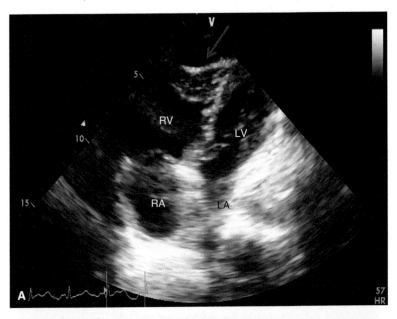

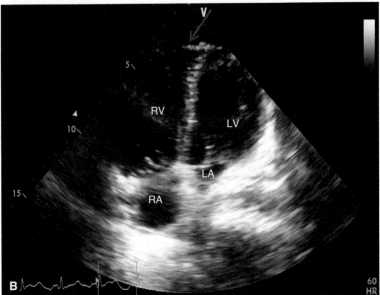

Figure 17-19. Apical four-chamber (A4C) view in (**A**) systole and (**B**) diastole showing right ventricular enlargement and McConnell sign with apical hyperkinesis (*arrow*) and right ventricle (RV) basal to mid free wall hypokinesis in a patient with a pulmonary embolism. LA, left atrium; LV, left ventricle; RA, right atrium.

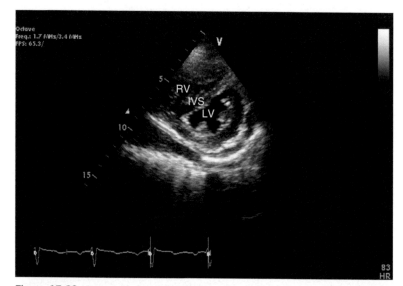

Figure 17-20. Parasternal short-axis (PSAX) at the papillary muscle level demonstrating enlarged right ventricle (RV) and "D-shaped" left ventricle (LV) with interventricular septal (IVS) flattening in a patient with severe pulmonary hypertension.

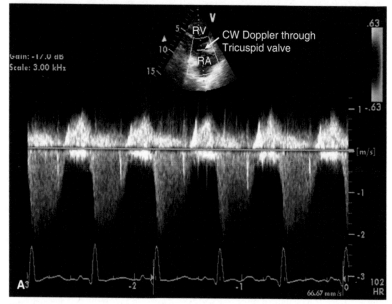

Figure 17-21. "60/60" sign in patient with acute pulmonary embolism. **A:** Continuous-wave (CW) Doppler through the tricuspid valve demonstrates a peak tricuspid regurgitant gradient <60 mm Hg.

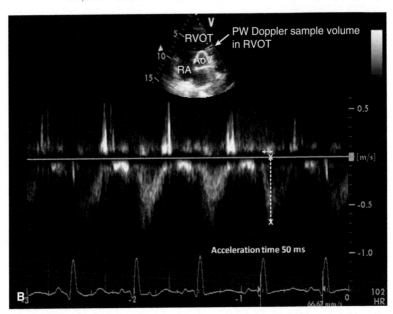

Figure 17-21. (*Continued*) **B:** Parasternal short-axis (PSAX) pulsed-wave (PW) Doppler in the right ventricular outflow (RVOT) shows an acceleration time (*double-headed arrow*) <60 msec. RA, right atrium; RV, right ventricle.

18

Congenital Heart Disease

Tyson E. Turner, Kathryn J. Lindley, and Majesh Makan

In recognizing the complexity of this topic, this chapter is intended to give an introduction to congenital abnormalities that may be seen in the adult population. As many of these patients undergo surgical repair during childhood, this chapter will attempt to highlight the echocardiographic characteristics of both unrepaired congenital heart disease and residual lesions that can arise following repair or palliative procedures.

SEGMENTAL ECHOCARDIOGRAPHIC EXAM

- *Establish situs:* Using a standard subcostal view of the aorta (Ao) and inferior vena cava (IVC) in cross section with color Doppler (probe perpendicular to spine with indicator pointing to the patient's left hip), determine whether the Ao (red) is to the left and IVC (blue) to the right (**situs solitus** – normal) or opposite (**situs inversus**) of the spine (Fig. 18-1). Atrial situs (morphologic right atrium [RA] to the right and morphologic left atrium [LA] to the left) follows abdominal situs in ~80% of patients.
- *Establish ventricular orientation:* Using a standard subcostal view (probe indicator points to patient's left shoulder), if the apex of the heart is pointing to the right of the patient's body = **dextrocardia,** if to the left = **levocardia** (normal).
- *Identify ventricular morphology:* The morphologic right ventricle (RV) will be trabeculated, and it will have a moderator band, an apically displaced tricuspid valve (TV) compared to the mitral valve (MV), and septal attachment of TV. The morphologic left ventricle (LV) has a smoother endocardial surface and two papillary muscles.
- *Establish the great vessels:* In the normal heart, the morphologic LV gives rise to the Ao and the RV gives rise to the pulmonary artery (PA). This results in an anterior and leftward PA and a posterior and rightward Ao. The orientation of the great arteries is best appreciated on the short-axis view at the base of the heart by echocardiography. Also identify the arch (left sided vs. right sided).

> • Key Point: *Atrioventricular (AV) valves always stay with their respective ventricle. The apically displaced TV establishes its ventricle as the morphologic RV.*

SHUNTS

Key Concepts

- L → R shunt: Blood returning to the left side of heart from the pulmonary veins (PVs) is shunted into the right side of heart, reducing cardiac output by the amount of the shunted volume.

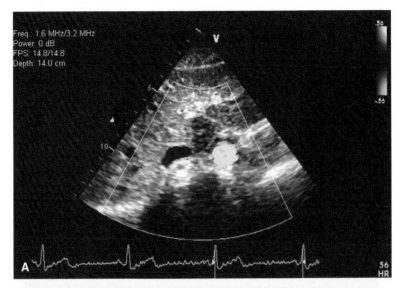

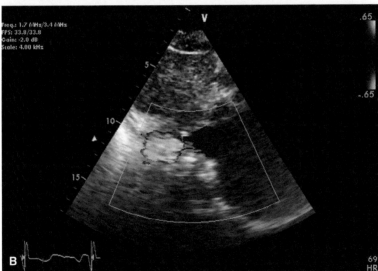

Figure 18-1. Subcostal cross-sectional view with color Doppler to establish atrial situs. **A:** Inferior vena cava (IVC) (blue) to the right and abdominal aorta (yellow) to the left in situs solitus (normal) of the spine. **B:** IVC to the left and abdominal aorta to the right in a patient with situs inversus.

- R → L shunt: Blood is shunted directly from the right side of the heart to the left side, bypassing the lungs and decreasing oxygen content of systemic arterial blood in proportion to the shunted volume.
- To calculate shunt fraction (pulmonary flow/systemic flow = Qp/Qs), measure the cross-sectional area (CSA) of both the left ventricular outflow tract (LVOT) and the right ventricular outflow tract (RVOT), trace pulsed-wave (PW) Doppler through each valve to get velocity time integral (VTI).

$$Qp/Qs = CSA_{RVOT} \times VTI_{RVOT}/CSA_{LVOT} \times VTI_{LVOT}$$

- Qp/Qs >1:1 indicates pulmonary flow exceeds systemic flow and defines a net L → R shunt as volume of shunted oxygenated blood + venous blood entering the pulmonary circuit exceeds amount of blood leaving the systemic circuit.
- Qp/Qs <1:1 indicates net R → L shunt as venous deoxygenated blood mixes with oxygenated systemic blood.
- **Qp/Qs >1.5:1 is considered a significant L → R shunt *especially if right heart chamber dilation is present.***

Atrial Septal Defect (ASD)

See Figure 18-2.

Types

- *Secundum:* 75% of ASDs; located near the foramen ovale (mid-interatrial septum [IAS])

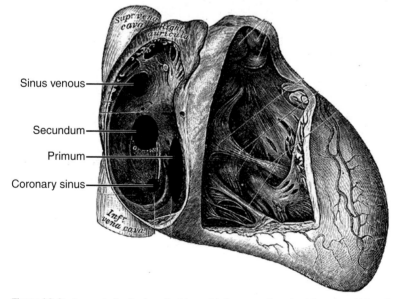

Figure 18-2. Anatomic distribution of atrial septal defect as seen from the right atrium. (Adapted from Gray, H. *Anatomy of the Human Body.* 20th ed. Philadelphia, PA: Lea & Febiger; 1918.

- *Primum:* 15% of ASDs; associated with atrioventricular septal defects (AVSD; base of IAS)
- *Sinus venosus:* 10% of ASDs; posterior edge of IAS; usually associated with partial anomalous pulmonary venous return (typically right superior PV); typically not visualized in standard transthoracic echocardiography (TTE) views
- *Coronary sinus defects:* Rare; absence of the common wall that separates the LA from the coronary sinus as it courses in the AV groove to the RA; associated with persistent left superior vena cava

Hemodynamics
- Flow across an ASD is determined by the difference in compliance and capacity of both ventricles.
- The LA has decreased compliance and higher pressures than the RA, favoring L → R shunting.
- This leads to increased pulmonary blood flow and **RV volume overload** (dilated RV, diastolic flattening of interventricular septum [IVS]).
- **Eisenmenger syndrome** occurs when right heart pressures exceed left heart pressures, promoting R → L shunt and hypoxemia.

- **Key Points:**
  1. *Best views to locate ASD are the parasternal short axis (PSAX), apical four chamber (A4C), and subcostal. Beware of "drop-out" of the IAS in the A4C view related to reduced lateral resolution of the ultrasound beam that may mimic a secundum ASD. The presence of an ASD should be confirmed in the subcostal view (where the IAS is perpendicular to ultrasound beam) and by color and PW Doppler. Typically, ASD flow begins in systole and continues throughout the cardiac cycle with a broad peak in late systole and early diastole (Fig. 18-3).*
  2. *The subcostal and "off-axis" subcostal views are typically the only views in which a sinus venosus ASD may be visualized (Fig. 18-4). A transesophageal echocardiogram (TEE) should be performed to assess for sinus venosus ASD in patients with unexplained right heart volume overload, especially if the agitated saline study is markedly positive without a shunt location identified.*

Echocardiography
- TTE and TEE should document the type and size of ASD (ASD diameter) as well as direction (color and spectral Doppler), degree of shunt fraction Qp/Qs ratio), and presence of any associated congenital lesions.
- Conduct post transcatheter closure assessment for the maintenance of position of the occluder and any residual shunt (Fig. 18-5). Often a small residual shunt is noted immediately after occluder placement. This should eventually resolve due to endothelialization of the occlude device.
- Identify AV valve defects (e.g., cleft MV [commonly seen in AVSD, typically affecting the anterior leaflet]) that can lead to residual mitral regurgitation (MR).

- **Key Point:** *Injection of agitated saline results in a quick (<3 to 4 beats), intense opacification of the LV that clears with subsequent beats.*

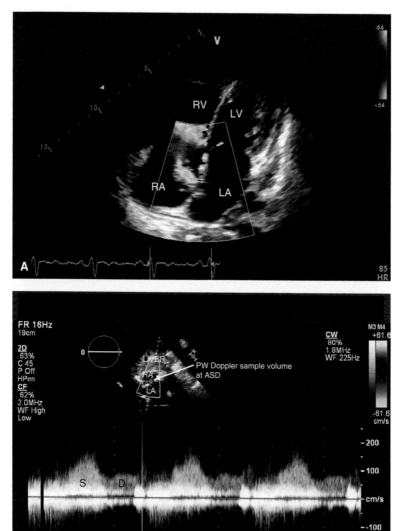

Figure 18-3. A: Apical four-chamber view with color Doppler demonstrating L → R flow across a secundum atrial septal defect (ASD). **B:** Pulsed-wave (PW) Doppler across the secundum ASD in a subcostal view demonstrating the characteristic broad peak flow in late systole and early diastole. LA, left atrium; LV, left ventricle; RA, right atrium; RV, right ventricle.

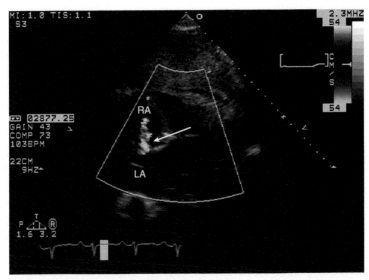

Figure 18-4. An off-axis subcostal image with color Doppler demonstrating L → R flow (*arrow*) at the posterior aspect of the interatrial septum consistent with a sinus venosus atrial septal defect. LA, left atrium; RA, right atrium.

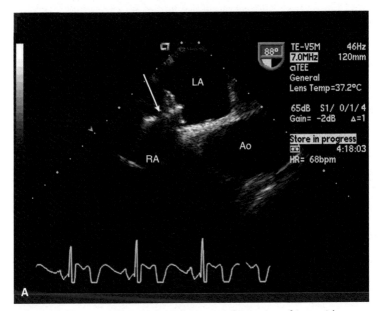

Figure 18-5. Transesophageal echocardiogram 90-degree view of interatrial septum during placement of the clam-shell occluder device. **A:** The occluder is positioned across the interatrial septal defect and is still attached to the guiding catheter (*arrow*). (*continued*)

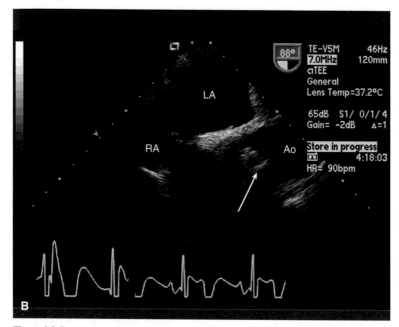

Figure 18-5. (*Continued*) **B:** A few minutes later, after occluder release, the device has migrated through the left atrium (LA) and left ventricle to the aorta (Ao) (*arrow*). RA, right atrium.

Ventricular Septal Defect (VSD)

See Figure 18-6.

Types

- *Perimembranous:* 80% of VSDs, located near the septal leaflet of the TV and below the aortic valve (AoV)
- *Muscular:* Either single or multiple ("Swiss cheese" septum) involving the septum (Fig. 18-7)
- *Inlet:* Involves inflow portion of the septum; associated with atrioventricular canal defect (AVCD)
- *Supracristal or outflow tract:* Involves RVOT (above crista supraventricularis) and near the outflow valves; frequently occluded by a cusp of the AoV causing aortic regurgitation; also have a chance of spontaneous closure

Hemodynamics

- As a result of higher pressures in LV compared to RV, there is a L → R shunt. Significant shunting leads to increased flow in pulmonary circulation and eventual LV volume overload and dilation (in congenital VSD).
- "Restrictive" VSDs are small diameter and high velocity/gradient jets (typically >75 mm Hg). These rarely lead to increased pulmonary pressures or left heart dilation as they are typically low volume (Fig. 18-8).

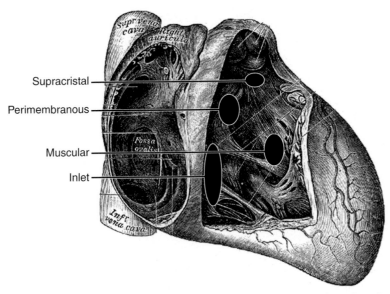

Figure 18-6. Anatomic distribution of ventricular septal defect as seen from the right ventricle. (Adapted from Gray, H. *Anatomy of the Human Body*. 20th ed. Philadelphia, PA: Lea & Febiger; 1918.)

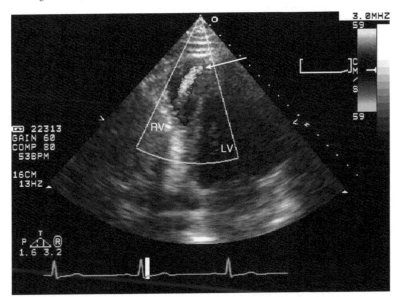

Figure 18-7. Off-axis apical four-chamber view tilted toward the apex to reveal a congenital apical ventricular septal defect with L → R flow (*arrow*) on color Doppler in a 23-year-old male with a loud systolic murmur. LV, left ventricle; RV, right ventricle.

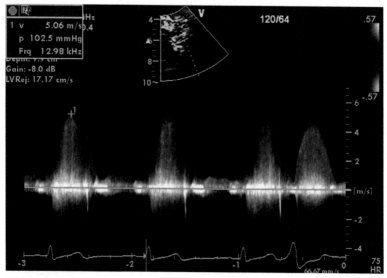

Figure 18-8. Systolic flow velocity seen on continuous-wave Doppler with a peak velocity (~5 m/sec) and gradient (~103 mm Hg), suggestive of a restrictive ventricular septal defect.

- "Nonrestrictive" VSDs are characterized by large defects with low peak velocity/ gradient noted on spectral Doppler (typically <25 mm Hg), suggesting that there is minimal pressure difference between the LV and RV.
- Thus, **nonrestrictive** VSDs can result in a large transmission of volume to the pulmonary circulation and LV, leading to pulmonary hypertension and **left heart dilation.** Late in the natural history of this disease, *Eisenmenger syndrome* may occur.
- In the absence of pulmonic stenosis or RVOT obstruction, pulmonary artery systolic pressure (PASP) can be estimated if the systolic blood pressure (SBP) is known $(PASP = SBP - 4V_{VSD}^2)$.

- **Key Point:** *Significant congenital VSD shunt leads to LV, not RV, volume overload.*

Echocardiography

- The PSAX at the AoV level is a key view to differentiate between perimembranous VSD (typically noted between 9 and 12 o'clock) and supracristal VSD (between 12 and 3 o'clock) (Fig. 18-9).
- Muscular VSDs are best seen in the A4C and subcostal views. Because of the complex path of these VSDs, "off-axis" imaging is often required. They may be **easily missed.**
- Evaluate LV dilation, size of defect in systole, gradient across defect, and presence of pulmonary hypertension.
- Perimembranous VSD may be partially covered by the septal TV leaflet, whereas supracristal VSD may be partially covered by an aortic leaflet, leading to valvular regurgitation.
- **Gerbode defect** is a VSD with flow from the LV to RA. The defect occurs in the region between the RA and LV as a result of the more apical location of the septal

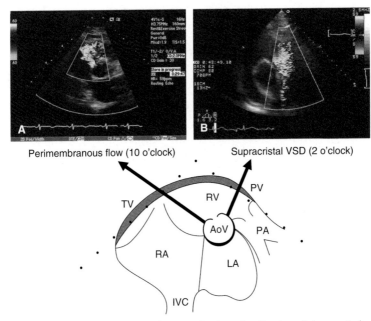

Perimembranous flow (10 o'clock)

Supracristal VSD (2 o'clock)

Figure 18-9. Diagram (bottom) demonstrating how the direction of the ventricular septal defect (VSD) jet in the parasternal short-axis view at the aortic level differentiates between perimembranous VSD (**A**) and supracristal VSD (**B**).

TV leaflet. On TTE, one must be careful not to confuse this flow with the tricuspid regurgitation (TR) jet.
- During VSD evaluation, look for other anomalies commonly associated with VSD, such as patent ductus arteriosis (PDA), ASD, coarctation, tetralogy of Fallot, truncus, and transposition of the great arteries. Of all VSDs, 25–30% occur as isolated defects.
- Postoperatively evaluate the VSD patch for residual shunt.

Patent Ductus Arteriosus
- PDA is defined as persistent patency of the ductus arteriosus (present in fetal circulation) connecting the Ao and main PA.
- It arises from the anterior surface of the proximal descending thoracic Ao, distal to the origin of the left subclavian artery and enters the main PA.
- Most large PDAs are repaired in childhood, and usually unrepaired PDAs seen in adulthood are small and insignificant. Large, unrepaired defects eventually lead to Eisenmenger syndrome.

Hemodynamics
- PDA normally results in **L → R shunting** and **LV volume overload** and has the potential for developing pulmonary hypertension (such as in a VSD).
- **Continuous shunt flow** is seen because of the large pressure difference between the Ao and PA.
- PASP can be estimated if the SBP is known (PASP = SBP – $4V_{PDA}^2$).

Echocardiography
- Identify PDA by color Doppler flow in the PSAX at the level of the AoV with the probe tilted toward the pulmonic valve and main PA.
- Continuous-wave (CW) Doppler through the PDA will identify continuous flow and allows for measurement of peak velocity.
- Evaluate size and gradient across the PDA with identification of flow by color Doppler (Fig. 18-10).
- Evaluate for volume and pressure overload by identifying right ventricular hypertrophy (RVH), LA and LV dilation, and elevated PA pressures.

- **Key Point:** *Best view to identify and measure velocity of PDA flow is PSAX at the level of the AoV with probe tilted toward the pulmonic valve and main PA.*

Endocardial Cushion Defect

- This is defined as a failure of the embryonic endocardial cushions to fuse and form the common AV canal.
- It is a commonly seen defect in trisomy 21.
- Endocardial cushion defects include partial AVCD, complete AVCD, and isolated inlet VSD.
- Abnormalities associated with AVCDs are cleft anterior MV leaflet, inlet VSD, and ostium primum ASD.

Hemodynamics
- Hemodynamics of endocardial cushion defects depend on which components of the defect predominate.
- Combination of ASD and VSD in complete AVSD results in marked volume overload of the pulmonary circulation.
- Abnormalities of AV valves result in significant AV valve regurgitation.

Echocardiography
See Figure 18-11.
- AV valves are on the *same plane* – the TV is NOT apically displaced.
- Evaluate for primum ASD and inlet VSD (A4C).
- Identify a common AV valve connection between the atria and ventricles, with bridging leaflets overriding the IVS and chordal attachments in both ventricles.
- In partial AVCD, the common valve is separated by a ridge of tissue into two AV valve orifices.
- Due to the common valve structure, the MV is *cleft,* most commonly in the anterior leaflet, and may lead to MR.
- LVOT is abnormally elongated ("goose-neck" deformity) and obstruction may be present.
- Evaluate PA pressures and look for the evidence of RVH.
- Identify associated anomalies (PDA, coarctation, hypoplasia of RV and LV).
- Post surgery, evaluate for residual shunts and MR.

OBSTRUCTIONS

Bicuspid AoV

Key Concepts
- Found in 1% to 2% of the population, this is the most common cause of congenital aortic stenosis (AS) (95% of cases). Unicuspid valve is rare.

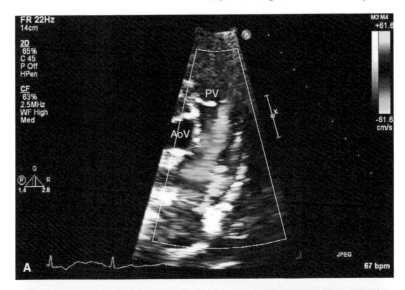

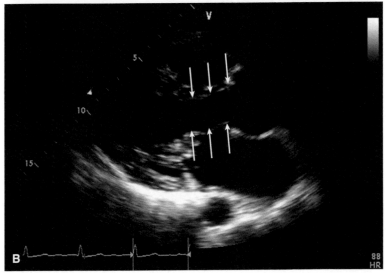

Figure 18-10. A: A zoomed parasternal short-axis view tilted toward the pulmonary vein (PV) and main pulmonary artery shows a high velocity jet directed back toward the probe and PV (red jet) consistent with patent ductus arteriosus flow. **B:** Continuous-wave Doppler shows classic high velocity continuous flow.

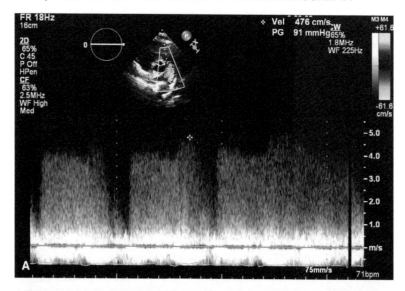

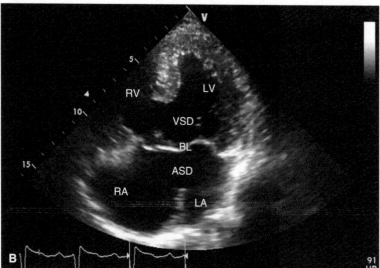

Figure 18-11. Characteristic findings suggestive of atrioventricular canal defect (AVCD). **A:** "Goose-neck" deformity or abnormal elongation of the left ventricular outflow tract seen in the parasternal long-axis view (*arrows*). **B:** Complete AVCD seen in the apical four-chamber view with large primum atrial septal defect (ASD) and inlet ventricular septal defect (VSD) with common bridging atrioventricular leaflets (BL).

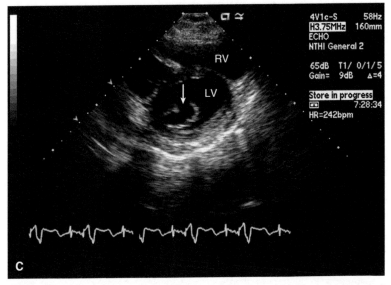

Figure 18-11. (*Continued*) **C:** Parasternal short-axis view showing "cleft" mitral valve (*arrow*) in patient with partial AVCD. LA, left atrium; LV, left ventricle; RA, right atrium; RV, right ventricle.

- Biscuspid AoV occurs as a result of fusion of left and right coronary cusps (70–85%) or fusion of noncoronary and right coronary cusps (15–30%) (Fig. 18-12).
- A raphe, or line of fusion, between the two cusps is often seen and gives the valve a "tricuspid appearance" when viewed in diastole.
- Calcification leads to stenosis (more commonly) or regurgitation.
- Aortic root dilation occurs in up to 50% of patients.
- Commonly associated lesions include coarctation of the Ao and Shone syndrome (multiple left-sided obstructive lesions).

Echocardiography
- Parasternal long-axis (PLAX) view: Shows doming of valve leaflets in systole. Occasionally prolapse and eccentric regurgitation is identified.
- High PLAX: Evaluate for aortic root dilation.
- PSAX: Shows ellipsoid opening in systole. Evaluate for raphe and identify which cusps are fused.
- Suprasternal notch: CW Doppler is used to evaluate proximal descending thoracic Ao for coarctation.
- AS gradients should be evaluated in multiple views due to eccentric opening and aortic jet.

Cor Triatriatum and Congenital Mitral Stenosis (MS)

- Cor triatriatum and congenital MS are very rare congenital disorders that have usually been surgically corrected by adulthood, unless mild in severity (Fig. 18-13).
- Cor triatriatum describes the division of the LA into two chambers (distal chamber where the PVs enter LA and proximal LA and LA appendage).

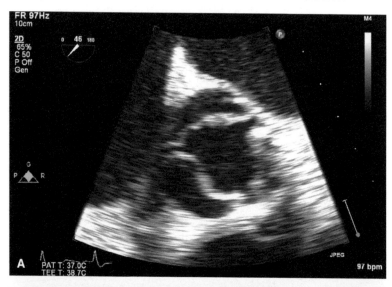

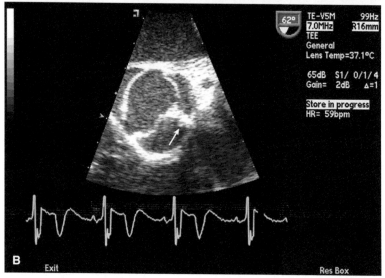

Figure 18-12. Transesophageal echocardiogram short axis of the aortic valve showing normal triangular opening of a tri-leaflet valve (**A**) and ellipsoid opening of a bicuspid valve with fusion of the right and left cusps (raphe seen, *arrow*) (**B**). (**C**) Unicuspid aortic valve with slit-like opening.

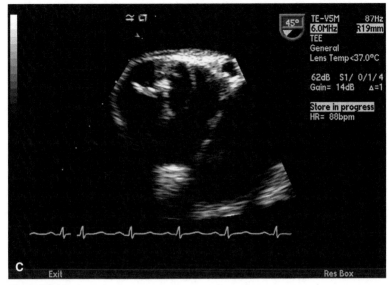

Figure 18-12. (*Continued*)

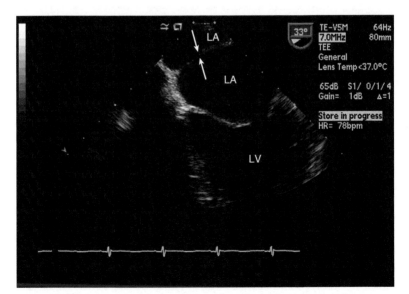

Figure 18-13. Transesophageal echocardiogram "home" view showing cor triatriatum membrane in the left atrium (LA) (*arrows*) separating the pulmonary veins from the proximal LA (mitral valve and LA appendage). LV, left ventricle.

- Congenital MS describes a broad range of disorders causing obstruction at the valvular level that includes parachute MV and double-orifice MV (Fig. 18-14).

Aortic Coarctation

- Congenital obstructive lesion that accounts for 5–8% of congenital heart disease
- Occurs distal to the origin of the left subclavian artery at the site of the aortic ductal attachment (ligamentum arteriosum)
- 50% of patients with coarctation have **bicuspid AoV.**

Hemodynamics
- **Collateral flow often develops via mammary and intercostal arteries** and may mask the severity of obstruction between upper and lower segments.
- Results in **arterial hypertension**

Echocardiography
- Suprasternal notch: CW Doppler of the descending Ao identifies **classic sawtooth flow pattern (elevated peak systolic velocity and persistent diastolic forward flow)** (Fig. 18-15).
- If significant collateralization has developed, peak systolic gradient may only mildly increase.
- Dual velocity envelopes can be seen, representing pre- and post-coarctation blood flow velocities.
- Subcostal: PW Doppler of the abdominal Ao reveals persistent diastolic forward flow.
- Evaluate for associated anomalies (bicuspid AoV, Shone syndrome).

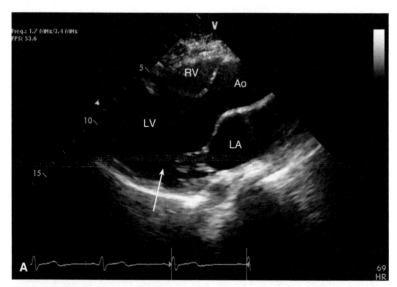

Figure 18-14. Parasternal long-axis view (**A**) and apical four-chamber view (**B**) showing tethering of the mitral leaflet to a single papillary muscle (*arrow*) restricting the opening orifice as seen in (**C**), the parasternal short axis consistent with parachute mitral valve. Ao, aorta; LA, left atrium; LV, left ventricle; RA, right atrium; RV, right ventricle.

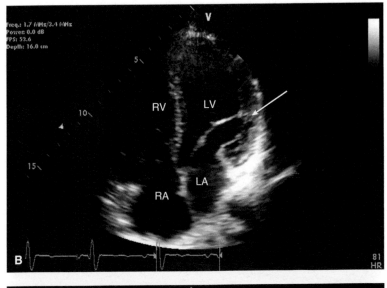

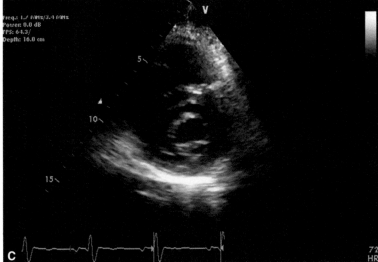

Figure 18-14. (*Continued*)

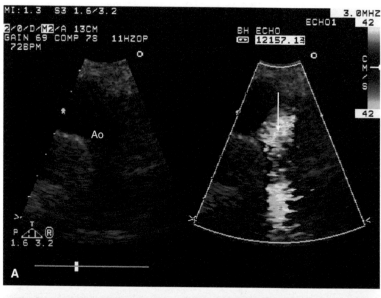

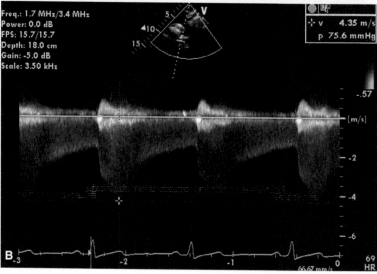

Figure 18-15. A: Suprasternal notch view with turbulence and flow acceleration (*arrow*) secondary to narrowing of the proximal descending aorta (Ao). **B:** Classic "shark-tooth" spectral Doppler demonstrating increased peak velocity and slow diastolic decrease in velocity consistent with aortic coarctation where significant collateral circulation is present.

- Postoperative evaluation may show pericoarctation repair aneurysmal dilation or residual stenosis or recoarctation as evidenced by increased peak velocities and turbulence in the proximal descending thoracic Ao. Diastolic run-off may or may not be seen and is dependent on the presence of collateral flow.

> - **Key Point:** *Shone syndrome describes the presence of multiple left-sided obstructive lesions (congenital MS – parachute MV and/or supravalvular membrane; AS – subvalvular, valvular, or supravalvular; aortic coarctation).*

TRANSPOSITION OF THE GREAT ARTERIES (TGA)

D-TGA

- D-TGA is defined as abnormal **ventricular–arterial connection** with preserved AV concordance.
- The AV valve always *stays with its ventricle* (TV is always associated with RV; MV is always associated with LV).

Hemodynamics/Physiology

1. Prerepair

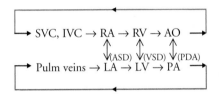

- A **parallel circulation** is formed with two closed circuits:
  - The systemic circuit: Venous blood returns from the IVC/superior vena cava (SVC) to the RV and then recirculates through the Ao and systemic circulation back to the IVC/SVC.
  - The pulmonic circuit: Oxygenated blood returns from the PVs to the LV and then recirculates in the pulmonary circulation back to the PVs.
- **Survival prior to surgery is dependent on the presence of a shunt** (ASD, VSD, PDA) that allows mixing of systemic and pulmonary blood.

2. Post repair—*atrial switch – Mustard or Senning*

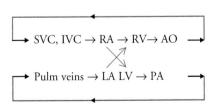

- *Atrial switch* procedures involve creation of a tunnel or **baffle** to redirect blood from the RA → LV and LA→RV, connecting the ventricles *in series*. **The RV remains the systemic ventricle.**

- Postoperative complications include baffle malfunction (leaks and stenoses) and systemic ventricular failure.

3. Post repair—*arterial switch*

```
        ┌─────────────────────────────◄──────────────────────┐
        │                                                     │
        └──► Pulm veins → LA → LV → AO ──► SVC, IVC → RA → RV → PA ──►
```

- The more recent and preferred Jatene *arterial switch* procedure allows for complete anatomic and physiologic correction. **The LV is now the systemic ventricle**.
- The Ao and PAs are excised from their native roots and reimplanted on the opposite roots respectively (i.e., pulmonary native root becomes neoaortic root and aortic native root becomes neopulmonic root).
- The coronary arteries are reimplanted into the neoaortic root.
- Postoperative complications include ostial coronary artery stenosis, narrowing of the RVOT, and supravalvular AS and pulmonic stenosis (PS).

Echocardiography—Post Repair
- Great artery positioning: Normally the PA is anterior and perpendicular to the Ao, but in D-TGA the great arteries are parallel with the Ao located anteriorly and rightward.
- PLAX view is used to evaluate for possible baffle leaks and stenosis using color, PW Doppler and agitated saline injection.
- PSAX view is used to evaluate for Ao located anteriorly and rightward ("D" for "dextro") to the centrally located PA (Fig. 18-16).
- A4C is a useful view to evaluate for possible baffle leaks and stenosis as detailed previously (Fig. 18-17).
- In patients with *atrial switch procedures,* evaluate for dilation/dysfunction of the pressure-overloaded systemic RV.
- Evaluate for residual shunts (ASD, VSD, or PDA) with color Doppler.
- Patients with *arterial switch procedures* can be difficult to distinguish from normal patients. Focal "brightness" may be seen at the anastomosis site of the great arteries (just superior to outflow valves). Evaluate for supravalvular AS and LV regional wall motion abnormalities secondary to coronary artery ostial stenosis.

L-TGA (congenitally corrected transposition)

- **Ventricular–arterial discordance** and **AV discordance.** The morphologic RV and associated TV are located under the LA on the left side of the heart, whereas the morphologic LV with associated MV are located under the RV on the right side of the heart.
- Ao arises from the **morphologic RV (systemic ventricle)** and is parallel, anterior, and leftward ("L" = Levo) of the PA.
- The AV valve always *stays with its ventricle* (TV is always associated with RV; MV is always associated with LV).
- These patients often have not had any corrective surgical procedures.

Hemodynamics
- Although there is ventricular inversion, normal blood flow through the systemic and pulmonic circulatory systems is preserved.

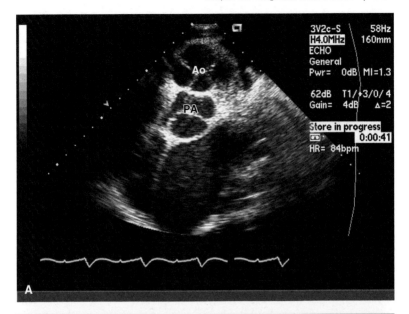

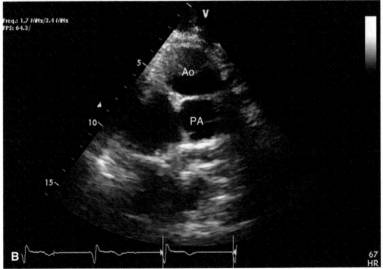

Figure 18-16. Parasternal short-axis view demonstrating (**A**) congenitally corrected transposition of the great arteries with the aorta (Ao) anterior and toward the left side of the patient compared to the pulmonary artery (PA), and (**B**) complete transposition of the great arteries with the Ao anterior and toward the right side of the patient compared to the PA.

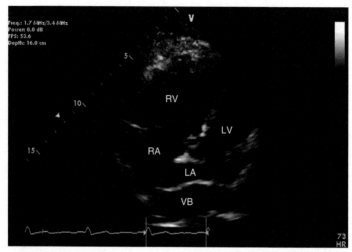

Figure 18-17. Apical four-chamber view in patient with complete transposition of the great arteries with history of atrial switch surgery. The venous baffle (VB) can be seen directing blood from the right atrium (RA) to the pulmonic ventricle (morphologic left ventricle [LV]). LA, left atrium; RV, right ventricle.

Echocardiography

- A4C: Identify the morphologic RV by the apically displaced TV, trabeculations, and moderator band.
- PLAX and PSAX: Identify Ao arising from the morphologic RV. It is parallel (PLAX), anterior and leftward (PSAX) (L = Levo) of the PA.
- Evaluate size and function of the pressure-overloaded systemic RV.

TETRALOGY OF FALLOT

Tetrad of defining features (Fig. 18-18):
1. RVH
2. VSD
3. Overriding Ao
4. Sub-PS or PS

Hemodynamics

- **VSD is usually large and nonrestrictive.** Patients **rarely develop pulmonary hypertension,** as sub-PS and/or PS protects pulmonary circuit.
- The greater the degree of the Ao overriding septum, the greater the degree of pulmonic obstruction.

Surgical Repair

- Most adults will have had either palliative or reparative surgery.
- *Palliative surgeries* are designed to **augment pulmonary blood flow** (which is markedly reduced by PS) and allow normal PA development prior to reparative surgery. These include:

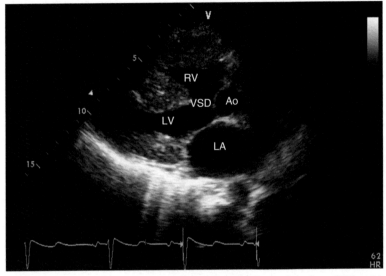

Figure 18-18. Parasternal long-axis view of a patient with unrepaired tetralogy of Fallot with large nonrestrictive ventricular septal defect (VSD), overriding aorta (Ao), and marked left ventricular (LV) and right ventricular (RV) hypertrophy. LA, left atrium.

- Blalock–Taussig shunt—subclavian artery to PA anastomosis
- Waterston shunt—ascending Ao to main or right PA anastomosis
- Potts shunt—descending Ao to left PA anastomosis
- *Reparative surgery* involves patch closure of the VSD and relief of PS.
- A variety of options to relieve subpulmonic obstruction are available, depending on the clinical presentation and anatomy. These may involve resection of subpulmonic muscle bundles, subpulmonic or transannular patch, PV valvotomy or replacement (homograft or bioprosthetic), or Rastelli procedure (conduit from RV to PA).
- Transannular patch repair results in severe pulmonary regurgitation (PR) with accompanying RV volume overload and failure. A limited patch repair with the "trade-off" of residual stenosis may also be performed.
- Common late postoperative complications include severe PR with RV dilation and failure as well as residual or recurrent PS. LV dysfunction, usually mild, may also occur as a late complication.
- Patients with persistent palliative shunts are prone to develop pulmonary hypertension.

Echocardiography

- PLAX and PSAX: Evaluate for stenosis or regurgitation of the pulmonary valve/conduit with color flow and CW Doppler.
- A4C: Evaluate size and function of LV and RV. Also evaluate RV for the evidence of pressure or volume overload.

TRUNCUS ARTERIOSUS

- Origin of single great artery from the heart giving rise to both PA and Ao
- Absence of pulmonary valve
- Cardiac anatomy similar to tetralogy of Fallot with large perimembranous VSD and overriding great vessel
- The "truncal" valve often dysplastic with varying degrees of cusp stenosis and insufficiency
- Commonly associated lesions: interrupted aortic arch or coarctation of the Ao

Surgical Repair

- Separation of PAs from Ao with placement of an extracardiac conduit from RV to PA with VSD closure
- Common postoperative complications: stenosis and regurgitation of truncal and conduit valves, pulmonary hypertension, ventricular dysfunction, residual VSD, branch PA stenosis

Echocardiography

- PLAX: Aortic root often enlarged and not necessarily pathologic
- PSAX, used to evaluate:
  - Pulmonary conduit stenosis/regurgitation
  - For branch PA stenosis with color, CW, and serial PW Doppler
  - Morphology and function of truncal valve
- A4C, used to evaluate:
  - Biventricular function
  - For truncal valve stenosis or regurgitation
  - For the evidence of pulmonary hypertension
- Suprasternal notch: Evaluate for associated coarctation of the Ao
- Evaluate for evidence of residual VSD

EBSTEIN ANOMALY

- This is defined as an abnormality of the TV in which the septal and posterior leaflets are markedly apically displaced and the anterior leaflet is elongated ("sail-like") and attached to the RV free wall.
- TV coaptation is apically displaced, causing significant regurgitation and "atrialization" of the RV.
- It is typically associated with interatrial communication (e.g., ASD, patent foramen ovale [PFO]).
- Surgical repair, when appropriate, includes reconstruction or replacement of the TV.

Hemodynamics

- Most patients have at least moderate TR secondary to leaflet malcoaptation.
- Right heart failure may be due to the small RV with diminished filling and contractile capacity as well as significant TR.
- Associated ASD/PFO allows for R → L shunting, which leads to hypoxemia when right heart pressures are elevated.

Echocardiography

- A4C:
  - Apical displacement of TV compared to MV >0.8 cm/m^2 (indexed to body surface area)
  - Assess leaflet mobility, attachments of anterior leaflet to RV free wall
  - Assess TR severity and pulmonary pressures
  - Assess size and function of nonatrialized RV
- Identify the presence and direction of interatrial shunts

FONTAN PROCEDURE FOR SINGLE VENTRICLE PHYSIOLOGY

- This is a palliative procedure for children with single ventricle physiology (e.g., hypoplastic LV or RV, TV atresia). Figure 18-19 shows short-axis view of Fontan conduit in a case of hypoplastic right heart.
- The procedure is performed in two stages. Initially blood from the SVC is directed to the PAs, which have been surgically disconnected from the subpulmonic ventricle (bi-directional Glenn procedure). In the final stage, the IVC blood is also directed to the PAs, resulting in total caval flow bypassing the subpulmonic ventricle (Fontan completion). This may be done via direct connection of the RA to the PA, or more commonly via a tunneled or extracardiac prosthetic conduit. A fenestration may be placed in the conduit to augment cardiac output at the expense of some R → L shunting and desaturation.

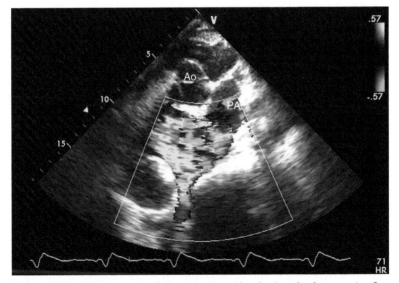

Figure 18-19. Off-axis parasternal short-axis view with color Doppler demonstrating flow in the Fontan conduit, behind the left atrium, directing caval blood to the pulmonary artery (PA). Ao, aorta.

- Common cardiovascular complications include arrhythmias, pulmonary arteriovenous malformations (AVMs), ventricular dysfunction, baffle leaks, and thrombus formation.

Echocardiography

- The Fontan conduit is best visualized in the subcostal location.
- Fontan flow is low velocity, venous flow.
- Subcostal view:
  - Dilated hepatic or IVC veins suggest elevated Fontan pressures and/or Fontan obstruction.
  - Both two-dimensional and color flow and spectral Doppler should be used to assess for conduit obstruction. The color scale should be lowered to adequately assess disturbances in the low velocity flow.
- A4C view:
  - The Fontan conduit can often be visualized coursing posterior to the RA or within in the posterior portion of the RA (in the case of a lateral tunnel conduit).
  - Color flow and spectral Doppler can be used to assess the presence of fenestration and estimation of pulmonary pressures.
  - Evaluate ventricular and valvular function.
  - Assess IAS for presence of residual shunt
- Saline contrast bubble study can be performed to assess for intrapulmonary AVMs.

Cardiac Masses

Justin S. Sadhu

ARTIFACTS

- Interactions of ultrasound waves with matter and the subsequent processing of the reflected waves may produce artifacts that give the appearance of masses within the heart.
- Imaging from multiple planes, interrogation with color Doppler, and contrast administration can be helpful where artifacts are suspected; however, use of alternative imaging modalities may be needed to exclude important pathology.
- Examples of common ultrasound artifacts are shown in Figure 19-1.
- *Side-lobe artifact:* These secondary, oblique "lobes" of ultrasound energy occur off the main beam axis. In general, because of the lower energy of the side lobes, this does not commonly affect the image that is displayed. However, when there is a bright reflector (e.g., catheter, wire, or pericardium) detected by the side lobe, the reflected wave may occasionally be misassigned to the central beam and projected in the echo-free spaces of the heart or its surroundings.
- *Reverberations:* These secondary reflections occur when the ultrasound beam meets two parallel highly reflective surfaces. The returning ultrasound wave may be reflected between the two surfaces multiple times before returning to the transducer. The delay in detection of the returning wave is interpreted as a greater distance from the probe to the matter that was detected. This artifact may be displayed as a trail of bright echoes behind the reflector (e.g., mechanical valve) or as a distinct duplication of the reflector (e.g., duplicate mitral valve [MV] or posterior pericardium seen in echo-free space posterior to the heart), often at a multiple of the true distance from the ultrasound probe.

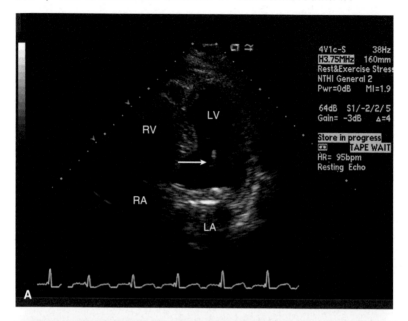

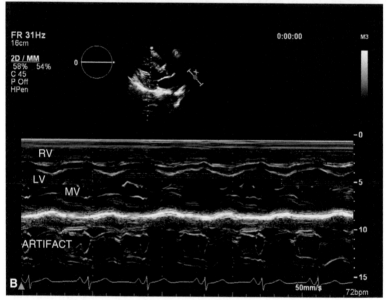

Figure 19-1. Ultrasound artifacts. **A:** Side-lobe artifact places the image of the right ventricular (RV) pacing wire in the left ventricle (LV) (*arrow*). Note reverberation artifact below mechanical mitral valve (MV). **B:** Parasternal long-axis (PLAX) M-mode shows duplication artifact of MV in the echo-free space behind the LV.

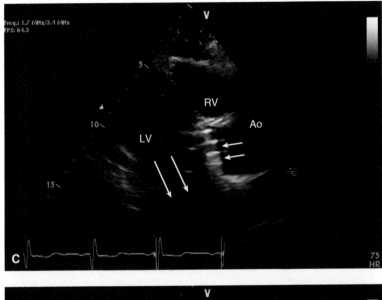

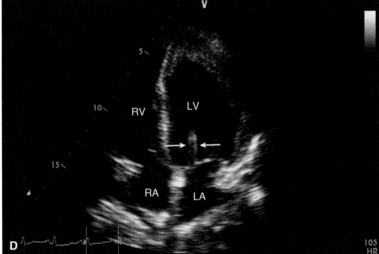

Figure 19-1. (*Continued*) **C:** PLAX in patient with mechanical bileaflet valve in the aortic position exhibiting shadowing or attenuation artifact (*long arrows*) as well as reverberation (*short arrows*). **D:** Comet-tail artifact (*arrows*) in patient with pleural effusions and pulmonary edema (note apical thrombus secondary to hypereosinophilic syndrome). Ao, aorta; LA, left atrium; RA, right atrium.

- *"Comet-tail" artifact:* This is a form of reverberation where the two reflective surfaces are closely spaced, leading to a series of microreflections displayed as a triangular band, or "comet-tail," extending from the object. This may be seen with very strong reflectors (e.g., metal or calcification) or at the interface between two materials with marked difference in acoustic impedance (i.e., tissue and fluid, such as with ascites or pleural effusions).
- *Ring-down artifact:* Also known as "near field clutter," this occurs when high amplitude oscillations are produced by the transducer. It usually appears as a thrombus in the LV apex in the apical four-chamber (A4C) views.
- *Shadowing/attenuation:* When the majority of ultrasound energy is reflected back to the transducer because of a strong reflector, there is "shadowing" of the structures behind the reflector. This area is displayed as an echo-free space. This may give an appearance of a hypoechoic mass (e.g., thrombus) and requires the use of additional views to find a path that is not "blocked" by the strong reflector to interrogate the area of interest. Prosthetic valves and heavily calcified structures are common sources of shadowing artifact.

- **Key Points:**
  1. *Echocardiographic artifacts may arise from the interaction of ultrasound waves with tissue and the way in which reflected waves are processed to produce an image.*
  2. *All suspected masses should ideally be visualized in more than one plane.*
  3. *Use color flow Doppler and/or IV contrast to evaluate whether a mass is artifactual.*

NORMAL VARIANTS AND PATHOLOGIC VARIATIONS IN NORMAL STRUCTURES

Normal Variants

- **LV false tendons:** These are fibromuscular bands that extend across the LV and may attach to the septum, free wall, and/or the papillary muscles (Fig. 19-2A). They may be distinguished from other structures by an echo-free space seen on both sides of the false tendon.
- **Moderator band:** Defined as a muscular band that contains conduction tissue and extends across the right ventricle (RV) from the septum to the base of the papillary muscles of the RV. In addition, RV trabeculations (unlike LV trabeculations) are normal structures seen at the RV apex.
- Prominent or calcified **papillary muscles** of the MV or tricuspid valve
- **Crista terminalis:** Defined as a vertical ridge of smooth myocardium in the posterior right atrium (RA) that divides the smooth muscle of the RA from the trabeculated RA appendage. It extends from the orifice of the superior vena cava to the right side of the valve of the inferior vena cava (IVC). It may be visualized on A4C views and can be mistaken for a RA mass. The crista terminalis may play a role in RA arrhythmias.
- **Eustachian valve:** This is a valve flap at the distal end of the IVC that directs blood into the RA and toward the interatrial septum. When prominent and filamentous, it is called a **Chiari network** (see Fig. 19-2B). Presence of a Chiari network may be associated with patent foramen ovale, atrial septal aneurysm, and paradoxical embolism.
- **"Coumadin ridge":** This prominent fold of tissue separates the left superior pulmonary vein and the left atrial (LA) appendage and may be confused on transesophageal echocardiography with a thrombus.

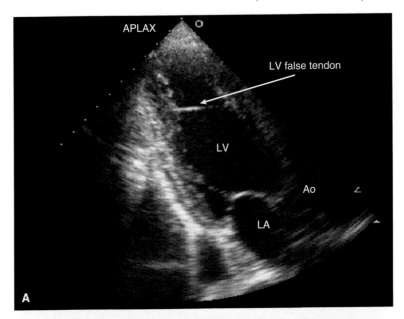

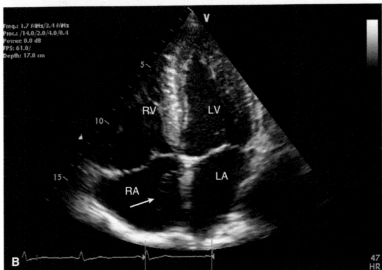

Figure 19-2. A: Apical parasternal long-axis (APLAX) view with bright linear echodensity seen in distal left ventricle (LV) consistent with false tendon. **B:** Apical four-chamber view with bright, echodense, webbed network seen in right atrium (RA) consistent with a Chiari network (*arrow*). Ao, aorta; LA, left atrium; RV, right ventricle.

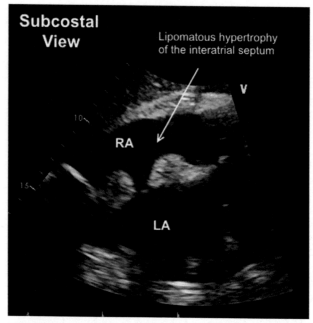

Figure 19-3. Subcostal view showing the typical "dumbbell" appearance of lipomatous interatrial septal hypertrophy. LA, left atrium; RA, right atrium.

Pathologic Variations in Normal Structures

- **Dense mitral annular calcification**
- **Lipomatous infiltration/hypertrophy of the interatrial septum** (Fig. 19-3): Benign fatty deposits that spare the fossa ovalis, producing a characteristic "dumbbell" shape with narrow central waist; most often seen in older adults
- **Epicardial fat:** Echo-lucent space between the outer myocardium and the visceral pericardium; may be mistaken for a pericardial effusion
- **LV trabeculations:** Recesses within the LV wall that may be seen with dilated cardiomyopathies or LV noncompaction; contrast may be needed to distinguish trabeculations from complex thrombi
- **Lambl's excrescences:** Filiform strands (typically small, linear, mobile, homogeneous, echo-dense structures <1 cm) that originate at valve closure sites, most often on the aortic valve (AoV) and MV; usually thought of as a normal variant (found in 40–50% of adults). Associated embolism has been reported, but a true causal relationship remains controversial. When large and associated with embolism, examine carefully to rule out a papillary fibroelastoma.

- **Key Points:**
  1. *Normal variants: LV false tendons, moderator band, crista terminalis, Eustachian valve, Chiari network, coumadin ridge.*
  2. *Pathologic structures: dense mitral annular calcification, lipomatous hypertrophy of the interatrial septum, epicardial fat, LV trabeculations, Lambl's excrescence.*

TRUE CARDIAC MASSES

Thrombus

- Intracardiac thrombi may be one of two varieties: **thrombus in situ** or **thrombus in transit**.
- Fresh thrombus is homogenous, has irregular borders, and often has mobile components.
- Old thrombus can be more calcified and is generally less mobile.
- **In situ thrombus occurs at sites of low flow.**
  - In the LA, this occurs most often in the LA appendage, best viewed in the apical two-chamber (A2C) view and in the parasternal short-axis view at the level between the MVs and AoVs. However, the LA appendage is difficult to visualize adequately with a transthoracic approach, and transesophageal examination is required if clinical suspicion of thrombus is high.
  - In the LV, thrombus is found almost exclusively at the site of a wall motion abnormality. This can be an akinetic, dyskinetic, or aneurysmal segment resulting from any etiology (infarction, nonischemic cardiomyopathy, myocarditis, etc.). An exception to this general rule is Loeffler endocarditis (i.e., **eosinophilic myocarditis**), where LV or RV thrombi may occur without a corresponding wall motion abnormality (see Fig. 19-1D). Scanning across the apex in multiple, nonforeshortened views and using IV contrast increases sensitivity and specificity for detecting thrombi (Fig. 19-4). Contrast enhancement is also important to distinguish an apical thrombus from **apical–variant hypertrophic cardiomyopathy** (Fig. 19-5).

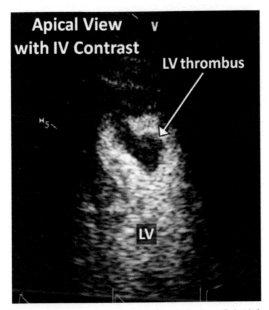

Figure 19-4. Zoomed contrast enhanced view of the left ventricular (LV) apex showing an echolucent pedunculated mass consistent with thrombus.

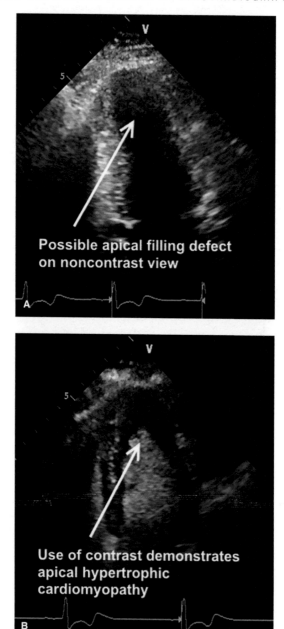

Figure 19-5. A: Noncontrast apical view suspicious for an apical filling defect. **B:** After administration of contrast, apical hypertrophy is readily appreciated.

- In situ thrombi in the RA and RV are less common, but may occur at the site of instrumentation and have also been described with Behçet disease. Giant RA thrombi may occur in patients with a history of univentricular congenital heart disease status post-Fontan operation.
- Thrombus can also occur on foreign bodies in any chamber (e.g., valve prostheses, catheters, pacing wires).
- **Thrombus in transit is typically due to deep venous thrombus that migrates toward the pulmonary arteries or across an interatrial shunt.** In a patient with a known pulmonary embolus, thrombus in transit may be an indication for thrombolytics or thrombectomy (Fig. 19-6).

Vegetations

- **Vegetations can be infectious or noninfectious,** and are typically irregularly shaped and **attached to the upstream side of the valve** (e.g., atrial side of the MV and ventricular side of the AoV).
- Noninfectious vegetations occur as a result of formation of sterile platelet and fibrin thrombi on cardiac valves in response to trauma, circulating immune complexes, vasculitis, or a hypercoagulable state.
  - Libman–Sacks lesions: These are verrucous masses associated with systemic lupus erythematosus and antiphospholipid antibodies. They typically have irregular borders, heterogeneous echodensity, and no independent motion, and they most

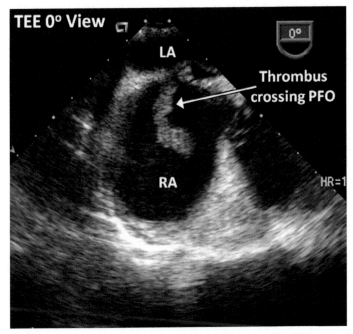

Figure 19-6. An upper-esophageal transesophageal echocardiographic (TEE) view of the right atrium (RA) showing a thrombus in transit crossing the interatrial septum. LA, left atrium; PFO, patent foramen ovale.

often involve the basal or mid portions of the MV and AoV. Diffuse valve thickening can be observed and represents the chronic healed phase of the disease process. These are most often clinically silent, but emboli and valvular abnormalities (usually regurgitation) can occur.

- **Infectious vegetations** may be bacterial or fungal and are **frequently associated with valvular regurgitation** (see Chapter 14).

Tumors

- In the case of a suspected tumor, it is important to describe the mass and also investigate any associated hemodynamic significance.
  - **Pericardial tumors can cause pericarditis or pericardial effusion,** impair ventricular filling, and lead to cardiac tamponade.
  - **Intracavitary tumors can impair normal flow** through the heart and produce the same obstructive physiology as valvular stenosis.
  - Extracardiac tumors (such as mediastinal masses) can also displace normal structures and may impair normal intracardiac flow.

Benign Tumors

- **Myxomas** account for the majority of benign cardiac tumors. These are most often single masses that arise from the fossa ovalis of the interatrial septum and protrude into the **LA (75% of cases),** but they can also be seen in the RA, LV, or RV. The Carney complex is an autosomal dominant disorder that may be associated with multiple myxomas. Myxomas have the following characteristics:
  - Often are heterogeneous and have an irregular shape
  - Often are asymptomatic—found incidentally on imaging—but can embolize, be associated with constitutional symptoms, or cause symptoms of right or left heart failure as a result of significant impairment of ventricular filling (i.e., "pseudo mitral stenosis") (Fig. 19-7).
- **Papillary fibroelastomas** are the most common primary tumors of the cardiac valves. They may be seen on either side of the MV and AoV, although they can also be subvalvular or rarely attached to the ventricular free wall. They are usually <1 cm in diameter, typically pedunculated with high-frequency oscillations during the cardiac cycle, and may appear "frondlike" (have a stippled/shimmering edge). Papillary fibroelastomas have been associated with cardioembolic events (Fig. 19-8).
- Other benign cardiac tumors include fibromas, lipomas, rhabdomyomas, and hemangiomas.

Malignant Tumors

- **Secondary cardiac tumors are far more common than primary cardiac tumors. A cardiac mass in a patient with known malignancy should raise the suspicion of metastatic disease.**
- Tumors can involve the heart through direct extension, hematogenous spread, lymphatic spread, or intracavitary extension from the IVC.
- Cardiac involvement from metastatic malignancies most often involves the pericardium and epicardium, presenting as pericardial effusion (Fig. 19-9). Other signs of cardiac involvement include arrhythmias, elevated cardiac biomarkers, and ST-T wave changes on electrocardiogram.
  - **Lung, breast, and hematologic malignancies** comprise the majority of cardiac metastases.
  - **Melanoma** has the highest rate of pericardial metastases.

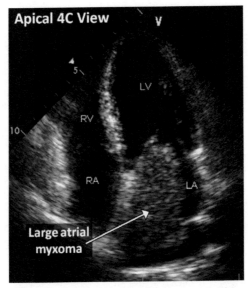

Figure 19-7. Apical four-chamber view showing a large obstructing left atrial (LA) myxoma extending from the interatrial septum and filling the mitral valve inflow area. LV, left ventricle; RA, right atrium; RV, right ventricle.

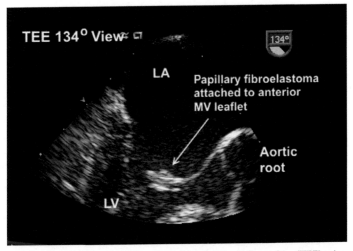

Figure 19-8. Midesophageal transesophageal echocardiographic (TEE) view demonstrating a sessile, frondlike mass attached to the anterior leaflet of the mitral valve (MV) in a patient with recurrent cerebrovascular accident (CVA)/transient ischemic attack (TIA). Surgical pathology confirmed papillary fibroelastoma. LA, left atrium; LV, left ventricle.

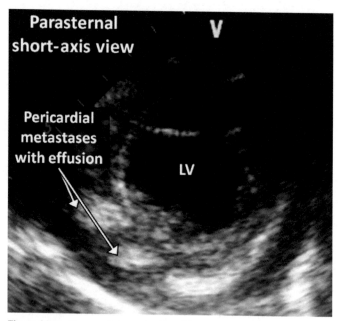

Figure 19-9. Parasternal short-axis view of the left ventricle (LV) showing bright ovoid echodensities in the pericardial space found to be metastatic breast cancer.

- **Renal cell carcinoma** (and less commonly uterine leiomyoma or hepatocellular carcinoma) **can extend from the kidney up through the IVC** and into the RA. The tumor can appear similar to a thrombus in transit (Fig. 19-10).
- Primary malignant tumors of the heart are exceptionally rare and are most often sarcomas. These are usually intramural, may involve any cardiac chamber, grow rapidly, and are destructive (can even cause myocardial rupture). They are associated with a high mortality.

Establishing a Differential Diagnosis

When an intracardiac mass is seen, providing a full description is the most important step to developing a differential diagnosis. That description should include the following:

- **Location:** Where is the mass attached (pericardial, intramural, intracavitary, interatrial septal, valvular)?
- **Mobility:** Mobile/pedunculated versus sessile (fixed, with a broad base), independent versus dependent movement with cardiac cycle.
- **Visual appearance:** Solid versus hollow, homogeneous versus heterogeneous, echogenic (bright) versus echolucent (dark), irregular versus regular borders, linear versus globular.

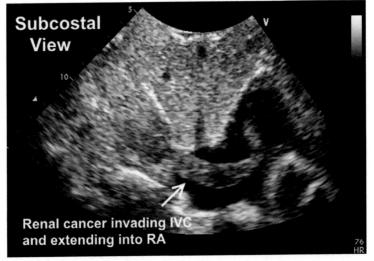

Figure 19-10. Off-axis subcostal view that demonstrates a large serpiginous mass extending from the inferior vena cava (IVC) into the right atrium (RA); this represented direct intravenous extension from a renal adenocarcinoma.

- **Effect on other structures:** Impairment in chamber filling, valvular stenosis, or regurgitation.

- **Key Points:**
  1. *Thrombi usually occur in areas of low flow—for example, adjacent to an akinetic LV wall.*
  2. *Vegetations are typically located on the upstream side of the valve.*
  3. *A cardiac mass in a patient with known malignancy should raise the suspicion of metastatic disease.*
  4. *Assess tumors for size, shape, and physiologic significance (i.e., disruption of flow, displacement of normal structures).*
  5. *Describe the location, mobility, appearance, and effect on other structures of the mass to help develop a differential diagnosis.*

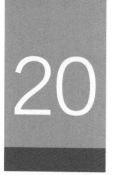

20 Cardiac Manifestations of Systemic Illness

Justin Hartupee and Justin M. Vader

Amyloidosis
- Biventricular hypertrophy
- Electrocardiogram voltage lower than expected for degree of hypertrophy on imaging
- Granular, "sparkling" pattern of myocardium
- Valvular thickening and insufficiency
- Interatrial septal thickening
- Apical sparing of longitudinal strain

Carcinoid
- Right heart valvulopathy
- Thickened, club-like appearance of tricuspid valve (TV) and pulmonary valve (PV) with regurgitation>>stenosis
- Subcostal views: may show liver metastases

Hypereosinophilic syndrome
- LV involvement normally in apex and inflow areas
- Apical obliteration with fibrosis and thrombus
- Papillary muscle involvement: possible cause of significant mitral regurgitation (MR) secondary to tethering

Marfan syndrome
- "Pear-shaped" aortic root with dilation of sinuses and effacement of sinotubular junction
- Aortic dissection
- Mitral valve (MV) prolapse

Sarcoidosis
- Focal "bite"-like aneurysms of basal septum, lateral, and inferior walls
- Valvular thickening
- Pulmonary hypertension

Scleroderma
- Pericardial effusion
- Pulmonary hypertension with right ventricular (RV) failure

Systemic lupus erythematosus
- Libman–Sacks endocarditis
- Pericarditis
- Pericardial effusion
- Myocarditis

Radiation-induced cardiac disease
- Generalized valvular thickening
- Pericardial effusion
- Constrictive pericarditis
- Restrictive cardiomyopathy

Cancer therapeutics-related cardiac dysfunction
- Drop in left ventricular ejection fraction (LVEF) ≥10% (asymptomatic) or 5% (symptomatic)
- Changes in longitudinal strain precede fall in EF

AMYLOIDOSIS

Classifications

Primary (AL)
- Most common form: Plasma cell dyscrasia results in light-chain protein deposition.
- Typical age of onset is >40 years.

- Multiple organs typically are involved. Cardiac involvement is common (approximately 1/3 to 1/2 of cases).
- Mean survival is ~4 months after development of heart failure.

Secondary (AA)
- Amyloid fibrils result from accumulation of acute phase reactant, serum amyloid A.
- This classification is secondary to underlying chronic inflammatory conditions.
- Cardiac involvement is uncommon and rarely significant.

Familial (ATTR)
- ATTR is secondary to autosomal dominant mutation of transthyretin.
- Cardiac and peripheral nerve involvement is common.
- Age of onset varies, from 30s to 70s.

Senile
- This type is age-related, secondary to accumulation of wild-type transthyretin.
- Onset is usually >70 years.
- This classification can have significant cardiac involvement.

Atrial (AANF)
- This type is related to age and valvulopathy.
- Protein is atrial natriuretic peptide and released in response to wall stretch.

Hemodialysis
- In long-term hemodialysis patients, this is related to accumulation of β2-microglobulin.

Echocardiographic Findings (Fig. 20-1)
- Early manifestations include progressive diastolic dysfunction and increasing biventricular wall thickness.
- The LV cavity is normal to slightly reduced in size, although it may become dilated late in the disease.
- A granular **"sparkling"** pattern may be noted in the myocardium (see Fig. 20-1):
  - This is not specific for cardiac amyloidosis with harmonic imaging and can be seen in severe hypertensive heart disease, hypertrophic cardiomyopathy, and glycogen storage disease.
- Amyloid deposits on cardiac valves with **valvular thickening and insufficiency** are likely.
- Advanced cardiac involvement from amyloid may show LV dilation, LV failure, restrictive diastolic pattern, biventricular thickening, **atrial septal thickening** (specific for amyloid), bi-atrial dilation, and pericardial effusion.
- May be characterized by restrictive mitral filling pattern with markedly reduced mitral annular peak velocities.
- Speckle-tracking derived longitudinal strain imaging often demonstrates preserved apical longitudinal strain and reduced strain in the basal segments (Fig. 20-2).

- **Key Points:**
  1. *Atrial septal thickening is specific for cardiac amyloidosis in the correct clinical context.*
  2. *Impaired basal segment longitudinal strain with preserved apical strain should prompt consideration of cardiac amyloidosis.*

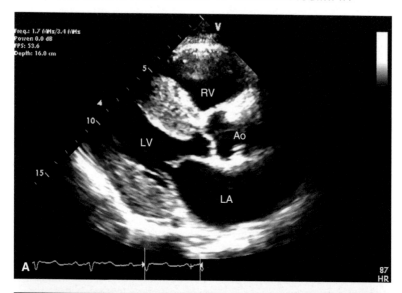

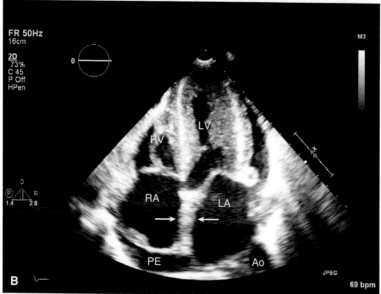

Figure 20-1. Patient with amyloid heart disease. (**A**) Parasternal long-axis view and apical four-chamber view (**B**) show biatrial enlargement marked left ventricular hypertrophy (LVH) with "granular" appearance as well as interatrial septal infiltration (*arrows*).

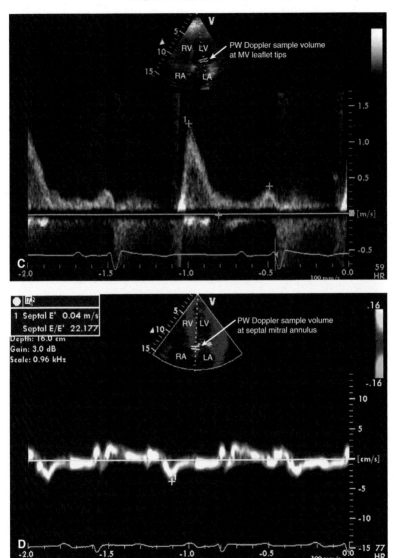

Figure 20-1. (*Continued*) (**C**) Restrictive mitral inflow pattern and marked reduction in peak tissue Doppler velocity (**D**) of the mitral annulus. Ao, aorta; LA, left atrium; LV, left ventricle; MV, mitral valve; PE, pericardial effusion; PW, pulsed wave; RA, right atrium; RV, right ventricle.

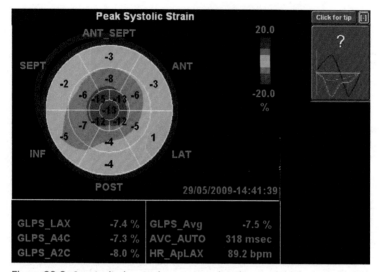

Figure 20-2. Longitudinal strain demonstrates relatively preserved left ventricular (LV) apical strain with abnormal strain of the LV mid and basal segments.

CARCINOID

Background

- Slow-growing neuroendocrine tumor often arises from enterochromaffin cells in the gastrointestinal tract.
- Cardiac involvement occurs following metastasis to the liver and exposure of the heart to active substances such as serotonin and bradykinin.
- Generally symptoms are **limited to the right heart** as the lungs clear carcinoid-related substances.
- Left-sided involvement can be seen when there is an interatrial communication (i.e., patent foramen ovale or atrial septal defect).

Echocardiographic Findings

- Carcinoid substances often cause valvular thickening and restricted leaflet movement resulting in a **"club"-like appearance of the leaflets** (Fig. 20-3).
- This in turn results in severe tricuspid regurgitation (TR) and possibly even tricuspid stenosis.
- The pulmonic valve may be similarly affected.
- These valvular changes lead to RV volume overload and eventually failure.
- Subcostal views may reveal liver metastases.
  - Check for hepatic vein systolic flow reversal in this view as a marker of severe TR.

- **Key Points:**
  1. *Left-sided valvulopathy may occur in a patient with carcinoid disease if an intracardiac right-to-left shunt is present.*
  2. *Look for markedly thickened and restricted TV leaflets with possible PV involvement.*

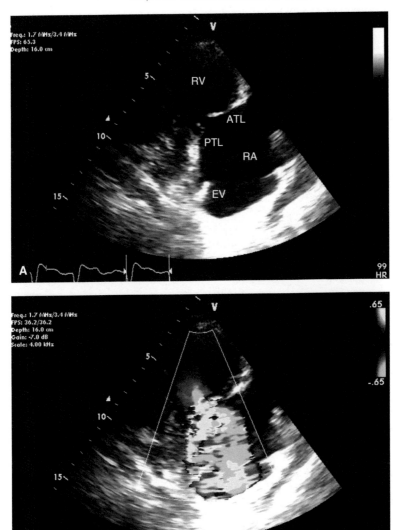

Figure 20-3. Patient with carcinoid heart disease. (**A**) Parasternal right ventricular (RV) inflow view shows shortened, thickened, "club-like" posterior (PTL) and anterior (ATL) tricuspid valve leaflets with severe tricuspid regurgitation (TR) seen on color Doppler (**B**). (*continued*)

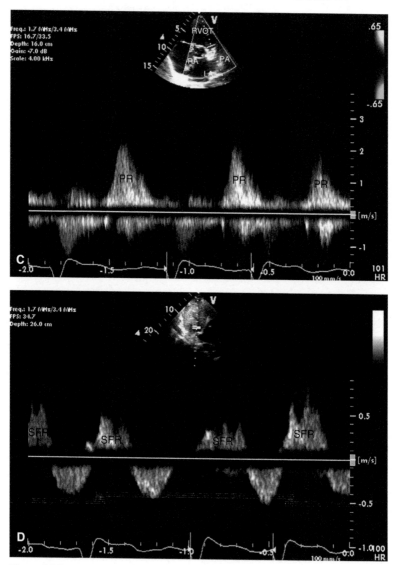

Figure 20-3. (*Continued*) (**C**) Continuous-wave Doppler across the pulmonic valve in the parasternal short-axis view shows a dense, diastolic jet with a short deceleration time consistent with severe pulmonary regurgitation (PR). (**D**) Hepatic Doppler exhibits systolic flow reversal suggestive of severe TR. EV, eustachian valve; LA, left atrium; PA, pulmonary artery; RA, right atrium; RVOT, right ventricular outflow tract.

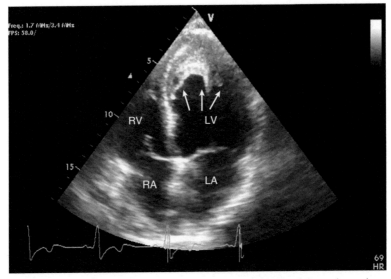

Figure 20-4. Apical four-chamber view of patient with hyperesosinophilic syndrome shows obliteration of the left ventricular (LV) apex by thrombus (*arrows*). LA, left atrium; RA, right atrium; RV, right ventricle.

HYPEREOSINOPHILIC SYNDROME

Background

- This is a proliferative disorder characterized by a peripheral eosinophilia (>1500 eosinophils/mm^3) without any identifiable etiology and with organ involvement.
- Organ dysfunction arises from eosinophilic infiltration and consequent fibrosis.
- Although several systems can be affected, **mortality is often secondary to myocardial fibrosis and heart failure**.

Echocardiographic Findings

- Echocardiographic findings may involve one or both ventricles.
- Endomyocardial fibrosis shows a predilection for the **LV apex and inflow areas.**
- Apical obliteration with **LV thrombus** can be seen (Fig. 20-4).
- Generally, the thrombus is hypoechoic with punctate calcification.
- Basal ventricular hypercontractility may be seen (Merlon sign).
- Papillary muscle involvement can cause significant MR.
- Posterior wall thickening can be noted and autopsy series suggest the possibility of adhesion of the mitral leaflet to the posterior wall, thus leading to MR.
- Tricuspid involvement with concomitant regurgitation may also occur.
- Advanced cases may demonstrate nearly obliterated ventricles with restrictive filling and marked biatrial enlargement.

- **Key Point:** *Patients with hypereosinophilic syndrome may develop apical thrombus despite normal underlying myocardial contractility. This is an exception to the rule that thrombus forms adjacent to an akinetic or aneurysmal myocardial segment.*

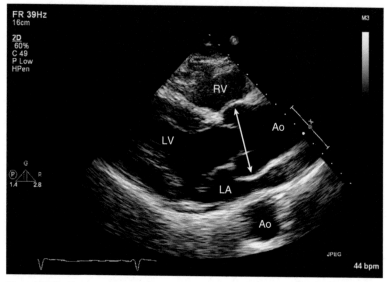

Figure 20-5. Parasternal long-axis view of patient with Marfan syndrome with dilation of the sinus of Valsalva (*double-headed arrow*), giving a "pear-shaped" appearance to the aortic root. Ao, aorta; LA, left atrium; LV, left ventricle; RV, right ventricle.

MARFAN SYNDROME

Background

- Marfan syndrome is a connective tissue disorder of the *FBN1* gene, which encodes fibrillin-1, a supporting protein for elastin and vascular smooth muscle.
- It is usually autosomal dominant, but can be a spontaneous mutation.
- Involved systems include cardiac, pulmonary (pneumothorax), musculoskeletal, ocular, and neurologic (dural ectasia).
- Aortic dilation, dissection, and cardiac valvulopathy (MV prolapse) are known to also occur.

Echocardiographic Findings

- Dilation of the aortic annulus, ascending aorta, and **sinus of Valsalva** are noted in 60–80% of Marfan patients (Fig. 20-5).
- Aortic dissection may occur secondary to intrinsic wall weakness and dilation.
- MV prolapse is also occasionally seen in this syndrome.

SARCOIDOSIS

Background

- Sarcoidosis is a systemic inflammatory condition characterized by the formation of noncaseating granulomas.
- Involvement includes the lungs, heart, skin, and reticuloendothelial system.
- A higher prevalence of this condition is seen in African Americans.

- Although cardiac involvement by sarcoid can be asymptomatic, complications include conduction abnormalities, arrhythmias, dilated cardiomyopathy, LV aneurysm, and pericardial effusion.

Echocardiographic Findings

- Progressive diastolic dysfunction is seen with an initially preserved EF.
- Systolic dysfunction occurs late in the disease.
- Regional areas of myocardial thickening are thought to be secondary to sites of active inflammation and granuloma formation.
  - These eventually progress to fibrosis and focal myocardial thinning, especially at the **basal septal, inferior, and lateral walls** (Fig. 20-6).
  - **These look like aneurysmal "bites" out of the myocardium.**
- Valvular thickening can occur, resulting in significant regurgitation.
- Pulmonary hypertension from sarcoidosis may result in RV hypertrophy.

> • **Key Point:** *Sarcoidosis is occasionally associated with aneurysms of the basal septal, inferior, and lateral walls.*

SCLERODERMA

Background

- This chronic autoimmune disease is characterized by arteriolar fibrosis and multi-organ involvement.
- Affected organs include the skin, esophagus, lungs, kidneys, and heart.

Echocardiographic Findings

- Reduction in systolic and diastolic ventricular function is seen, with the evidence of restrictive cardiomyopathy.
- Pulmonary hypertension and RV dysfunction may result from primary lung disease or secondary LV failure.
- Infrequently, pericardial effusion, and pericarditis may be seen.

SYSTEMIC LUPUS ERYTHEMATOSUS (SLE)

Background

- Systemic autoimmune disorder is characterized by the formation of auto-antibodies against certain nuclear antigens.
- The resultant formation and subendothelial deposition of immune complexes can cause inflammatory effects in a variety of organ systems, including the heart.
- Cardiac complications include valvulitis, vegetations, coronary artery disease, pericarditis, pericardial effusion, and systolic and diastolic ventricular dysfunction.

Echocardiographic Findings

- Valvulitis occurs from a secondary antiphospholipid syndrome. Affected leaflets become thickened and fibrotic, resulting in regurgitation.
- **Libman–Sacks vegetations may be noted with valvulitis.**
  - These vegetations are **irregular** and **cauliflower-shaped,** generally **less than 1 cm** in diameter, and heterogeneous in appearance.
  - Vegetations may exacerbate regurgitation and can also **embolize.**

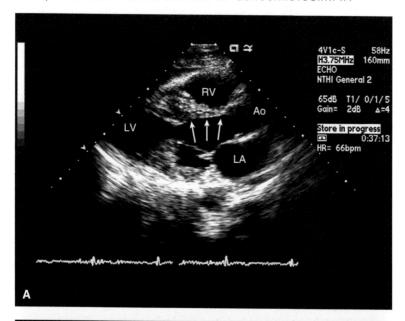

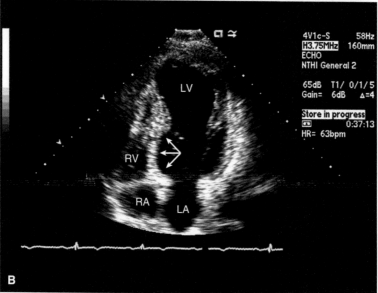

Figure 20-6. Patient with sarcoidosis and (**A**) basal anteroseptal and (**B**) inferoseptal aneurysms (*arrows*) secondary to myocardial fibrosis, seen in the parasternal long-axis and apical four-chamber views, respectively. Ao, aorta; LA, left atrium; LV, left ventricle; RA, right atrium; RV, right ventricle.

- Libman–Sacks vegetations may be mistaken for infective endocarditis and should be interpreted within the clinical presentation of the patient.
- **Left-sided valves are affected more frequently than the right.**
- **Pericarditis and pericardial effusions** may be seen; but rarely have tamponade physiology.
- Pericardial thickening with constrictive pericarditis is also a rare complication in SLE.

RADIATION-INDUCED CARDIOMYOPATHY

Background

- Mediastinal radiation can damage coronary arteries, valves, pericardium, and the myocardium leading to coronary stenosis, pericardial effusion, valvular disease, systolic dysfunction, and restrictive cardiomyopathy.
- **The time course of cardiac manifestations is variable.**

Echocardiographic Findings

- Systolic and diastolic dysfunction may occur and can progress to restrictive cardiomyopathy.
- The pericardium may also be involved, leading to constrictive physiology.
- Valves may be affected, leading to thickening and restriction, resulting in stenosis, regurgitation, or both.
- The TV is particularly affected secondary to its anterior location and proximity to the radiation source.

CHEMOTHERAPY-INDUCED CARDIOTOXICITY

Background

- Cardiac dysfunction resulting from treatment with cancer chemotherapeutics, particularly anthracyclines, is an important source of morbidity and mortality in cancer survivors.
- Optimal outcomes rely on early recognition that allows for timely withdrawal of the offending agent and initiation of treatment.

Echocardiographic Findings

- Various definitions of cardiotoxicity have been applied.
  - In general, chemotherapy-induced cardiotoxicity is diagnosed by a drop in LVEF of >10% to a value <50–55%.
- Simpson biplane technique is the most widely used method for assessing LVEF.
  - However, three-dimensional echocardiography has been shown to be a more accurate and reproducible method of determining LVEF.
- Changes in speckle-tracking–derived measures of LV strain have been shown to precede changes in LVEF.
  - Global longitudinal strain is likely the easiest deformation parameter to follow.
  - Measurements of strain should be compared to the patient's baseline.

- **Key Point:** *In patients receiving chemotherapy for cancer, particularly anthracycline-based chemotherapy regimens, serial assessment of longitudinal strain by two-dimensional speckle tracking may allow early detection of subclinical myocardial dysfunction.*

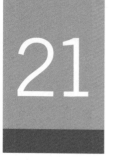

21 Transesophageal Echocardiography

Rafael S. Garcia-Cortes, Praveen K. Rao, and Nishath Quader

COMMON INDICATIONS
- Valvular endocarditis
- Cardiac source of embolism
- Mitral/aortic valve disease
- Prosthetic valve disease
- Aortic dissection/aneurysm
- Intracardiac masses

ABSOLUTE CONTRAINDICATIONS
- Perforated viscus
- Esophageal stricture
- Esophageal tumor
- Esophageal perforation, laceration
- Esophageal diverticulum
- Active upper gastrointestinal (GI) bleed

RELATIVE CONTRAINDICATIONS
- History of radiation to neck and mediastinum
- History of GI surgery, recent upper GI bleed, Barrett esophagus, or dysphagia
- Restriction of neck mobility (severe cervical arthritis, atlantoaxial joint disease)
- Symptomatic hiatal hernia
- Esophageal varices
- Coagulopathy, thrombocytopenia
- Active esophagitis
- Active peptic ulcer disease
- Severe respiratory distress

From Hahn RT, Abraham T, Adams MS, et al. Guidelines for performing a comprehensive transesophageal echocardiographic examination: recommendations from the American Society of Echocardiography and the Society of Cardiovascular Anesthesiologists. *J Am Soc Echocardiogr*. 2013;26:921–964.

BASIC PRINCIPLES

Transesophageal echocardiography (TEE) allows high-resolution imaging of posterior cardiac structures and thoracic great vessels closest to the esophagus.

- The TEE probe is a long (~100 cm), flexible tube with piezoelectric crystals at its tip capable of high frequency (3–7 Hz) imaging. Because of the small depth of imaging using this approach, the highest frequency is most often used to obtain high spatial resolution.
- The tip of the probe may be bent in an anterograde (flexion) and retrograde (extension) orientation by rotating a large wheel at the base of the probe. The leftward and the rightward movement can also be performed by rotating an adjacent smaller wheel (Fig. 21-1). Levers that lock the wheels and therefore the orientation of the probe are available, but in general should not be used so as to minimize potential risk of esophageal trauma.
- The orientation of the piezoelectric crystal and therefore the imaging plane can be rotated around the long axis of the ultrasound beam by a toggle at the base of the probe. The resulting alteration in angle (in degree increments to a maximum of 180 degrees) is indicated by a semicircle icon on the machine screen. This feature allows multiple planes of a structure to be viewed without moving the probe. At 0 degrees, the crystal or imaging plane is horizontal, with the patient's right side appearing on the left side of the display. As the angle increases, the beam rotates in a clockwise fashion. The view at 180 degrees is a mirror image of the 0-degree view.

- **Key Points:**
  1. *TEE is best suited to assess posterior structures and structures closest to the esophagus.*
  2. *TEE allows imaging at higher frequencies.*
  3. *The echocardiographer should be familiar with basic manipulation of the TEE probe.*

PATIENT EVALUATION AND PREPARATION

Adequate patient evaluation and preparation prior to probe intubation reduces procedural complications and inappropriate studies. In answering the referring physician's question, it is important to decide whether TEE, transthoracic echocardiography (TTE), or a combined approach is most suitable.

- TEE is superior to TTE for evaluating possible valvular endocarditis, left atrial (LA) masses, mitral valve (MV) disease, prosthetic valves, or aortic pathology such as proximal aortic dissections.
- There is benefit in a *combined* approach where Doppler-based hemodynamic assessment may be more accurate by TTE because of better orientation with blood flow. This data complements the increased anatomic detail provided by TEE.
- TTE is superior to TEE when imaging structures closer to the chest wall, such as the left ventricle (LV), to measure function or assess for apical pathology.

Patient preparation includes the following:
- In nonemergent cases, patients should be NPO for >6 hours to prevent aspiration. Patients who are intubated should have feeding stopped for this period of time.
- A history focused on the reason for the study, medication allergies, and prior anesthesia-related complications should be reviewed.
- Absolute and relative contraindications for a TEE should be thoroughly reviewed.

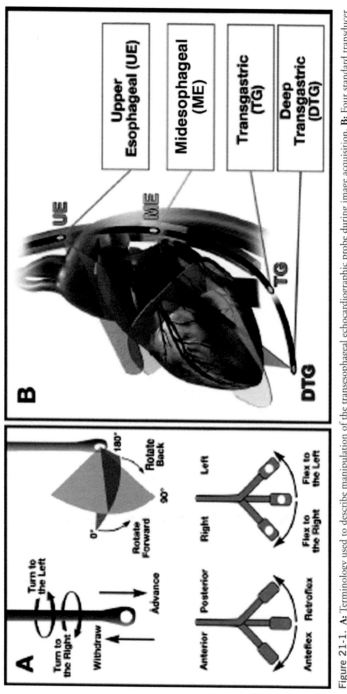

Figure 21-1. A: Terminology used to describe manipulation of the transesophageal echocardiographic probe during image acquisition. **B:** Four standard transducer positions within the esophagus and stomach and the associated imaging planes. (From Hahn RT, Abraham T, Adams MS, et al. Guidelines for performing a comprehensive transesophageal echocardiographic examination: recommendations from the American Society of Echocardiography and the Society of Cardiovascular Anesthesiologists. *J Am Soc Echocardiogr*. 2013;26:921–964.)

- Physical examination and history should assess the following:
  - Current hemodynamic status of the patient
  - Poor dentition, loose teeth, removable bridges
- Anesthesia airway score will help identify patients at high risk of airway complications. This is determined by the amount of space in the posterior pharynx.
- The following studies and their findings should be reviewed prior to the procedure:
  - Past TTE/TEE studies
  - Other imaging studies pertinent to the indication for TEE
  - Severe anemia (Hb <7 g/dL) in the setting of active bleeding
  - Supratherapeutic International Normalized Ratio (>4) (postpone the procedure or treat with fresh frozen plasma if urgent to prevent bleeding from contact of the probe with the esophagus)
  - Platelet count <50,000, especially if there has been a recent decline (administer IV platelets to prevent bleeding during the procedure)
  - Significant liver dysfunction (and its possible effect on the pharmacodynamics of sedatives used for the procedure)
    - History of esophageal varices (in patients with liver disease)

A description of the procedure and the following procedure-related risks should be explained to the patient prior to consent:

- Mortality close to zero in several large-population studies
- 1 in 10,000 risk of esophageal perforation
- 3 in 10,000 risk of esophageal bleeding
- 3 in 1,000 risk of dental injury (higher if poor dentition)
- 1 in 1,000 risk of severe odynophagia, more commonly mild if present

---

- **Key Points:**
  1. *Understand the advantages of TEE over TTE.*
  2. *Understand when these studies are complementary.*
  3. *A thorough history and physical should be obtained.*
  4. *Know the contraindications to a TEE.*
  5. *Know the procedure-related risks.*

TEE PROCEDURE

Machine Settings
- The probe is inserted into the machine and is selected on the machine control panel as the probe for imaging.
- In general, the examiner alters the probe power with higher frequencies used in the esophageal views for high resolution of adjacent cardiac structures.
- Lower frequencies are used in the transgastric views for improved penetration to see cardiac structures that are now farther from the transducer.
- Gain settings and focus are altered to optimize the image.
- Acquisition is set to capture number of beats or time if the triggering electrocardiogram is unstable or irregular, such as in atrial fibrillation.

Patient Settings and Positioning
- A recently placed, functional IV (20 gauge or higher) should be present to allow safe administration of sedation and fluid resuscitation if required.

- Patient vitals (heart rate, blood pressure, oxygen saturation) should be monitored every 3–5 minutes during and after the administration of sedation.
- Wall-mounted suction via a Yankauer tube should be available to clear the airway of secretions.
- The patient is typically in a left lateral decubitus position with chin tucked to chest (best position to prevent aspiration and align the esophagus for easy intubation).
- Other positions include the patient sitting up in a 90-degree position with head bent forward.
- Mechanically ventilated patients are intubated lying flat. A bite-block is placed to protect the probe.
- Dentures/plates are removed from the mouth and the oropharynx is locally anesthetized with topical benzocaine spray and lidocaine gel to reduce the gag reflex. Despite adequate local anesthesia, anxious patients may still gag; therefore reassurance and a clear explanation of what to expect is important.
- **Rarely benzocaine spray can cause methemoglobinemia. This is cyanosis secondary to an increase in the methemoglobin fraction of blood (normal <2%) and subsequent reduction in oxygen-carrying capacity. Treatment is IV methylene blue 2 mg/kg.**
- A nurse or anesthesiologist should be present to administer sedation and monitor patient vital signs during and after the procedure. In most cases IV opioid and benzodiazepines are used for "conscious sedation." Elderly patients often need only a small dose of these medications, which act in a synergistic manner.
- **A rare, idiosyncratic, paradoxical reaction may occur with benzodiazepines causing the patient to have uncontrollable weeping, depression, agitation, aggression, or disinhibited behavior. This has been mostly described in younger patients and resolves with stopping the administration of the medication.**

Esophageal Intubation

- Ensure that there is no damage to the probe casing and that movement with the wheels at the base and alteration of the transducing beam angle are functional prior to intubation. Coat the probe with lubricant to minimize friction. Excessive lubricant may result in the patient coughing during the procedure.
- Flex the probe slightly to follow the curve of the tongue and the palate. Advance the probe to the back and center of the mouth and then straighten it and pass it into the esophagus. If difficulty is encountered, place a finger alongside the probe to help gently guide the tip over the base of the tongue.
  - NEVER push against resistance.
  - If the patient is awake, encourage swallowing when ready to pass the probe into the esophagus.
  - Typically the most uncomfortable locations for the patient are when the probe is at the back of the oropharynx, in the high esophageal position, and at the gastroesophageal junction. Limit time in these areas when possible.
- **Usually assistance with a forward "jaw-thrust" is required to allow easier esophageal intubation of patients with an endotracheal tube, small oropharynx, and/or large tongue. Removal of nasogastric and oral feeding tubes may aid intubation and image quality. If not removed, the position of these tubes should be checked postprocedure by chest radiograph as movement may occur with manipulation of the TEE probe.**

• **Key Points:**
  1. *Familiarize yourself with machine settings.*
  2. *Recognize adverse effects of sedatives, topical anesthetics.*
  3. *Familiarize yourself with safe practices for esophageal intubations.*

THE TEE EXAM AND BASIC VIEWS

The TEE Exam

• The instructions described are for an operator standing to the patient's left, holding the probe controls with the right hand and the probe near the patient's mouth with the left hand.

• Most structures can be obtained by the movement of the probe itself, with the use of the wheels at the base of the probe optimizing image definition.

• Small movements of the probe outside of the patient translate to large movements within the patient at the transducer level.

• Movements of the probe are made with the operator's hand closest to the patient's mouth.

• Clockwise rotation of the probe images right heart structures, and counterclockwise rotation images left heart structures.

• Flexion of the probe angles the ultrasound beam superior while extension angles the beam inferior.

• The operator should rely on the image obtained rather than the depth of the probe to produce the views detailed in Section II. If the probe is deeply advanced without producing the expected image, the operator should consider coiling the probe (resistance should be felt) or tracheal intubation (associated patient dyspnea, coughing, and hypoxia).

• Structures of interest should be stored with a focused ultrasound beam at standard and "zoomed" views.

• For image orientation, the LA is the most posterior structure and is therefore displayed at the top of the screen closest to the probe.

• For proximal isovelocity surface area (PISA) assessment of mitral regurgitation (MR) severity, the Nyquist baseline is moved down (opposite to TTE) to increase or optimize visualization of the MR flow convergence distance. The baseline should always be moved in the direction of flow of interest to allow for earlier aliasing and increased PISA radius for measurement.

• Reducing imaging depth and color box sector width will help acquire images at correct Nyquist limits and detect higher velocity jets with pulsed-wave (PW) Doppler.

Basic Views

The examination described is an angle-based TEE assessment where all structures in a given view are studied. An alternative assessment (not described here) is a structure-based system where structures of interest are imaged sequentially at different angles.

Midesophageal 0-degree View
• Position 30–40 cm from the incisors with imaging power at 7 MHz and depth set to allow all four cardiac chambers to be seen (Fig. 21-2).

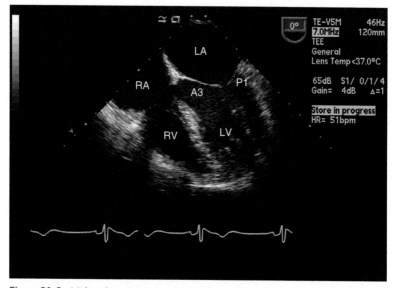

Figure 21-2. Midesophageal 0-degree view. The P2 and A2 scallops are visualized at the mitral leaflet tips. LA, left atrium; LV, left ventricle; RA, right atrium; RV, right ventricle.

- Ideally slight extension provides a nonforeshortened view, but "contact" with the esophagus may be lost, compromising the image. The right ventricle (RV) anterior wall and LV inferoseptal and anterolateral walls are seen in this view.
- Mitral valve anterior leaflet is seen arising from the septum. Mitral valve A2 and P2 scallops are seen at the leaflet tips in 0-degree view.
- Advancement of the probe demonstrates A3 and P3 scallops of the MV. Rotation of the probe clockwise at this level shows the septal and anterior tricuspid leaflets and often the coronary sinus.
- The probe is then pulled back to the *left ventricular outflow tract (LVOT) and aortic valve leaflets.* In this higher esophageal position, MV A1 and P1 scallops are seen.

Midesophageal 30-degree View
- The aortic valve is seen in cross-section at the base of the heart by withdrawing the probe to a higher esophageal position or flexion of the probe tip (Fig. 21-3).
- The left atrial appendage (LAA) can be evaluated in this higher esophageal position next to the aortic valve. Color and PW Doppler velocities (normal >40 cm/sec) should also be obtained.
- The left superior pulmonary vein is seen by further counterclockwise rotation with color and PW Doppler. PW Doppler shows continuous flow (with systolic and diastolic peak velocities) as opposed to Doppler obtained in the LAA.

Midesophageal 60-degree View ("bicommissural view")
- Clockwise rotation of the probe shows the RV inflow/outflow view with visualization of the anterior and posterior tricuspid valve leaflets. This view is typically best

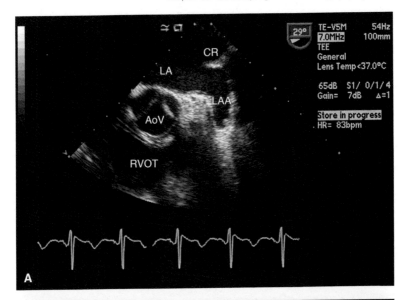

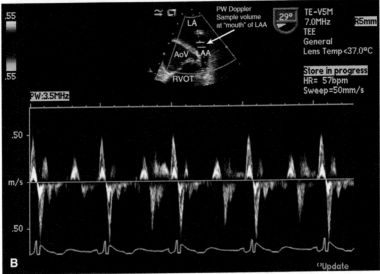

Figure 21-3. A: Short-axis view of the aortic valve (AoV). **B:** Normal pulsed-wave (PW) Doppler pattern in the left atrial appendage (LAA). **C:** Normal PW Doppler pattern in the left superior pulmonary vein. aR, atrial reversal; CR, coumadin ridge; D, diastolic; LA, left atrium; RVOT, right ventricular outflow tract; S, systolic. *(continued)*

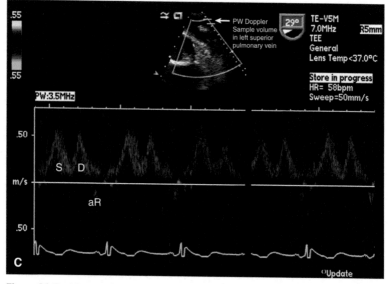

Figure 21-3. (*Continued*)

for obtaining Doppler-based assessment of peak systolic pulmonary pressures from the TR jet (Fig. 21-4).

- Note, as the piezoelectric crystal moves past 60 degrees, a **transition** occurs whereby the posterior MV leaflet is now displayed on the left and the anterior MV leaflet on the right side of the screen.
- Counterclockwise rotation develops the bicommissural view, so named because the ultrasound beam bisects the saddle-shaped MV commissures at two locations. This is one reason multiple regurgitant jets may be noted in this view. From left to right, P1-A2-P3 MV cusps are seen.
- Further counterclockwise rotation shows the entire posterior leaflet (P1, P2, P3), whereas clockwise rotation can show the entire anterior leaflet (A1, A2, A3).
- The mitral subvalvular apparatus (chordae, papillary muscles) is best assessed in this view.
- The LAA is reassessed in this view.

Midesophageal 90-degree View ("bicaval view")

- The probe is rotated clockwise and withdrawn to demonstrate the interatrial septum (IAS). Color Doppler is used to assess for patent foramen ovale or atrial septal defect (ASD). Clockwise rotation with deeper probe placement shows the inferior vena cava (IVC) entrance, and counterclockwise rotation and withdrawal of the probe shows the superior vena cava (SVC). This is especially important in the assessment of sinus venosus ASD and pacing wires and intracardiac catheters (Fig. 21-5).
- Further clockwise rotation shows the entrance of the right superior pulmonary vein using color Doppler and PW Doppler.
- Counterclockwise rotation and advancement of the probe shows a two-chamber view with the anterior and inferior walls of the LV seen. Different depth settings and focus should be used to evaluate the LA, LV, and MV.

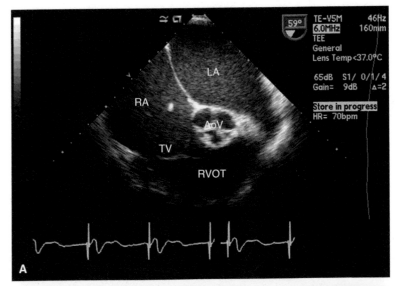

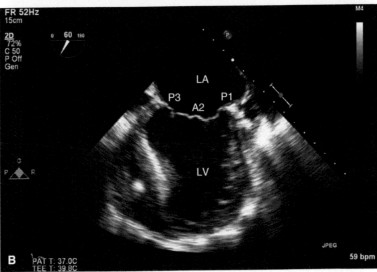

Figure 21-4. A: Midesophageal right ventricular inflow/outflow view. **B:** Midesophageal mitral bicommissural view. AoV, aortic valve; LA, left atrium; LV, left ventricle; RA, right atrium; RVOT, right ventricular outflow tract; TV, tricuspid valve.

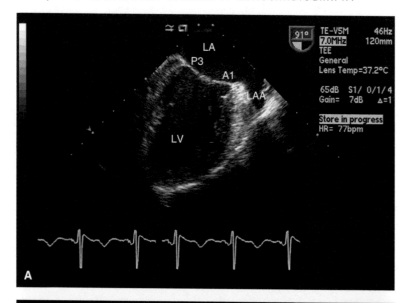

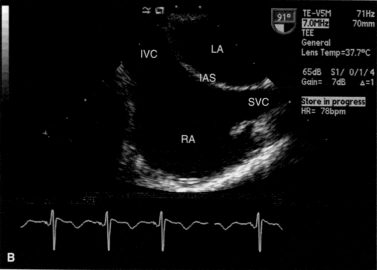

Figure 21-5. A: 90-degree two-chamber view (left atrium [LA] and left ventricle [LV]). **B:** 90-degree bicaval view. IAS, interatrial septum; IVC, inferior vena cava; LAA, left atrial appendage; RA, right atrium; SVC, superior vena cava.

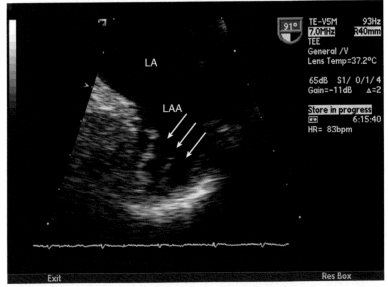

Figure 21-6. Pectinate muscles (normal finding, *arrows*) projecting from the apex of the left atrial appendage (LAA). LA, left atrium.

- The LAA is once again assessed in this view. *The LAA should be assessed in multiple nonforeshortened views as often it is multilobed. Do not mistake the fine fingerlike projections at the apex for thrombi. These are pectinate muscles and represent normal LAA anatomy (Fig. 21-6). Also, fibrinous material lying in the transverse sinus behind the LAA may also be occasionally mistaken for LAA thrombus.*

Midesophageal 120-degree View ("long-axis view")
- Inferolateral and anteroseptal walls of the LV are seen.
- P2–A2 MV scallops are seen.
- The aortic valve is seen with counterclockwise rotation (typically noncoronary cusp and right coronary cusp) (Fig. 21-7).
- The aortic root (sinus of Valsalva, sinotubular junction, and proximal ascending aorta) is assessed by withdrawing the probe to a higher esophageal position. The angle should be reduced to ~110 degrees with rotation and slight flexion to visualize the ascending aorta.
- The true long-axis of the LV is ~135 degrees, which can usually show both the mitral and aortic valves in the same view.

Transgastric 0-degree View
- The probe is advanced without resistance into the stomach. The ultrasound power is decreased to 5 MHz to allow better penetration and the imaging depth is increased for better visualization.
- Advancing and flexing the probe just past the gastroesophageal junction, the MV *en face* view is seen with all cusps visualized (note the posterior leaflet is closest to the probe). This is a good view for confirmation of the location of a regurgitant jet. Clockwise rotation at this level shows the coronary sinus (Fig. 21-8).

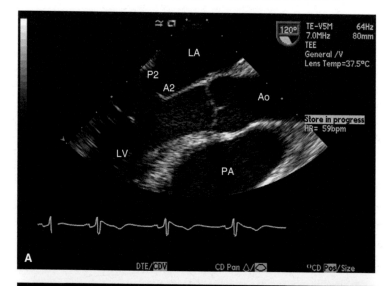

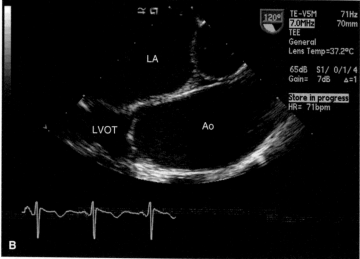

Figure 21-7. A: 120-degree left ventricular (LV) long-axis view. **B:** Evaluation of aorta (Ao) by withdrawing the probe in the LV long-axis view. LA, left atrium; LVOT, left ventricular outflow tract; PA, pulmonary artery.

- Deeper probe placement shows the cross-section of the LV at the midpapillary muscle level. Flexion again brings the MV into view and subvalvular apparatus while extension or advancing the probe shows the apex of the LV. This is a good view to assess LV wall motion and interventricular septal motion or defects.
- Clockwise rotation shows the *en face view of* the tricuspid valve.

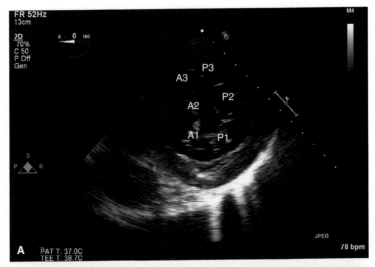

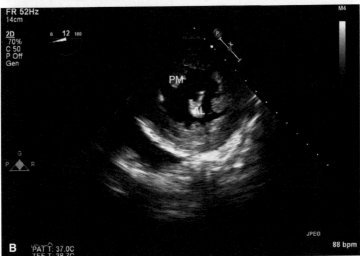

Figure 21-8. A: Transgastric left ventricular (LV) short-axis view at the level of the mitral valve. **B:** Transgastric LV short-axis view at the papillary muscle level. AL, anterolateral papillary muscles; PM, posteromedial.

Transgastric 90-degree View
- LV anterior and inferior walls and MV are seen (Fig. 21-9).
- Clockwise rotation shows the tricuspid valve in the RV inflow view with posterior and anterior leaflets seen.
- **Transgastric 140-degree view**
  - A long-axis view of the LV is seen particularly for the assessment of the aortic valve.

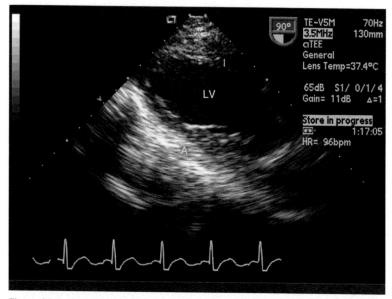

Figure 21-9. Transgastric 90-degree view of the left ventricle (LV) (anterior [A] and inferior [I] walls).

Deep Transgastric 0-degree View

- The probe is advanced until the apical portion of the LV is seen. The large wheel at the base is then rotated to provide maximal flexion. The probe is carefully withdrawn until the LVOT and aortic valves are seen.
- This is the best view for Doppler alignment for aortic valve stenotic and regurgitant jets.

Aortic Examination at 0 and 90 Degrees

- The probe is rotated posteriorly and the imaging depth is reduced and power increased to 7 MHz for high-resolution visualization of the thoracic aorta. If the probe is deep, often withdrawal of the probe is required to see the thoracic aorta.
- As the probe is withdrawn, 0- and 90-degree images are taken to evaluate aortic size and presence of pathology. If pathology such as aortic atheroma or hematoma is noted, views at both orientations with and without color Doppler are recommended to best define the structures seen.
- A high esophageal view of the aorta and pulmonary artery (PA) can be seen prior to the aortic arch views (Fig. 21-10).
- At the aortic arch, the arch vessels and the right PA are seen.
- Color and PW Doppler are used to assess aortic flow.
  - *PW Doppler in the proximal descending thoracic aorta should be performed in patients with moderate or greater aortic valve regurgitation to assess for holodiastolic flow reversal.*

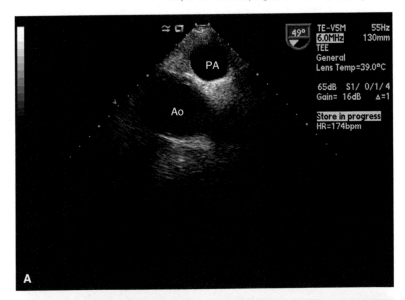

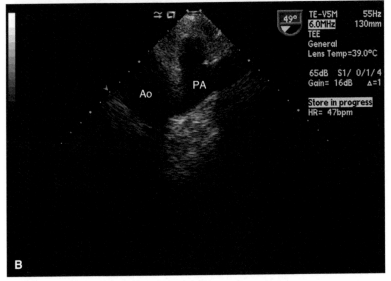

Figure 21-10. (**A**) High esophageal views of the thoracic aorta (Ao) and pulmonary artery (PA), with clockwise rotation of the probe showing the main PA bifurcation (**B**).

Mitral Valve Scallops at Different Angles (Fig. 21-11)

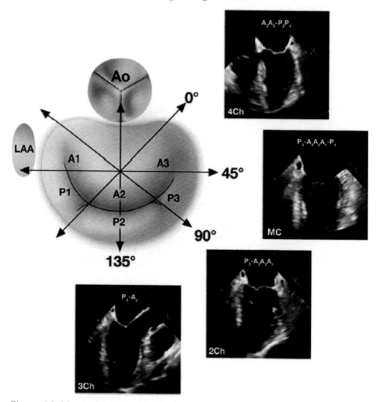

Figure 21-11. Schematic of the mitral valve (MV) with leaflet scallops (or segments) labeled. Corresponding images from different standard imaging views are labeled with the respective scallops and segments. Although this labeling scheme is applicable in the majority of cases, the exact regions of the MV leaflets image vary on the basis of the relation of the heart to the esophagus as well as transesophageal echocardiography probe position within the esophagus. Ao, aorta; LAA, left atrial appendage; MC, mitral commissural; 2Ch, two-chamber; 3Ch, three-chamber; 4Ch, four-chamber. (From Hahn RT, Abraham T, Adams MS, et al. Guidelines for performing a comprehensive transesophageal echocardiographic examination: recommendations from the American Society of Echocardiography and the Society of Cardiovascular Anesthesiologists. *J Am Soc Echocardiogr.* 2013;26:921–964.)

THREE-DIMENSIONAL TEE

- The applications of three-dimensional (3D) TEE are rapidly growing. Compared to two-dimensional (2D) imaging, 3D TEE can be used to:
  - Accurately diagnose specific valvular disorders (especially MV), including endocarditis and prolapse/flail, as well as identifying specific leaflets or scallops and mitral clefts that may be involved. Figure 21-12 demonstrates a 3D image of the mitral valve in the "surgeon's view". Figure 21-13 demonstrates a mitral valve with clefts.
  - Localize regurgitant jets (Fig. 21-14)

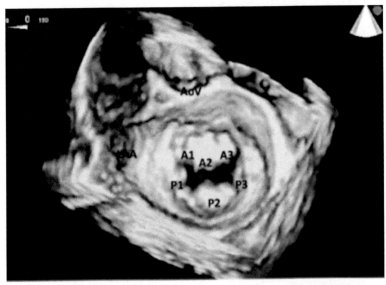

Figure 21-12. Three-dimensional (3D) view of the mitral valve in the surgeon's view with the aortic valve (AoV) at the 12 o'clock location and the left atrial appendage (LAA) at the 9 o'clock location. The anterior mitral leaflet is made up of the A1, A2, and A3 scallops, while the posterior mitral leaflet is made up of the P1, P2, and P3 scallops.

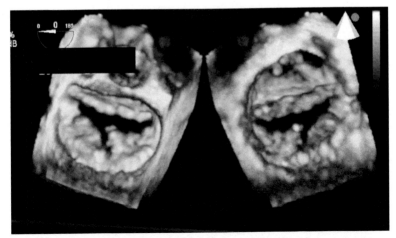

Figure 21-13. The left sided image demonstrates the mitral valve viewed from the left atrial aspect (surgeon's view) with an indentation extending from the mitral tips to the annulus. This is also well visualized when the mitral valve is viewed from the left ventricular aspect (right sided image). This indentation is a mitral cleft.

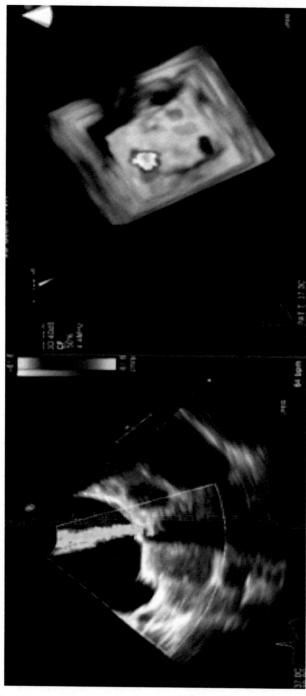

Figure 21-14. Three-dimensional (3D) echocardiography can be very useful in identifying locations of perivalvular regurgitation. On the left hand image is a two-dimensional view of the perivalvular regurgitation. The right hand side demonstrates this on 3D in the surgeon's view of the mitral valve. When 3D imaging is utilized, one can see that the perivalvular regurgitation is located at the 11 o'clock location.

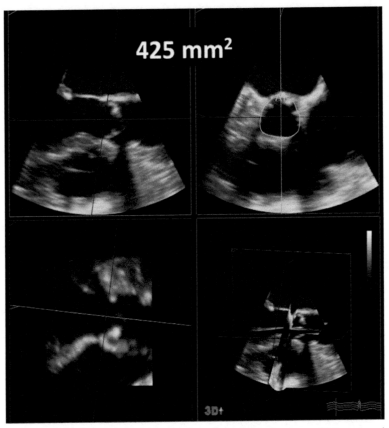

Figure 21-15. Three-dimensional (3D) echocardiography can be very useful in structural heart disease procedures. In this case, 3D echocardiography was utilized to size the aortic annulus using a 3D multiplanar reconstruction mode. The annulus measurement is shown on the image that is then used to determine which size valve is implanted in the patient. This is an extremely useful technique in patients who have chronic kidney disease and cannot undergo a computed tomography with contrast for annulus sizing.

- Better visualize prosthetic valves, including localizing and sizing perivalvular leaks
- Perform structural heart disease and percutaneous valvular procedures (Fig. 21-15) (Also see video library for TEE guidance during MitraClip and Transcatheter aortic valve replacement).
- **Technique**
  - Must have good 2D images, or 3D images will be poor.
  - Using the matrix transducer, start with "real time" or "live" acquisition using single-beat mode. One can use multiple beats for a higher frame rate if rhythm is stable and patient can cooperate with a breath hold (Fig. 21-16).

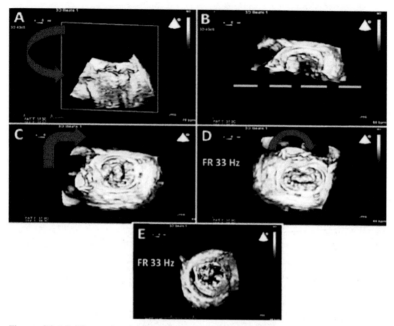

Figure 21-16. Steps taken in three-dimensional (3D) acquisition of mitral valve. **A:** The image sector is focused on the mitral valve. Note that a one beat full volume acquisition has been performed. **B:** The image is then rotated towards the viewer. Once part of the mitral annulus is in view, the green plane is extended so that the entire mitral annulus can be viewed. **C,D:** The image is then rotated to position the aortic valve at the 12 o'clock position. Here the mitral valve is seen from the left atrial side. **E:** The image can also be rotated so as to visualize the mitral valve from the LV side. This view can be useful to identify mitral clefts. Quader N, Rigolin VH. Cardiovasc Ultrasound. 2014 Oct 25;12:42 (Needs permission from publisher)

MINI ATLAS OF TEE IMAGES

(Fig. 21-17A,B)
(Fig. 21-18A,B)
(Fig. 21-19A,B)
(Fig. 21-20A–C)
(Fig. 21-21A–C)
(Fig. 21-22A–C)
(Fig. 21-23)
(Fig. 21-24A,B)
(Fig. 21-25)
(Fig. 21-26)

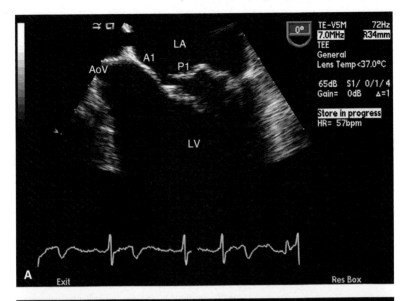

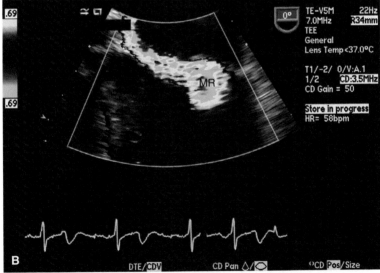

Figure 21-17. A: Flail P1 scallop of the mitral valve seen in this "superior" midesophageal 0-degree view. **B:** Severe eccentric anteriorly directed mitral regurgitation. AoV, aortic valve; LA, left atrium; LV, left ventricle.

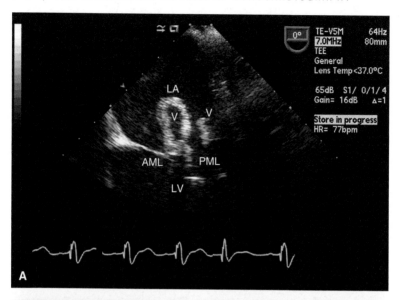

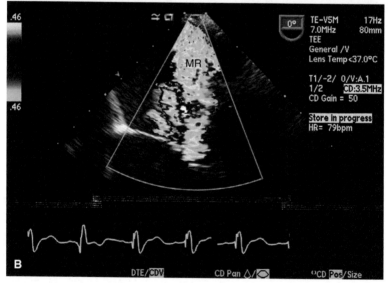

Figure 21-18. A: Midesophageal 0-degree view with vegetations (V) visible on the atrial surface of the anterior (AML) and posterior (PML) mitral valve leaflets. **B:** Severe mitral regurgitation is seen secondary to leaflet malcoaptation and destruction. LA, left atrium; LV, left ventricle.

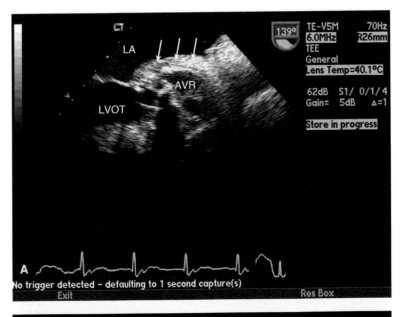

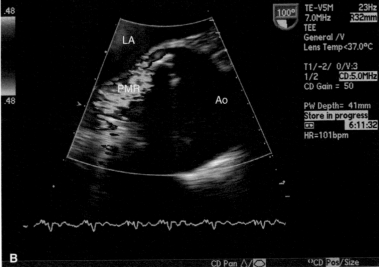

Figure 21-19. A: 120-degree long-axis view showing an aortic mechanical valve with abnormally thickened aortic root suggestive of abscess. **B:** Perivalvular regurgitation. Ao, aorta; AVR, mechanical aortic valve LA, left atrium; LVOT, left ventricular outflow tract; PVR, perivalvular regurgitation.

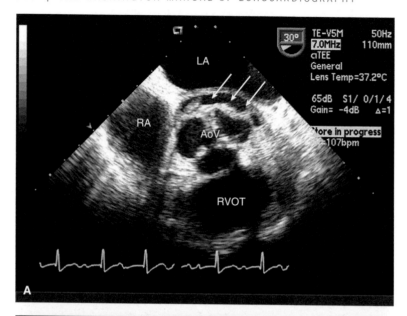

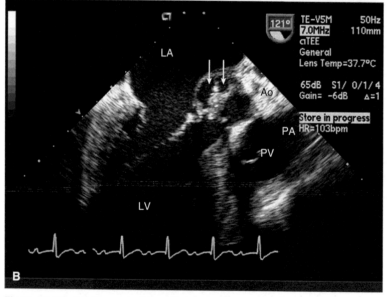

Figure 21-20. (**A**) Short-axis view of the aortic valve (AoV) with thickened leaflets and abnormal fluid (*arrows*) seen in the supporting aortic root tissue. (**B**) Long-axis left ventricular (LV) view confirms aortic root abscess (*arrows*) with severe aortic regurgitation (AR) (**C**). Ao, aorta; LA, left atrium; PA, pulmonary artery; PV, pulmonary vein; RA, right atrium; RVOT, right ventricular outflow tract.

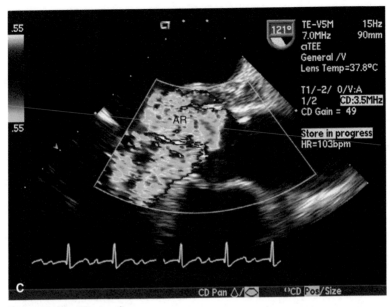

Figure 21-20. (*Continued*)

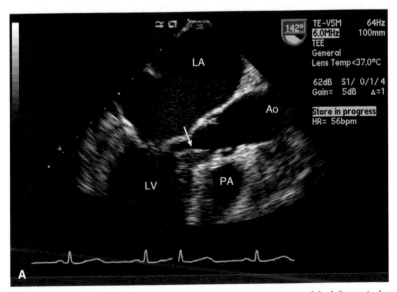

Figure 21-21. (**A**) Long-axis left ventricular (LV) view with narrowing of the left ventricular outflow tract (LVOT) secondary to tunnel-type subaortic membrane (*arrow*). (*continued*)

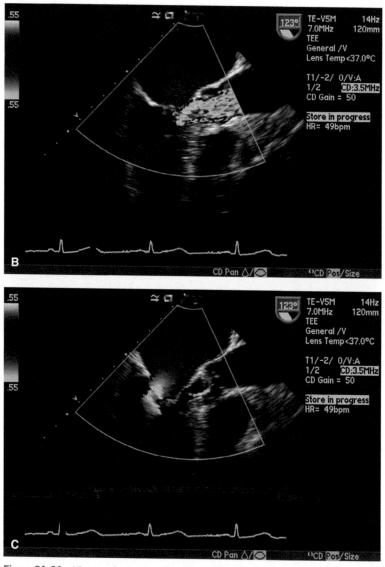

Figure 21-21. (*Continued*) (**B**) Marked systolic turbulence is seen in the LVOT (**C**) and mild aortic regurgitation. Ao, aorta; LA, left atrium; PA, pulmonary artery.

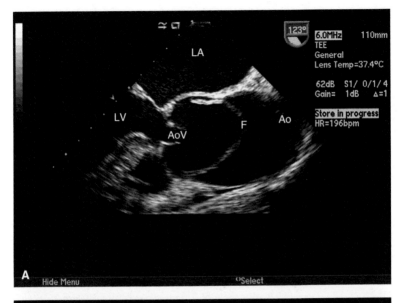

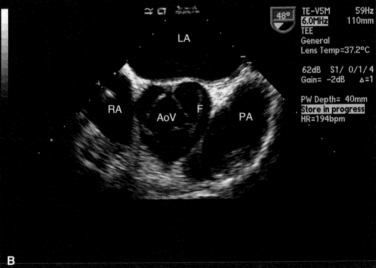

Figure 21-22. Dissection flap (F) seen in the aortic root on long-axis (**A**) and short-axis (**B**) views. (*continued*)

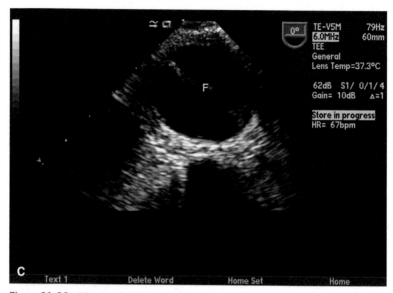

Figure 21-22. (*Continued*) (**C**) The dissection flap extended to the descending thoracic aorta. Ao, aorta; AoV, aortic valve; LA, left atrium; LV, left ventricle; PA, pulmonary artery; RA, right atrium.

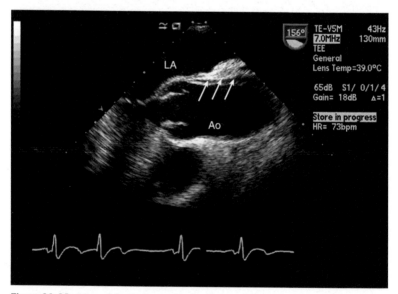

Figure 21-23. View of the aortic root showing abnormal echodensity in the wall of the proximal ascending aorta consistent with intramural hematoma (*arrows*). Ao, aorta; LA, left atrium.

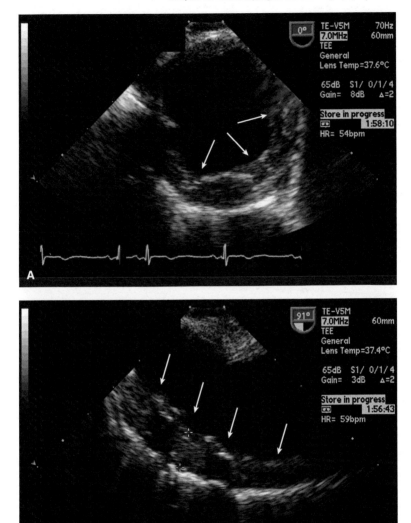

Figure 21-24. Short-axis (**A**) and long-axis (**B**) views of significant aortic atheroma seen in the descending thoracic aorta (*arrows*).

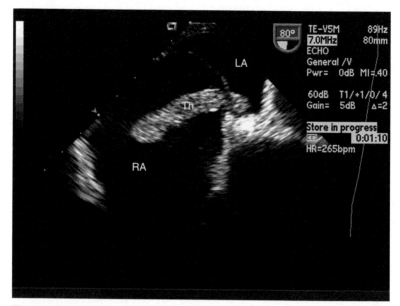

Figure 21-25. Thrombus (Th) seen crossing the interatrial septum at the fossa ovalis. LA, left atrium; RA, right atrium.

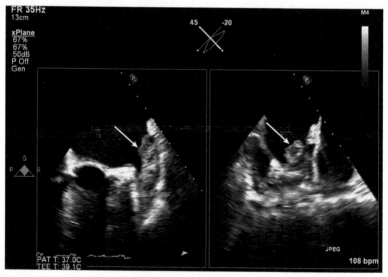

Figure 21-26. Biplane view of left atrial appendage thrombus (*arrows*). Spontaneous echo contrast can be seen in the left atrium.

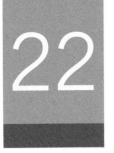

22

Cardiac Devices in Heart Failure

Michael E. Nassif and Justin M. Vader

HIGH-YIELD CONCEPTS

- Comprehensive transthoracic echocardiography (TTE) imaging of durable left ventricular assist devices (LVADs) consists of all the routine TTE measures with added attention to aortic valve (AoV) opening, apical and aortic cannula positioning and Doppler flow, and interventricular septal (IVS) position.
- LVADs provide benefit by reducing left heart filling pressures and augmenting cardiac output. Inadequate LVAD support results in the persistence of typical left heart failure signs and symptoms. Excessive LVAD support may compromise the right ventricle (RV) by increasing preload and altering IVS positioning, resulting in right heart failure signs and symptoms.
- LVAD speed change studies have utility in the confirmation of pump dysfunction resulting from thrombosis and may be useful in optimizing speed settings in certain individuals.
- Transesophageal echocardiography (TEE) and TTE imaging are useful adjuncts to management of temporary mechanical support modalities, including intraaortic balloon pump (IABP), Impella, and extracorporeal membrane oxygenation (ECMO).

KEY VIEWS

LVADs

- Parasternal long axis (PLAX)—Overall LV volume assessment is the first objective. Color Doppler evidence of mitral regurgitation (MR) and aortic regurgitation (AR) is key to estimating appropriateness of current level of support. M-mode through the AoV is helpful to determine frequency and degree of opening.
- Parasternal short axis (PSAX)—Pulsed-wave (PW) Doppler at the level of the pulmonic valve for velocity time integral (VTI) measurement allows estimation of changes in cardiac output.
- Apical four chamber (A4C)—Midline position of the IVS generally indicates appropriate LVAD speed settings. Assessment of left atrial (LA) volume along with mitral inflow parameters, including E-wave to A-wave ratio, E-wave deceleration time, and E-wave velocity provide context to the degree of left heart unloading.
- RV focused A4C—Assessment of RV function (tricuspid annular plane systolic excursion [TAPSE], RV tissue Doppler [RVS'], RV strain, fractional area change [FAC]), tricuspid valve (TV) coaptation, and tricuspid regurgitation (TR) determine degree of RV function in the face of LVAD support.

- LVAD cannula flow can be oriented in either direction depending on scanning angle and insertion angle.
- LV apical (inflow) cannula flows are best seen in off-axis PLAX view or PSAX apex. Off-axis views are often required to visualize cannula flows. Cannula Doppler waveform profiles should not look like mitral inflow.
- Aortic (outflow) cannula flow is best seen in right sternal border or high PLAX views of the ascending aorta. Use color Doppler to locate continuous flow in right sternal border view.
- Artifacts are common—VAD hardware obstructs color Doppler and continuous-wave (CW) Doppler in apical views. Off-axis, medial views may offer a better signal.

DURABLE MECHANICAL CIRCULATORY SUPPORT

Although temporary mechanical support of the RV is practiced widely, durable mechanical circulatory support is, with rare exceptions, a matter of isolated LVAD support.

- LVADs are indicated for patients with advanced systolic heart failure (ACC/AHA Stage D, NYHA Class IV), either as a bridge to future heart transplant (BTT) or as destination therapy (DT) in those patients ineligible for transplant.
- Two durable LVADs are currently approved for commercial use in the United States: Thoratec HeartMate II (HM II) and HeartWare HVAD (HeartWare Corp., Framingham, MA). Other durable LVADs remain investigational.
  - The HM II uses axial flow technology, similar to an Archimedes screw, to energize blood drawn from an LV apical inflow cannula, through the motor unit, and out to the ascending aorta through a tubular conduit. The LVAD pump itself is placed within a preperitoneal pocket, and the housing structure is implanted below the diaphragm (Fig. 22-1).
  - The HVAD utilizes centrifugal flow, as opposed to axial flow, to energize blood drawn through a similar circuit configuration to the HMII. This device is smaller and implanted intrapericardially, without a separate pump pocket. In contrast to HM II, this device's housing structure is implanted above the diaphragm (Fig. 22-2).

Echocardiography in Preimplantation Assessment
LV Assessment
- Patients with severe systolic dysfunction (e.g., left ventricular ejection fraction [LVEF] <25%), large LV volumes, and elevated left-heart filling pressures are the optimal candidates for LVAD support.
- Left ventricular internal end-diastolic diameter (LVIDd) should be measured and compared to the postoperative LVIDd as a marker of unloading after LVAD placement.
- Left ventricular end-diastolic volume (LVEDV) should also be used and perhaps would be a better marker of LV unloading; however, it is difficult to obtain LVEDV after LVAD placement as a result of limited apical views.
- Larger LVEDV predicts better response LVAD therapy and smaller LV volumes maybe associated with post-VAD complications.
- The presence of LV thrombus influences surgical planning and may be associated with increased risk of stroke during the LV cannulation portion of the procedure.

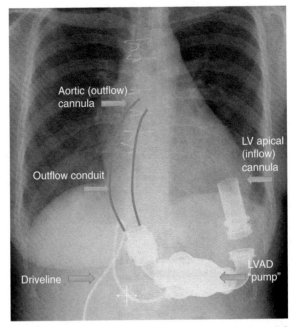

Figure 22-1. Chest radiograph of a patient with HeartMate 2 left ventricular assist device (LVAD) with radiopaque inflow cannula, pump, and driveline. Outflow conduit course is traced. Note the position of the pump.

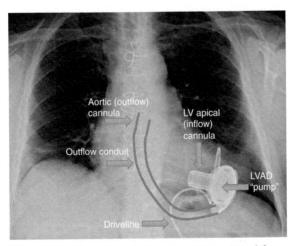

Figure 22-2. Chest radiograph of a patient with HeartWare left ventricular assist device (LVAD) with radiopaque inflow cannula, pump, and driveline. Outflow conduit course is traced. Compare the position of the pump from the HeartWare LVAD to the HeartMate 2 LVAD.

RV Assessment

- Failure of the mechanically unsupported RV is a major cause of morbidity in LVAD recipients and affects ~20–30% of LVAD recipients, with an incidence of 0.2 events per patient-year of support.
- In addition to clinical and demographic predictors, numerous echocardiographic parameters have been suggested to predict clinical RV failure after LVAD implant, including TAPSE, RV tissue Doppler, RV strain, right index of myocardial performance (RIMP), and RV fractional area change (FAC).
- Besides RV systolic function, RV size, estimation of RA pressure, and degree of TR should be assessed.

Valvular Assessment

- Aortic valve
  - Moderate or greater AR represents a major limitation to success with LVAD support resulting in a "futile loop" of circulation between the aortic root, LV, and LVAD.
  - Moderate or greater AR must be addressed at the time of surgery with AoV replacement, valve plication, or valve oversewing.
  - Aortic stenosis (AS) does not present an impediment to LVAD implant, as a normal AoV is frequently closed completely in LVAD-supported patients.
  - Mechanical aortic prostheses are a nidus for thrombus in the setting of LVAD support and minimal leaflet excursion. Mechanical AoVs are often replaced with bioprosthetic valves or are oversewn.
- Mitral valve (MV)
  - MR resulting solely from dilation of the LV and mitral annulus (functional MR) improves with LVAD support, while MR resulting from structural abnormalities and displacement of the MV leaflets often persists.
  - Mechanical mitral prostheses represent a higher thrombotic risk and require aggressive anticoagulation, but do not represent a complication to LVAD implant.
  - Severe mitral stenosis (mean pressure ≥10 mm Hg) should be addressed surgically at the time of LVAD implant.
- Tricuspid valve
  - Severe TR prior to LVAD implantation may result in continued right heart failure and reduced effectiveness of LVAD support. Recent guidelines suggest TV repair at the time of LVAD implantation.

Shunts

- Atrial septal defects and patent foramen ovale with significant shunting should be noted and closed during the LVAD surgery.
- Similarly, VSD should be identified and located.

- **Key Points:**
  1. *Echocardiographic assessment prior to LVAD implantation must include LVIDd, degree of AR, AS, MR, MS, and TR.*
  2. *RV size and function should be assessed and reported.*
  3. *Assess for interatrial and interventricular shunts.*

Intraoperative TEE in Guiding LVAD Placement

- TEE is useful to LVAD cannula placement and initial LVAD settings.
  - Speeds are set to decompress the LV, with close attention to midline septal positioning, as well MR, AR, TR, and RV function.

- LVAD conduit flows can be assessed through off-axis views for the detection of kinking or conduit malposition.
- LVAD inflow cannula position is usually seen in the midesophageal views. (Note that the cannula should not be excessively oriented toward the IVS.)
- LVAD outflow cannula is imaged in the mid-ascending aorta close to the right pulmonary artery (PA).
- The cannula positions and velocity should be interrogated before and after chest closure.
- Acute RV dysfunction may suggest air embolism down the right coronary artery.
- Acute RV dysfunction with severe TR may also suggest excessive LVAD pump speed (from LV "suck-down" and shifting of the IVS to the left).
- Use color Doppler and agitated saline to detect an interatrial shunt.
- Assess for AoV opening and degree of AR.

Routine Echocardiographic Assessment of the Normal Functioning LVAD

- The type of LVAD and pump speed must be noted in the TTE exam and report.
- Blood pressure should be noted.
- LVIDd from PLAX should be recorded in every patient so that the LV diameter can be tracked serially over studies.
- As noted previously, LV volumes may be difficult to assess in these patients because of technical limitations.
- If microbubble contrast is not used, a visual estimate of LVEF should be reported.
- Although mitral inflow and LA volume should be recorded, how these parameters can be used in the clinical management of these patients is unclear at present.
- IVS position should be noted (whether the septum is midline).
- RV size and function should be reported along with degree of TR and pulmonary regurgitation.
- Degree of MR should be assessed. Significant MR may suggest inappropriate LV unloading or interference of the cannula with the mitral apparatus.
- Refer to Figure 22-3 for routine echocardiographic assessment of LVAD patients.
- AoV function
  - AoV opening should be noted.
  - AoV is best assessed either by two-dimensional (2D) Doppler or with M-mode from the PLAX or PSAX view with 10–15 beats of acquisition sweep speed of 25–50 mm/sec (Fig. 22-4).
  - An AoV that does not open at all may be associated with thrombus formation on the valve and the aortic root should be carefully assessed.
  - Degree of AR should be assessed.
- Cannula imaging
  - LV apical (inflow) may be seen in off-axis PLAX views, PSAX apical views, or A4C views. Off-axis views are often required to visualize cannula flows. Both CW and PW Doppler of the cannula should be assessed (Fig. 22-5).
  - Aortic (outflow) cannula flow is best seen in right sternal border or high PLAX views of the ascending aorta. Use color Doppler to locate continuous flow in RSB view.
  - Typical inflow cannula peak velocity is <1.5 m/sec in HM2 LVAD. Higher velocities should prompt consideration of partial obstruction.
  - Outflow graft velocities >2 m/sec may be abnormal and warrants further assessment.

Aortic Valve

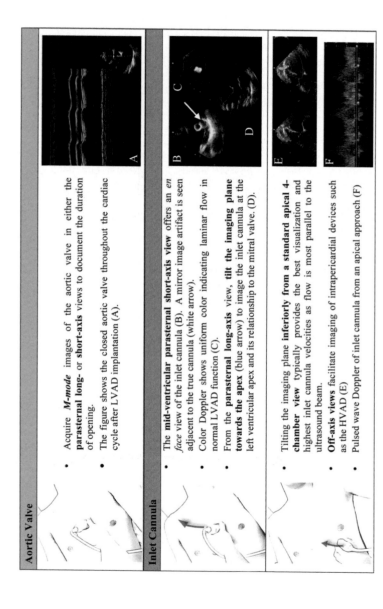

- Acquire **M-mode** images of the aortic valve in either the **parasternal long-** or **short-axis** views to document the duration of opening.
- The figure shows the closed aortic valve throughout the cardiac cycle after LVAD implantation (A).

Inlet Cannula

- The **mid-ventricular parasternal short-axis view** offers an *en face* view of the inlet cannula (B). A mirror image artifact is seen adjacent to the true cannula (white arrow).
- Color Doppler shows uniform color indicating laminar flow in normal LVAD function (C).
- From the **parasternal long-axis** view, **tilt the imaging plane towards the apex** (blue arrow) to image the inlet cannula at the left ventricular apex and its relationship to the mitral valve. (D).

- Tilting the imaging plane **inferiorly from a standard apical 4-chamber view** typically provides the best visualization and highest inlet cannula velocities as flow is most parallel to the ultrasound beam.
- **Off-axis views** facilitate imaging of intrapericardial devices such as the HVAD (E)
- Pulsed wave Doppler of inlet cannula from an apical approach (F)

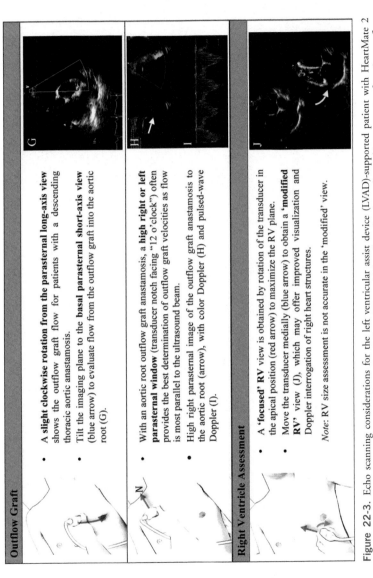

Outflow Graft

- **A slight clockwise rotation from the parasternal long-axis view** shows the outflow graft flow for patients with a descending thoracic aortic anastamosis.

- Tilt the imaging plane to the **basal parasternal short-axis view** (blue arrow) to evaluate flow from the outflow graft into the aortic root (G).

- With an aortic root outflow graft anastamosis, **a high right or left parasternal window** (transducer notch facing "12 o'clock") often provides the best determination of outflow graft velocities as flow is most parallel to the ultrasound beam.

- High right parasternal image of the outflow graft anastamosis to the aortic root (arrow), with color Doppler (H) and pulsed-wave Doppler (I).

Right Ventricle Assessment

- A **'focused' RV** view is obtained by rotation of the transducer in the apical position (red arrow) to maximize the RV plane.

- Move the transducer medially (blue arrow) to obtain a **'modified RV'** view (J), which may offer improved visualization and Doppler interrogation of right heart structures.

Note: RV size assessment is not accurate in the 'modified' view.

Figure 22-3. Echo scanning considerations for the left ventricular assist device (LVAD)-supported patient with HeartMate 2 LVAD. (Reprinted from Rasalingam R, Johnson SN, Bilhorn KR, et al. Transthoracic echocardiographic assessment of continuous-flow left ventricular assist devices. *J Am Soc Echocardiogr.* 2011;24:135–48.)

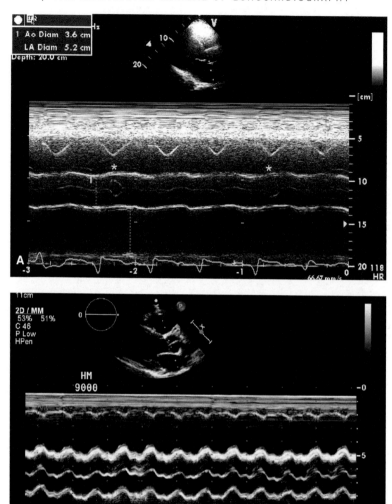

Figure 22-4. M-mode imaging of aortic valve in a patient with a left ventricular assist device. **A:** The intermittent aortic valve opening is denoted by the asterisks. **B:** In comparison, there is no aortic valve opening.

- Assessment of cardiac output
  - In the absence of significant AoV opening and significant AR, the LVAD cardiac output is the same as the right-sided cardiac output: where the right-sided cardiac output is calculated by using (RVOT PW VTI × cross-sectional area RVOT) × HR (Fig. 22-6) where RVOT = right ventricular outflow tract and HR = heart rate.

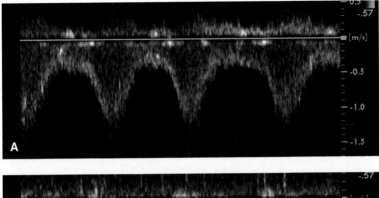

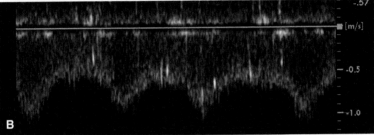

Figure 22-5. Left ventricular assist device aortic (outflow) cannula pulsed-wave Doppler. Shown at 8400 rpm (**A**) with greater pulsatility than at 9600 rpm (**B**).

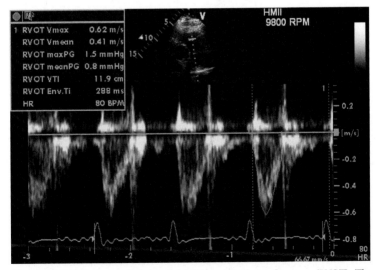

Figure 22-6. Pulsed-wave Doppler of the right ventricular outflow tract (RVOT). The velocity time integral (VTI) is then used to calculate right-sided cardiac output using the formula: (RVOT VTI × RVOT area) × HR. HR, heart rate.

- When the AoV opens in the absence of significant AR, the LVAD cardiac output = RVOT cardiac output—LVOT cardiac output.
- In cases of significant AR, the LVAD cardiac output is greater than the right-sided cardiac output.
- The estimated cardiac output should be reported.

- **Key Point:** *In addition to the standard reporting performed in all TTEs, the following parameters should be included in a LVAD TTE report: pump speed, type of LVAD, LVEF, LVIDd, IVS position, comment on AoV opening, degree of valvular regurgitation, RV size and function, estimation of cardiac output, inflow/outflow cannula velocities.*

Echocardiographic Assessment of LVAD Complications

- LVAD pump alarms and console readouts (Table 22-1)
  - High power and high flow—pump thrombosis, severe AR, peripheral vasodilation (e.g., sepsis), and normalization of LV systolic function
  - Low flow—overall intravascular volume depletion, mechanical obstruction to LV cannula inflow or aortic cannula outflow, right heart failure (producing low LV preload), cardiac tamponade (usually in the early postoperative setting), and very high afterload states

TABLE 22-1	Differential Diagnosis of Left Ventricular Assist Device Pump Alarms and Echo Correlations	
Alarm	**Problem**	**Echo correlate**
Low flow	Volume depletion	Collapsible IVC
	Mechanical obstruction to inflow or outflow	High cannula velocities Thrombus/pannus
	Right heart failure	RV dilation Small LV cavity Dilated IVC
	Cardiac tamponade	Pericardial effusion Dilated IVC
	High afterload states	Worsening AR
High power, high flow	Pump thrombosis	Dilated LV with MR Ramp study with failure of LV size to reduce
	Severe AR	Color Doppler findings of AR Progressive LV dilation
	Peripheral vasodilation	Increased LV contractility Collapsible IVC
	LV recovery	Increased LV contractility Normal unloading parameters

AR, aortic regurgitation; IVC, inferior vena cava; LV, left ventricle; MR, mitral regurgitation; RV, right ventricle.

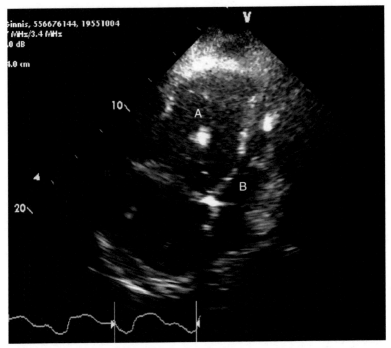

Figure 22-7. Right ventricular (RV) failure. Note dilated RV (**A**) and compressed left ventricle (**B**) in a patient with a history of RV failure and an acute pulmonary embolism when the echocardiographic images were obtained.

- RV failure (Fig. 22-7)
  - Assess RV size and function: TAPSE, RVS', RV strain, RIMP, and RV FAC.
  - Close attention should be paid to IVS position, tricuspid leaflet coaptation, and TR as these may be altered by pump speed settings. Higher speeds result in deformation of the IVS toward the LV, impairing tricuspid leaflet coaptation and worsening TR.
- AR
  - LVADs in general lower LV diastolic pressure and increase aortic root diastolic pressure. This may lead to AR, whether as an exacerbation of pre-LVAD AR or as a de novo phenomenon.
  - Severe AR creates a futile loop of circulation between LV, LVAD, and aortic root. Surgical correction of AR may be required.
  - Neither pressure half-time nor holodiastolic flow reversal in the distal aorta is reliable for determining AR severity in LVAD.
    - One may need to rely on vena contracta, AR jet width to LVOT, color Doppler to assess AR severity (Fig. 22-8).
- Suck-down
  - Excessive LVAD support, particularly in a small LV, may result in contact between the LV cannula and the LV wall or septum (i.e., so-called "suck-down").

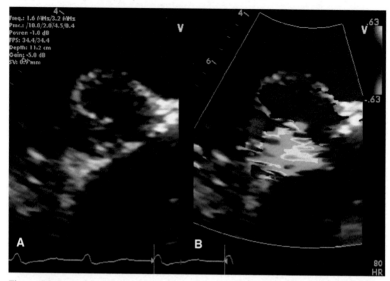

Figure 22-8. A: Parasternal short axis of the aortic valve demonstrating prolapse of the non-coronary cusp. **B:** Severe aortic regurgitation in a left ventricular assist device patient due to the prolapsed aortic valve cusp.

- Clinically this may manifest as dizziness or hypotension, ventricular arrhythmias as a result of irritation of the LV wall, or asymptomatic device-registered low pulsatility index events.
- Echocardiography to assess the LV volume and cannula position with regard to the septum may be useful. Serial changes in pump speed with echo imaging may be used to determine a more optimal pump speed less likely to produce suck-down.
- Pump thrombosis
  - Pump thrombosis occurs in approximately 5–10% of LVAD implants.
  - Thrombus in the LVAD most commonly manifests as impaired pump function and intravascular hemolysis.
  - Impaired pump function may range from subtle changes to full pump stoppage.
  - Hemolysis may manifest as a rise in serum lactate dehydrogenase or as hemoglobinuria.
  - Prompt assessment of the degree of pump dysfunction is important for clinical decision-making regarding the next therapeutic maneuver, which may include device exchange, urgent prioritization for transplant, or lytic therapy.
  - Assessment of changes in LV unloading with progressive increase in LVAD pump speed in the HeartMate II can be used to confirm pump thrombosis.
    ○ As speeds increase in a thrombosed pump, the LV chamber dimension fails to decrease and signs of high LV filling pressures such as functional MR persist. The AoV opens more frequently and may require very high speeds to remain closed, or it may continue to open despite high speeds.
    ○ Echocardiographic assessment of the LVIDd) over a range of increasing pump speeds demonstrating minimal change in LV dimension has a high predictive accuracy for pump thrombosis (Fig. 22-9).

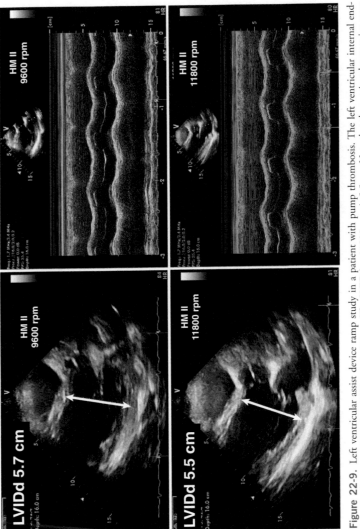

Figure 22-9. Left ventricular assist device ramp study in a patient with pump thrombosis. The left ventricular internal end-diastolic diameter (LVIDd) at 9600 rpm is 5.7 cm. The LVIDd at 11800 rpm is 5.5 cm. Note that the aortic valve remains open at both pump speeds as demonstrated with M-mode (*right side panels*).

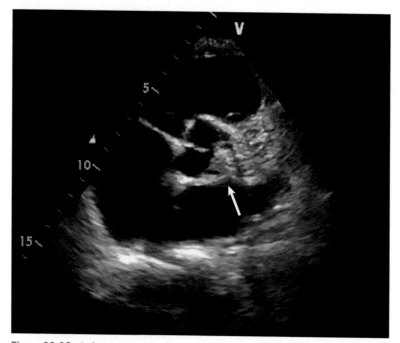

Figure 22-10. Left ventricular assist device patient presented with a ST-elevation myocardial infarction. A transthoracic echocardiography in the parasternal short-axis view at the level of the aortic valve demonstrates a large aortic root thrombus in the left coronary cusp (*yellow arrow*).

- Speeds are increased in increments of 200–400 rpm up to a maximum of 12000 rpm, with measures of LV dimensions at each speed.
- Limitation to speed ramp studies
  - False positives in AR or high mean arterial pressure states
  - False negatives in setting of concomitant inotropes
  - May not be generalizable to HeartWare LVADs—LVEDD changes with increased speed are less evident in normal functioning pumps.
- Thrombus formation in the aortic root may occur with LVAD support when there is minimal AoV opening (Fig. 22-10). It is unclear whether interventions to promote intermittent AoV opening are warranted. Complications may include growth of the clot into the coronary ostium and myocardial infarction.

TEMPORARY MECHANICAL CIRULATORY SUPPORT DEVICES

Abiomed Impella Devices

- Left-sided Impella devices are approved for use in high-risk revascularization or valve procedures in patients at risk of hemodynamic instability. These devices are also approved for short-term circulatory support in ongoing cardiogenic shock following acute MI and open heart surgery.

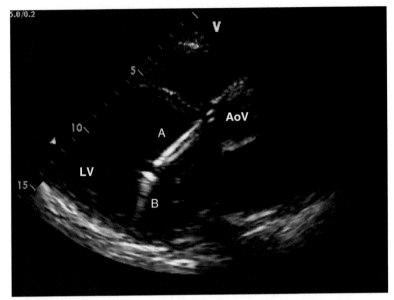

Figure 22-11. From parasternal long-axis view, an Impella device (**A**) seen crossing aortic valve (AoV), approximately 4 cm into the left ventricle (LV), beyond the mitral leaflet tips. Note the typical echo artifact (**B**).

- These devices are percutaneously inserted temporary LVADs that draw blood from the LV cavity via a pigtail catheter inserted retrograde across the AoV. Blood is drawn into the catheter, through a motor unit in the catheter, and out orifices in the ascending aorta.
  - Echocardiography is essential to the preinsertion assessment for candidacy. Contraindications include moderate-to-severe aortic insufficiency and moderate-to-severe AS.
  - Echocardiography (TEE or TTE) is helpful to confirm the placement of the device. From the PLAX view (Fig. 22-11), the catheter is seen traversing the AoV with:
    ○ Catheter inlet area in the LV midcavity (~4 cm from the AoV)
    ○ Pigtail angled toward the LV apex and free of chordae and papillary muscles
    ○ Outlet area well above the AoV
- A right-sided Impella device was recently approved for use in the setting of acute right heart failure following LVAD implantation, myocardial infarction, heart transplant, or open-heart surgery. This device essentially reverses the configuration of the left-sided device.
  Echocardiography may be adjunctive for confirming device positioning, but fluoroscopy is required to confirm proper seating of the device throughout its course.

• **Key Point:** *Assess for degree of AS and AR prior to placement of an Impella.*

Intra-aortic balloon pump (IABP)

- An IABP is a counterpulsation device that consists of an air-filled balloon-tipped catheter that rapidly inflates in diastole and deflates in systole, resulting in augmented coronary artery perfusion and modestly increased cardiac output.
  - TEE guidance can be useful for proper positioning of the IABP.
    - Preimplantation imaging should confirm the absence of severe aortic insufficiency or aortic pathology, including dissection, aneurysm, or severe atherosclerosis.
    - With implantation, TEE allows for the confirmation of proper wire position in the descending thoracic aorta, IABP catheter tip placement 1–2 cm distal to the origin of the left subclavian artery, typical diastolic inflation.

Extracorporeal membrane oxygenation (ECMO)

- ECMO is a mode of high level hemodynamic support consisting of:
  - Large bore cannula for venous drainage
  - Mechanical pump with controller
  - Oxygenator and temperature control unit in series with the pump for the oxygen of blood, removal of carbon dioxide, and regulation of temperature
  - Large bore return cannula for venous (veno-venous or VV ECMO) or arterial (veno-arterial or VA ECMO) return from the pump and oxygenator
- Anatomic sites of cannulation may vary by circumstance and need. Echocardiography, particularly TEE, is useful for determining positioning and flow of cannulae.
  - In VV ECMO, echo with Doppler imaging should confirm the position of the drainage cannula in the proximal IVC and the return cannula in the mid-right atrium (Fig. 22-12).
  - In peripheral VA ECMO, echo with Doppler imaging should confirm the position of the drainage cannula in the mid-right atrium. The cannula for oxygenated blood return to the arterial circulation is in the abdominal aorta of iliac arteries and cannot be echocardiographically visualized.
- Cardiac response to ECMO over time may be assessed by both TEE and TTE.
  - With peripheral VA ECMO, LV preload increases as a result of right heart drainage, but LV afterload increases as blood is injected retrograde into the arterial circulation.
    - Absence of AoV opening is indicative of very poor LV contractility or excessive ECMO support and may result in aortic root thrombosis if anticoagulation is inadequate.
    - LV overload as represented by progressive LV dilation and MR. In these cases, venting of the LV or use of a concomitant mechanical circulatory support device with drainage from the LV is required.
    - Weaning of ECMO may be assisted by echocardiographic assessment. As ECMO flow is reduced, signs of LV recovery, including improved contractility, reduced LV size, AoV opening, and improved MR, are indicative of possibility of weaning from ECMO.
    - TEE may be particularly useful for the assessment of ECMO cannulae for kinking, migration, or thrombus.

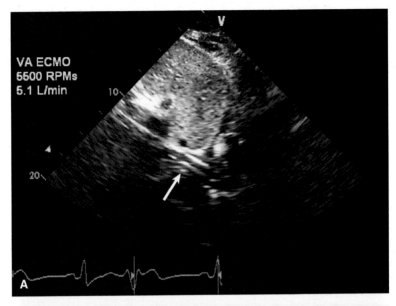

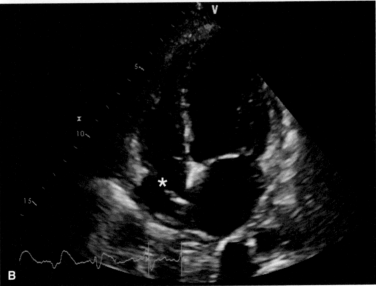

Figure 22-12. Venoarterial extracorporeal membrane oxygenation (VA ECMO). **A:** From the subcostal view, the venous drainage cannula is seen in the inferior vena cava (*yellow arrow*). **B:** From the apical four-chamber view, the venous drainage cannula tip is seen in the mid-right atrium (***).

Index

Note: Page numbers followed by f and t indicates figure and table respectively.